Burn Management

Editor

LEOPOLDO C. CANCIO

SURGICAL CLINICS OF NORTH AMERICA

www.surgical.theclinics.com

Consulting Editor
RONALD F. MARTIN

June 2023 • Volume 103 • Number 3

ELSEVIER

1600 John F. Kennedy Boulevard ● Suite 1800 ● Philadelphia, Pennsylvania, 19103-2899

http://www.surgical.theclinics.com

SURGICAL CLINICS OF NORTH AMERICA Volume 103, Number 3
June 2023 ISSN 0039–6109, ISBN-13: 978-0-443-18173-3

Editor: John Vassallo
Developmental Editor: Hannah Lopez

Surgical Clinics of North America (ISSN 0039–6109) is published bimonthly by Elsevier Inc., 360 Park Avenue South, New York, NY 10010-1710. Months of publication are February, April, June, August, October, and December. Business and Editorial Offices: 1600 John F. Kennedy Blvd., Suite 1800, Philadelphia, PA 19103-2899. Periodicals postage paid at New York, NY and additional mailing offices. Subscription prices are $479.00 per year for US individuals, $1045.00 per year for US institutions, $100.00 per year for US & Canadian students and residents, $575.00 per year for Canadian individuals, $1327.00 per year for Canadian institutions, $580.00 for international individuals, $1327.00 per year for international institutions and $250.00 per year for foreign students/residents. To receive student/resident rate, orders must be accompanied by name of affiliated institution, date of term, and the *signature* of program/residency coordinator on institution letterhead. Orders will be billed at individual rate until proof of status is received. Foreign air speed delivery is included in all *Clinics* subscription prices. All prices are subject to change without notice. POSTMASTER: Send address changes to *Surgical Clinics*, Elsevier Health Sciences Division, Subscription Customer Service, 3251 Riverport Lane, Maryland Heights, MO 63043. **Customer Service (orders, claims, online, change of address): Telephone: 1-800-654-2452 (U.S. and Canada); 314-447-8871 (outside U.S. and Canada). Fax: 314-447-8029. E-mail: journalscustomerservice-usa@elsevier.com (for print support); journalsonlinesupport-usa@elsevier.com (for online support)**.

Reprints. For copies of 100 or more, of articles in this publication, please contact the Commercial Reprints Department, Elsevier Inc., 360 Park Avenue South, New York, New York 10010-1710. Tel. 212-633-3874, Fax: 212-633-3820, E-mail: reprints@elsevier.com.

Surgical Clinics of North America is also published in Spanish by McGraw-Hill Interamericana Editores S.A., P.O. Box 5-237 06500 Mexico D.F. Mexico; and in Portuguese by Interlivros Edicoes Ltda., Rua Comandante Coelho 1085, CEP 21250, Rio de Janeiro, Brazil; and in Greek by Paschalidis Medical Publications, Athens Greece.

Surgical Clinics of North America is covered in *MEDLINE/PubMed (Index Medicus), EMBASE/Excerpta Medica, Current Contents/Clinical Medicine, Current Contents/Life Sciences, Science Citation Index,* and *ISI/BIOMED.*

Contributors

CONSULTING EDITOR

RONALD F. MARTIN, MD, FACS
Colonel (Retired), United States Army Reserve, Department of General Surgery, Pullman Surgical Associates, Pullman Regional Hospital and Clinic Network, Pullman, Washington, USA

EDITOR

LEOPOLDO C. CANCIO, MD, FACS, FCCM
Colonel (Retired), Medical Corps, US Army, Professor of Surgery (Adjoint), UT Health San Antonio, Director, US Army Institute of Surgical Research Burn Center, JBSA Fort Sam Houston, San Antonio, Texas, USA

AUTHORS

NIKKI ALLORTO, MBChB, MMed, FCS(SA)
Specialist Surgeon, Head Pietermaritzburg Metropolitan Burn Service, Pietermaritzburg, KwaZulu Natal, South Africa

EDWARD BITTNER, MD
Department of Anesthesia, Critical Care, and Pain Medicine, Shriners Hospital for Children, Department of Anesthesia, Massachusetts General Hospital, Boston, Massachusetts, USA

GARRETT W. BRITTON, DO
US Army Institute of Surgical Research, San Antonio, Texas, USA

KIMBERLEY C. BRONDEEL, BS
John Sealy School of Medicine, The University of Texas Medical Branch, Galveston, Texas, USA

JULIA BRYARLY, MD
Assistant Professor, Physical Medicine and Rehabilitation, The University of Texas Southwestern Medical Center, Dallas, Texas, USA

JILL M. CANCIO, OTD, OTR/L, CHT
US Army Institute of Surgical Research Burn Center, San Antonio, Texas, USA

LEOPOLDO C. CANCIO, MD, FACS, FCCM
Colonel (Retired), Medical Corps, US Army, Professor of Surgery (Adjoint), UT Health San Antonio, Director, US Army Institute of Surgical Research Burn Center, JBSA Fort Sam Houston, San Antonio, Texas, USA

JEFFREY E. CARTER, MD, FACS
Medical Director, University Medical Center Burn Center New Orleans, Professor of Surgery, Louisiana State University Health Sciences Center New Orleans, New Orleans, Louisiana, USA

RODNEY K. CHAN, MD, FACS, FRCSC
Associate Professor, Uniformed Services University of Health Sciences, Adjunct Professor, UT Health San Antonio, Metis Foundation, San Antonio, Texas, USA; United States Army Institute of Surgical Research, Fort Sam Houston, Texas, USA

ELIZABETH CHIPP, MBChB (Hons), FRCS (Plast)
Consultant Burns and Plastic Surgeon, University Hospital Birmingham, Birmingham, United Kingdom

KEVIN K. CHUNG, MD
Uniformed Services University of Health Sciences, Bethesda, Maryland, USA

WILLIAM S. DEWEY, BS, PT, CHT
US Army Institute of Surgical Research Burn Center, San Antonio, Texas, USA

MAXIMILIAN FETH, MD
Research Physician, US Army Institute of Surgical Research, Houston, Texas, USA; Anesthesiologist, Department of Anesthesiology and Critical Care Medicine, Armed Forces Medical Centre Ulm, Ulm, Germany

DAVID G. GREENHALGH, MD
Chief of Burns, Shriners Children's Northern California, Professor Emeritus, University of California, Davis, Sacramento, California, USA

BARRETT J. HALGAS, MD
US Army Institute of Surgical Research, San Antonio, Texas, USA

DAVID N. HERNDON, MD, FACS
CEO, Joseph M. Still Research Foundation, Augusta, Georgia, USA

WILLIAM L. HICKERSON, MD
Professor of Plastic Surgery, The University of Tennessee Health Science Center (Retired), Jesse Turner Burn Center, Memphis, Tennessee, USA

JAMES H. HOLMES IV, MD
Chair, Section of Burns, Department of Surgery, Director, AHWFB Burn Center, Professor of Surgery, Wake Forest University School of Medicine, Winston-Salem, North Carolina, USA

LINDA HONG, MD
Anesthesiologist, US Army Institute of Surgical Research, Houston, Texas, USA

CHELSEA L. INGLE, DO
Brooke Army Medical Center, Texas, USA

JAMES C. JENG, MD, FACS
Clinical Professor of Surgery, University of California Irvine, Orange, California, USA

MARC G. JESCHKE, MD, PhD, FCCM, FRCS(C)
Burn Program at Hamilton Health Sciences, Department of Surgery, McMaster University, TaAri Institute, Hamilton Health Sciences Research Institute, David Braley Research Institute, Hamilton, Ontario, Canada

RANDY D. KEARNS, DHA, MSA, FACHE, FRSPH
BS Health Care Management Program Director, Associate Professor of Healthcare Management and Disaster Management, University of New Orleans, New Orleans, Louisiana, USA

COREY KEENAN, DO
Metis Foundation, San Antonio, Texas, USA

JOHN L. KILEY, MD
Infectious Disease, Brooke Army Medical Center, Associate Professor, Uniformed Services University of the Health Sciences, Houston, Texas, USA

BOOKER KING, MD, FACS
Director, North Carolina Jaycee Burn Center, Clinical Professor of Surgery, The University of North Carolina at Chapel Hill, Chapel Hill, North Carolina, USA

KAREN KOWALSKE, MD
Professor, Physical Medicine and Rehabilitation, The University of Texas Southwestern Medical Center, Dallas, Texas, USA

JOSEPH K. MADDRY, MD, FACMT
Brooke Army Medical Center, US Army Institute of Surgical Research, Texas, USA; Uniformed Services University of the Health Sciences, Bethesda, Maryland, USA; JBSA Lackland, Texas, USA

SHANKAR MAN RAI, MD
Professor of Plastic Surgery, National Academy of Medical Sciences, Nepal Cleft and Burn Center at Kirtipur Hospital, Kathmandu, Nepal

CMD KWESI NSAFUL, MBChB, FWAS
Department of Plastic, Reconstructive Surgery and Burns Unit, Ghana Navy, Accra, Ghana

NOOR OBAIDI, MD, PhD
Metis Foundation, San Antonio, Texas, USA

ALEN PALACKIC, MD
Department of Surgery, University of Texas Medical Branch, Galveston, Texas, USA

KAITLIN A. PRUSKOWSKI, PharmD, BCPS, BCCCP, FCCM
Clinical Pharmacist, US Army Institute of Surgical Research, Houston, Texas, USA; Adjunct Assistant Professor of Medicine, Uniformed Services University, Bethesda, Maryland, USA

ANJU B. SARASWAT, MD
Department of Surgery, Associate Medical Director, AHWFB Burn Center, Assistant Professor of Surgery, Wake Forest University School of Medicine, Winston-Salem, North Carolina, USA

STEVEN G. SCHAUER, DO, MS
Brooke Army Medical Center, US Army Institute of Surgical Research, Texas, USA; Uniformed Services University of the Health Sciences, Bethesda, Maryland, USA

NIKHIL R. SHAH, MD
Department of Surgery, University of Texas Medical Branch, Galveston, Texas, USA

SHAHRIAR SHAHROKHI, MD, FRCSC
Burn Program at Hamilton Health Sciences, Department of Surgery, McMaster University, Hamilton, Ontario, Canada

ROBERT SHERIDAN, MD
Department of Surgery, Massachusetts General Hospital, Shriners Hospital for Children, Boston, Massachusetts, USA

JEFFREY W. SHUPP, MD, FACS
The Burn Center, MedStar Washington Hospital Center, Departments of Surgery and Plastic and Reconstructive Surgery, Georgetown University School of Medicine, Department of Biochemistry and Molecular and Cellular Biology, Georgetown University Medical Center, Washington, DC, USA

BARCLAY T. STEWART, MD, PhD
Assistant Professor of Trauma, Burn and Critical Care Surgery, University of Washington, Seattle, Washington, USA

SHAWN TEJIRAM, MD, FACS
The Burn Center, MedStar Washington Hospital Center, Department of Surgery, Georgetown University School of Medicine, Washington, DC, USA

STEPHEN P. TRANCHINA, BA
Georgetown University School, Washington, DC, USA

TARYN E. TRAVIS, MD, FACS
Burn Center, MedStar Washington Hospital Center, Departments of Surgery and Plastic and Reconstructive Surgery, Georgetown University School of Medicine, Washington, DC, USA

ELLIOT T. WALTERS, MD
Department of Surgery, The University of Texas Medical Branch, Galveston, Texas, USA

AMANDA R. WIGGINS, MD
Intensivist, US Army Institute of Surgical Research, Houston, Texas, USA

JASMINE M. WILLIAMS, MD
Brooke Army Medical Center, Texas, USA

STEVEN E. WOLF, MD, FACS
Department of Surgery, The University of Texas Medical Branch, Galveston, Texas, USA

Contents

With these many diverse functions, understanding normal anatomic composition of skin is pivotal to evaluating the extent of its disruption from burn injury. This article discusses the pathophysiology, initial evaluation, subsequent progression, and healing of burn wounds. By delineating the various microcellular and macrocellular alterations of burn injury, this review also augments providers' capacity to deliver patient-centered, evidence-based burn care.

Burn management has developed over time to encompass care that includes more than just survival but also quality of life and successful reintegration into society. Identification of burns that require timely operative intervention supports the goals of excellent functional and aesthetic outcomes in burn survivors. Appropriate patient optimization, detailed preoperative planning, and intraoperative communication are keys to success.

Hypermetabolism is a hallmark of larger burn injuries. The hypermetabolic response is characterized by marked and sustained increases in catecholamines, glucocorticoids, and glucagon. There is an increasing body of literature for nutrition and metabolic treatment and supplementation to counter the hypermetabolic and catabolic response secondary to burn injury. Early and adequate nutrition is key in addition to adjunctive therapies, such as oxandrolone, insulin, metformin, and propranolol. The duration of administration of anabolic agents should be at minimum for the duration of hospitalization, and possibly up to 2 to 3 years postburn.

Despite the fact that modern burn care has significantly reduced the mortality associated with severe burn injuries, the rehabilitation and community reintegration of survivors continues to be a challenge. An interprofessional team approach is essential for optimal outcomes. This includes early occupational and physical therapy, beginning in the intensive care unit (ICU). Burn-specific techniques (edema management, wound healing, and contracture prevention) are successfully integrated into the burn ICU. Research demonstrates that early intensive rehabilitation of critically ill burn patients is safe and effective. Further work on the physiologic, functional, and long-term impact of this care is needed.

The majority of hospitalized burn patients experience pain, agitation, and delirium. The development of each one of these conditions can also lead to, or worsen, the others. Providers, therefore, need to thoroughly assess the underlying issue to determine the most effective treatment. Multimodal pharmacologic regimens are often used in conjunction with non-pharmacologic strategies to manage pain, agitation, and delirium. This review focuses on the pharmacologic management of these complicated patients in a critical-care setting.

Julia Bryarly and Karen Kowalske

Better understanding of long-term outcomes after burn injury is essential for the burn clinician. Contractures are present in almost half of patients at discharge. Although less common, neuropathy and heterotopic ossification may be missed or go unaddressed. Close attention to psychological distress and to challenges with community reentry is essential. Obviously long-term problems with skin issues occur, but other issues must be addressed to maximize health and quality of life after injury. Facilitating access to community resources and providing long-term medical follow-up should be the standard of care.

Noor Obaidi, Rodney K. Chan, and Corey Keenan

This chapter highlights the importance of a comprehensive burn scar treatment plan in approaching a burn survivor. General concepts of burn scar physiology and a practical system to describe burn scars based on cause, biology, and symptoms are presented. Common scar management modalities including nonsurgical, surgical, and adjuvant therapies are further discussed.

Booker King, Leopoldo C. Cancio, and James C. Jeng

Mass-casualty incidents can occur because of natural disasters; industrial accidents; or intentional attacks against civilian, police, or in case of combat, military forces. Depending on scale and type of incident, burn casualties with a variety of concomitant injuries can be anticipated. The treatment of life-threatening traumatic injuries should take precedence but the stabilization, triage, and follow-on care of these patients will require local, state, and often regional coordination and support.

Randy D. Kearns, William L. Hickerson, and Jeffery E. Carter

Radiation-related injuries are rare. Yet the consequences of an event involving a radiation source can be substantial. As with any clinical emergency that rarely occurs, we are typically less prepared to deal with the situation. Compounding the crisis will be the "worried well" population who may believe that they too are contaminated or suffering from radiation poisoning and report to the hospital for evaluation. Identifying and triaging those who are sick or injured, managing the surge of patients, and knowing where resources can be accessed are all essential.

More than 95% of the 11 million burns that occur annually happen in low-resource settings, and 70% of those occur among children. Although some low- and middle-income countries have well-organized emergency care systems, many have not prioritized care for the injured and experience unsatisfactory outcomes after burn injury. This chapter outlines key considerations for burn care in low-resource settings.

SURGICAL CLINICS
OF NORTH AMERICA

SERIES OF RELATED INTEREST

Advances in Surgery
https://www.advancessurgery.com/
Surgical Oncology Clinics
https://www.surgonc.theclinics.com/
Thoracic Surgery Clinics
https://www.thoracic.theclinics.com/

THE CLINICS ARE AVAILABLE ONLINE!
Access your subscription at:
www.theclinics.com

Foreword

Burns

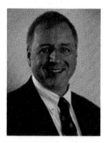

Ronald F. Martin, MD, FACS
Consulting Editor

As someone who has spent much of life dealing with pancreaticobiliary disorders, I can think of only one pathophysiologic state that has the range of injury and capacity to strike at the core of my clinical fears more than acute pancreatitis; that is the acutely burned patient. From a minor sunburn to the massive full-thickness burns, the potential for physiologic disruption is unparalleled in my knowledge. This capacity for harm coupled with the often frequently preventable nature of burns makes it even more frightening.

In this truly outstanding issue compiled by Dr Cancio and his colleagues, we are given a broad and deep overview of burns from basic physiology through rehab. We are guided from the most superficial level of treatment through the most complex systemic responses. It is a phenomenal collection. The issue begins with a discussion of the creation of burn units following the second World War. If one happened to train in my generation and in the New England area, we were all steeped in the story of the Cocoanut Grove nightclub fire that occurred in Boston, Massachusetts in November of 1942. That evening a group of people out for a night became trapped in a building on fire and could not escape. Part of the problem was exit doors that opened inward. The event had a huge impact on everything from building and fire codes to our understanding of salt and water metabolism to the fundamentals of transplantation. In fact, in the early days of trying to learn to transplant skin, many of the tools were studied to transplant other organs. This in some ways led to Dr Joseph Murray's (a pioneer plastic surgeon) receipt of the Nobel Prize for his role in the early renal transplants among twins at Brigham Hospital. Dr Francis Moore and many others made huge contributions to our understanding of salt and water metabolism, and others laid the beginning work for the science of nutritional metabolism that is the basis for much of what we know today.

The one common theme that insinuates through almost everything one can read about burn patients is the absolute necessity for a fully integrated team approach.

Surg Clin N Am 103 (2023) xiii–xiv
https://doi.org/10.1016/j.suc.2023.03.001
0039-6109/23/© 2023 Published by Elsevier Inc.

Whether in the intensive care unit, the operating room, rehabilitation environments, or anywhere else, the need for broad disciplinary integration and support remains paramount to achieve success.

The advances in the care of the burned patient in the last 80 years have been nothing short of remarkable. And those who contributed to them deserve their honored place in surgical history. That said, there is another side of the societal equation that also deserves enormous accolades but will likely never get them—those who have been instrumental in preventing burns in the first place. Changes in building materials and codes, development and enforcement of fire codes, improvements in fire-suppression systems, changes in automobile design, and even changes in clothing materials have all played outsized roles in diminishing our risks of becoming a burn patient.

There is clearly more to be done. We have environmental challenges to respond to for reduction in risk of wildfires. We have much to be done to reduce the risk of using devices of war, many of which achieve their effects through thermodynamic means, for the resolving of political disputes. And so on and so on. Obviously, the larger societal concerns are beyond the scope of what we at the *Surgical Clinics* attempt to cover directly. That said, we are all members of our communities, and we must appropriately participate in society and give our best counsel. This issue that Dr Cancio and his colleagues have put together for us is an excellent basis for understanding the needs of burn patients on many levels. I have had the privilege of following many of our contributors' work for many years and even had the opportunity to work with some of them directly. They all represent extremely outstanding clinicians who have made a valuable contribution to our surgical community. We hope you find this issue as valuable as we do at the *Surgical Clinic* series.

Ronald F. Martin, MD, FACS
Colonel (retired), United States Army Reserve
Department of General Surgery
Pullman Surgical Associates
Pullman Regional Hospital and Clinic Network
825 Southeast Bishop Boulevard, Suite 130
Pullman, WA 99163, USA

E-mail address:
rfmcescna@gmail.com

Preface

Burns: Recent Advances and Perennial Challenges

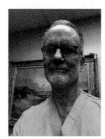

Leopoldo C. Cancio, MD, FACS, FCCM
Editor

In this issue of *Surgical Clinics*, we document advances and challenges across the entire spectrum of burn care–from prehospital, austere, and mass-casualty environments; to the intensive care unit (ICU) and operating room; all the way to postburn recovery and reintegration.

Postburn mortality has greatly improved in the United States since WW II. The lethal-area 50% for a thermally injured young person has doubled from about 40% to 80% of the total body surface area, meaning that half of such patients can now expect to survive. According to Dr Basil A. Pruitt Jr.—the US Army surgeon who led much of the effort to improve care—these advances were the result of a multidisciplinary team approach to the burn problem. For him, the successful burn team included not only clinicians from all the relevant specialties but also scientists, engaged in *integrated laboratory and clinical research*.[1,2] The Introduction to this issue by Dr David Herndon exemplifies this concept, as does the inclusion of authors from multiple specialties in the issue.

Much burn care can be safely performed on an outpatient basis, and outpatient follow-up of patients with larger burns is indispensable; thus, a multidisciplinary clinic is a core component of any burn center (article in this issue by Chipp). Successful care of the acutely injured begins in the prehospital setting and emergency department (article in this issue by Williams and colleagues). Fluid resuscitation of patients with large burns (those greater than about 10%–20% of the total body surface area) and balancing the risks of overresuscitation and underresuscitation challenge the team during the first 24 hours (article in this issue by Tejiram and colleagues). Following this, the critically ill burn patient enters a hypermetabolic phase, which places them at risk of multiple system organ failure and infection, at least until the wounds are healed (articles in this issue by Britton and colleagues and by Kiley and Greenhalgh).

Surg Clin N Am 103 (2023) xv–xvii
https://doi.org/10.1016/j.suc.2023.01.003
0039-6109/23/© 2023 Elsevier Inc. All rights reserved.

Patients with large burns and/or inhalation injury are at elevated risk of acute respiratory distress syndrome, mandating careful attention to mechanical ventilation and liberation strategies (article in this issue by Bittner and Sheridan).

The central problem in burn care is the wound—until it is successfully healed, systemic inflammation and immunosuppression will ensue (article in this issue by Shah and colleagues). Early excision and grafting is the standard of care for patients with large burns, and multiple technologies are available to support this effort (article in this issue by Saraswat and Holmes). Meanwhile, nutritional support to meet increased protein and calorie needs, and control of hypermetabolism/catabolism, are critical (article in this issue by Shahrokhi and Jeschke).

Today, we focus not on mere survival, but rather on functional survival: that is, on returning the patient to activities of daily living, to work, or to school. Rehabilitation must begin in the burn ICU and continue throughout the hospital stay and beyond (article in this issue by J. Cancio and Dewey). Burn care must holistically address the often-challenging problems of pain, anxiety, and delirium (article in this issue by Pruskowski and colleagues). A severe burn is a chronic disease with lifelong consequences, mandating attention to long-term outcomes (article in this issue by Bryarly and Kowalske). Initial wound closure is essential for survival, but long-term scar management and reconstructive plastic surgery are often equally essential for function (article in this issue by Obaidi and colleagues).

The advances we've made in burn care have occurred in large part because expertise has been concentrated in specialized centers. This has, unintentionally, decreased familiarity with burns outside of these centers. During normal operations such specialization increases the quality of care, but it could become problematic in a disaster, on the battlefield (article in this issue by King and colleagues), or (in a particularly worrisome scenario) following detonation of a nuclear device (article in this issue by Kearns and colleagues). One approach to disaster preparedness is to learn from how burn care is practiced in austere settings in low- and middle-income countries worldwide (article in this issue by Stewart and colleagues).

Although burns are considered a highly specialized area of surgery, in important ways they epitomize the problems seen in all surgical patients. Because of this, Dr Pruitt described burns as the *universal trauma model*.[3,4] Consistent with this philosophy, I believe that this issue of *Surgical Clinics* will be of broad value to all those who care for the injured.

Leopoldo C. Cancio, MD, FACS, FCCM
Colonel (retired), Medical Corps, US Army
US Army Institute of Surgical Research Burn Center
3698 Chambers Pass
JBSA Fort Sam Houston, TX, USA

E-mail address:
Leopoldo.c.cancio.civ@health.mil

REFERENCES

1. Pruitt BA Jr. Combat casualty care and surgical progress. Ann Surg 2006;243(6): 715–29.
2. Pruitt BA Jr. Multidisciplinary care and research for burn injury: 1976 presidential address, American Burn Association meeting. J Trauma 1977;17(4):263–9.
3. Pruitt BA Jr. The universal trauma model. Bull Am Coll Surg 1985;70(10):2–13.
4. Pruitt BA Jr. Forces and factors influencing trauma care: 1983 A.A.S.T. (American Association for the Surgery of Trauma) Presidential address. J Trauma 1984;24(6): 463–70.

Introduction
The Multidisciplinary Team Approach to Burn Care

David N. Herndon, MD

KEYWORDS

• Burns • Inhalation injury • Teams • Multidisciplinary • Outcomes

KEY POINTS

- Multidisciplinary teamwork, as practiced in modern burn units, is essential to successful care of burn patients.
- Since the first such units were established after World War II, postburn mortality has decreased by a factor of 50% in younger patients.
- Scientific progress and improved outcomes in burn patients is the product of closely integrated teams of researchers and clinicians, meeting frequently at the bedside.

INTRODUCTION: THE MULTIDISCIPLINARY TEAM APPROACH TO BURN CARE

Teamwork characterizes the modern approach to burn care. The first burn units in the United States to organize multidisciplinary teams to address this complex problem were the Medical College of Virginia in Richmond and the US Army Surgical Research Unit (later called the US Army Institute of Surgical Research) in 1949. The University of Texas Medical Branch in Galveston burn unit was formed following the 1947 fire disaster in neighboring Texas City, where an ammonium nitrate-carrying freighter, the *SS Grandcamp*, exploded in the port resulting in a mass fire disaster. There was a parallel development of burn centers and multidisciplinary burn teams in England and Europe during and immediately after World War II (WW II).

The leader of the burn team has been a burn surgeon, either a general or plastic surgeon, with expertise in critical care and skin grafting and flap techniques.

The team includes other general and plastic surgeons, intensivists, anesthesiologists, nurses, physical and occupational therapists, respiratory therapists, nutritionists, and psychosocial experts (social workers, psychiatrists, and psychologists). Other team members may include cardiologists, pulmonologists, gastroenterologists, nephrologists, hematologists, radiologists, pediatricians, pediatric surgeons, students, residents, fellows, spiritual therapists, music therapists, and exercise physiologists.

Joseph M. Still Research Foundation, Augusta, GA, USA
E-mail address: david@burnscare.org

Surg Clin N Am 103 (2023) 369–376
https://doi.org/10.1016/j.suc.2023.01.004
0039-6109/23/© 2023 Elsevier Inc. All rights reserved.

surgical.theclinics.com

Many burns units have incorporated basic scientists into their teams: physiologists, microbiologists, biochemists, statisticians, epidemiologists, and pathologists. The inclusion of scientists in burn teams has contributed to an explosion in scientific productivity.

Impact of the Team Approach

Great advances in understanding and treating burn shock, smoke inhalation injury, pneumonia, and invasive burn wound infections, and in achieving early coverage of the burn wound with cadaver graft or xenograft (and, more recently, biosynthetic skin substitutes), have decreased morbidity and mortality. In 1946, just before the early burn units were established, a 50% of total body surface area burn killed 50% of the young people who received it. Now a 90% total body surface burn can be survived half of the time it is received in younger individuals.[1–14]

Collaboration of basic scientists and clinicians allowed for retrospective and prospective examinations of large patient data sets from the burn units that led to the development of precise methodologies for fluid resuscitation.[15,16] Researchers and clinicians decreased mortality for major burns by better describing, understanding, and treating pathophysiologic changes related to pulmonary edema, smoke injury, and pneumonia.[17–34] Researchers and clinicians together developed techniques to measure, support, and modulate the hypermetabolic, and hypercatabolic response characteristic of significant burn injury.[35–46] Advances in the early coverage of burn wounds[38–47] included coverage of the newly excised wound with allograft,[48–53] amnion, a temporary synthetic skin substitute (Biobrane),[54–57] a dermal regeneration template (Integra),[58] or cultured human keratinocytes.[59,60] Further advances occurred in the treatment of infection and sepsis.[22,61–69]

The organization of the burn units responsible for these advances called for at least one weekly interaction between clinicians and scientists, in rounds and conferences that encourage interaction and development of new approaches for each burn-patient problem. Most units conduct full multidisciplinary rounds weekly. Daily rounds are conducted with at least the surgeons, fellows, residents, physician extenders, student nurses, therapists, dietitians, pharmacists, and respiratory therapists in most units. Interactions among the many disciplines develop ideas for improvement that result in advances in patient care.

Team Members and Roles

Present at burn-unit rounds and conferences are nurses, the largest single disciplinary segment of the care team. The nurse working at the bedside continuously throughout the day or night with each patient is truly the primary caregiver who translates the many complex treatments and therapies to clinical care. They provide emotional support, recognize changes in condition, and initiate therapeutic interventions. Burn nurses are sophisticated intensive-care nurses and wound experts who deliver critical medicine and treatment, change wound dressings, and provide psychosocial nurturing to treat pain, anxiety, and suffering.

The respiratory therapist treats smoke inhalation injury, pneumonia, and pulmonary edema by directing pulmonary toilet, ventilatory support strategies, and respiratory exercise.

Rehabilitation therapists, including occupational and physical therapists, treat patients from their initial admission through the recovery phase 2 to 6 years after injury. Initially, the burn patient requires special positioning and splinting, strengthening exercises, and early mobilization. Later, pressure garments and application of silicone and other materials to promote healing and retard scar formation are added.

Rehabilitation therapists must have a profound understanding of the psychosocial responses of patients to be able to encourage them to fight through the rigors of successful splint application, exercise, and rehabilitation.

Dietitians monitor daily caloric delivery, recommending dietary formulations and rates of administration to combat catabolism, and the appropriate amount and type of minerals, trace elements, and vitamins needed to allow appropriate recovery.[36]

Physician assistants, burn fellows, interns, residents, medical students, and nurse practitioners are key contributors to many teams. They participate in daily rounds, presenting aspects of critical care administered the previous day, and plans for the upcoming day or week. The assistant who participated in the last surgery, wound washing, or dressing change will describe in detail the characteristics of the burn at the current time. Ideally, photographs of the wound are displayed for the whole burn team to be able to appreciate any change that may have occurred in the wound. Of particular interest will be whether there are any signs of progression of infection—such as color changes (to include white, black, or purple dots), exudate, pus, or odor. An infection-control nurse and sometimes a representative of the microbiology laboratory will be present, and details regarding the last cultures of the wound and the culture results will be discussed. This will include whether bacteria, fungus, or viral elements have been identified, and the results of any quantitative cultures. The physician assistant, resident, or medical student will further discuss the laboratory findings of the day with a focus on electrolytes and liver function tests, blood coagulation parameters, signs of infection, or disruption of vital sign trends in the prior day. They will present daily fluid balance and reiterate the dietitian's reports of caloric balance, and the occupational and physical therapists' reports on splints and positioning, and the movement and exercise performed by the patient.

The social worker, psychologist, or psychiatrist will give reports on the methodologies of pain control, pharmaceutical interventions, distraction methodologies, and psychotherapeutic approaches and will characterize family interactions. If available, child life and music therapists will present techniques they have employed and advise on new plans in each of these areas. A clinical research nurse will comment on any research studies the patient might be eligible for or is participating in. A quality-assurance nurse will identify any quality issues raised in the presentation, focusing on nosocomial infections, central-line, and catheter issues, infection-control principles, and adherence to nutrition, fluid, and other protocols as applied to the individual patient being discussed.

In most units, intensivists will participate in care management, surgeons will comment on surgical procedures and wound progression. The pharmacist will discuss drugs being administered to an individual patient with particular attention to the variance in the metabolism of these agents in burn patients, adverse interactions of these agents, and the appropriateness in the given setting.

The pathologist will discuss any surgical pathological material that had been obtained on a patient. They can advise on whether rapid pathologic sections can be performed to immediately identify the presence of bacteria, fungi, virus, or signs of infection. The pathologist is also an expert in interpreting laboratory abnormalities and laboratory techniques that might be available for further diagnosis in particular circumstances. The pathologist also performs autopsies on as many patients who die in the burn unit as possible if permission can be obtained. In many states, burn deaths are coroner cases, and that pathologist can also direct autopsies. The pathologist's findings have profoundly improved burn care because clinical acumen is limited relative to the perspective of an adequately conducted autopsy.[2]

Education and Publication

Weekly educational presentations on specific topics often augment the daily and weekly conferences. A team-oriented curriculum discusses burn-wound care, shock, metabolism, nutrition, infectious disease and control, wound coverage, intensive care techniques, rehabilitation, and psychosocial support. Local and visiting experts delve in-depth into the area presented because it affects burn patients. Most units with active research programs will have a weekly research conference with many of the attendees who participate in daily and weekly clinical rounds. They focus on performing clinical and basic research projects; discuss consent issues, ethical considerations, and details of all protocols; and identify patients suitable for inclusion in the protocols. Participation in clinical research projects results in presentations and publications to improve burn care everywhere. All outside presentations are presented at the unit research or clinical meetings. These presentations are most frequently given at the American Burn Association (ABA) or the International Society for Burn Injuries meetings. These works are commonly published in the *Journal of Burn Care and Research* or in *Burns*, respectively. Publications to more general audiences are submitted to journals such as *Journal of Trauma and Acute Care Surgery*, *Shock*, *Annals of Surgery*, *Journal of the American College of Surgeons*, *Lancet*, and *New England Journal of Medicine*.

The role of professional organizations

The few burn units in existence in the late 1940s were joined by new units throughout the United States, Canada, Mexico, Central and South America, Australia, New Zealand, Britain, and Europe. The multidisciplinary teams of individual units came together to support organizations based on the team approach to burn care. First, the International Society for Burn Injuries was established in the early 1960s. Shortly after that, the ABA, the British Burn Association, the European Burn Association, and the Australian and New Zealand Burn Association were organized. The ABA established the *Journal of Burn Care and Research* for the publication of articles produced from the burn teams. The International Society for Burn Injuries developed the journal *Burns* for the same purpose. Special interest groups in each of these organizations meet independently for surgery, plastic surgery, psychosocial practitioners, rehabilitation therapies, dietitians, nurses, and burn survivors. However, most of the association's activities are focused on the products of teams, which are dedicated to the interaction between the different disciplines. Publications in both journals mentioned represent all disciplines in burn care with an emphasis on teamwork, team interactions, and production of advances in burn care. The stated goal of these combined teams includes prevention, education, research, and advancement of burn care throughout the world.

SUMMARY

The extraordinary progress achieved in burn outcomes since WW II did not occur by accident but rather by intentional efforts to build and support high-functioning multidisciplinary teams. These teams bring together not only the clinical personnel needed holistically to address the burn patient's complex physical and emotional needs but also the scientific personnel needed to advance care through basic and applied research. Such teamwork will be critical for continued advances in burn care, and furthermore can serve as a model for tackling other similarly challenging clinical problems.

DECLARATION OF INTERESTS

The author has no conflicts of interest relevant to this article.

REFERENCES

1. Bull JP, Fisher AJ. A study of mortality in a burns unit: a revised estimate. Ann Surg 1954;139(3):269–74.
2. Pereira CT, Barrow RE, Sterns AM, et al. Age-dependent differences in survival after severe burns: a unicentric review of 1,674 patients and 179 autopsies over 15 years. J Am Coll Surg 2006;202(3):536–48.
3. Porter C, Tompkins RG, Finnerty CC, et al. The metabolic stress response to burn trauma: current understanding and therapies. Lancet 2016;388(10052):1417–26.
4. Herndon DN, Voigt CD, Capek KD, et al. Reversal of growth arrest with the combined administration of oxandrolone and propranolol in severely burned children. Ann Surg 2016;264(3):421–8.
5. Lee JO, Herndon DN, Andersen C, et al. Effect of exercise training on the frequency of contracture-release surgeries in burned children. Ann Plast Surg 2017;79(4):346–9.
6. Chao T, Porter C, Herndon DN, et al. Propranolol and oxandrolone therapy accelerated muscle recovery in burned children. Med Sci Sports Exerc 2017;50(3):427–35.
7. Hundeshagen G, Wurzer P, Herndon DN. Life-long relationships? The future of pediatric burn care and research. Burns 2017;43(3):457–8.
8. Ojeda S, Blumenthal E, Stevens P, et al. The safety and efficacy of propranolol in reducing the hypermetabolic response in the pediatric burn population. J Burn Care Res 2018;39(6):963–9.
9. Cambiaso-Daniel J, Parry I, Rivas E, et al. Strength and cardiorespiratory exercise rehabilitation for severely burned patients during intensive care units: a survey of practice. J Burn Care Res 2018;39(6):897–901.
10. Reeves PT, Herndon DN, Tanksley JD, et al. Five-year outcomes after long-term oxandrolone administration in severely burned children: a randomized clinical trial. Shock 2015;45(4):367–74.
11. Finnerty CC, Jeschke MG, Branski LK, et al. Hypertrophic scarring: the greatest unmet challenge after burn injury. Lancet 2016;388(10052):1427–36.
12. Goverman J, Mathews K, Goldstein R, et al. Adult contractures in burn injury: a burn model system national database study. J Burn Care Res 2016;38(1):e328–36.
13. Goverman J, Mathews K, Goldstein R, et al. Pediatric contractures in burn injury: a burn model system national database study. J Burn Care Res 2016;38(1):e192–9.
14. Patel DD, Rosenberg L, Rosenberg M, et al. The epidemiology of burns in young children from Mexico treated at a U.S. hospital. Burns 2016;42(8):1825–30.
15. Evans EI, Purnell OJ, Robinett PW, et al. Fluid and electrolyte requirements in severe burns. Ann Surg 1952;135(6):804–17.
16. Carvajal HF. Fluid therapy for the acutely burned child. Comprehensive Therapy 1977;3(3):17–24.
17. Shirani KZ, Pruitt BA Jr, Mason AD Jr. The influence of inhalation injury and pneumonia on burn mortality. Ann Surg 1987;205(1):82.
18. Herndon DN, Barrow RE, Traber DL, et al. Extravascular lung water changes following smoke inhalation and massive burn injury. Surgery 1987;102(2):341–9.
19. Herndon DN, Barrow RE, Linares HA, et al. Inhalation injury in burned patients: effects and treatment. Burns Incl Therm Inj 1988;14(5):349–56.
20. Dehring DJ, Doty S, Kimura R, et al. Effect of preexisting inhalation injury on response to bacteremia in sheep. J Burn Care Rehabil 1988;9(5):467–71.

21. Linares HA, Herndon DN, Traber DL. Sequence of morphologic events in experimental smoke inhalation. J Burn Care Rehabil 1989;10(1):27–37.

22. Shangraw RE, Jahoor F, Miyoshi H, et al. Differentiation between septic and postburn insulin resistance. Metabolism 1989;38(10):983–9.

23. Abdi S, Herndon DN, Traber LD, et al. Lung edema formation following inhalation injury: Role of the bronchial blood flow. J Appl Physiol 1991;71(2):727–34.

24. Cox CS Jr, Zwischenberger JB, Traber DL, et al. Immediate positive pressure ventilation with positive end-expiratory pressure (peep) improves survival in ovine smoke inhalation injury. J Trauma 1992;33(6):821–7.

25. Gilpin DA, Rutan RL, Herndon DN. Recognition and treatment of burn sepsis. Clin Adv Crit Care 1993;2:1–3.

26. Herndon DN, Zeigler. ST Bacterial translocation after thermal injury. Crit Care Med 1993;21(2 Suppl):S50–4.

27. Zwischenberger JB, Cox CS Jr, Minifee PK, et al. Pathophysiology of ovine smoke inhalation injury treated with extracorporeal membrane oxygenation. Chest 1993; 103(5):1582–6.

28. Desai MH, Mlcak R, Richardson J, et al. Reduction in mortality in pediatric patients with inhalation injury with aerosolized heparin/n-acetylcystine [correction of acetylcystine] therapy. J Burn Care Rehabil 1998;19(3):210–2.

29. Enkhbaatar P, Herndon DN, Traber DL. Use of nebulized heparin in the treatment of smoke inhalation injury. J Burn Care Res 2009;30(1):159–62.

30. Lange M, Hamahata A, Traber DL, et al. Preclinical evaluation of epinephrine nebulization to reduce airway hyperemia and improve oxygenation after smoke inhalation injury. Crit Care Med 2011;39(4):718–24.

31. Cox RA, Jacob S, Zhu Y, et al. Airway obstruction and bacterial invasion in autopsy tissue of pediatric burn victims. J Burn Care Res 2014;35(2):148–53.

32. Peterson JR, De La Rosa S, Eboda O, et al. Treatment of heterotopic ossification through remote ATP hydrolysis. Sci Translat Med 2014;6(255):255ra132.

33. Sousse LE, Herndon DN, Andersen CR, et al. High tidal volume decreases ARDS, atelcstasis, and ventilator days compared to low tidal volume in pediatric burned patients without inhalation injury. J Am Coll Surg 2014;220(4):570–8.

34. Enkhbaatar P, Pruitt BA Jr, Suman O, et al. Pathophysiology, research challenges, and clinical management of smoke inhalation injury. Lancet 2016;388(10052): 1437–46.

35. Hildreth MA, Herndon DN, Desai MH, et al. Reassessing caloric requirements in pediatric burn patients. J Burn Care Rehabil 1988;9(6):616–8.

36. Curreri PW, Marvin J, Baxter CR. Dietary requirements of patients with major burns. J Am Diet Assoc 1974;65(4):415–7.

37. Wilmore DW, Long JM, Mason AD Jr, et al. Catecholamines: mediator of the hypermetabolic response to thermal injury. Ann Surg 1974;180(4):653.

38. Herndon DN, Barrow RE, Stein M, et al. Increased mortality with intravenous supplemental feeding in severely burned patients. J Burn Care Rehabil 1989;10(4): 309–13.

39. Rutan TC, Herndon DN, Van Osten T, et al. Metabolic rate alterations in early excision and grafting versus conservative treatment. J Trauma 1986;26(2):140–2.

40. Irei M, Abston S, Bonds E, et al. The optimal time for excision of scald burns in toddlers. J Burn Care Rehabil 1986;7(6):508–10.

41. Desai MH, Herndon DN, Broemeling L, et al. Early burn wound excision significantly reduces blood loss. Ann Surg 1990;211(6):753–62.

42. Barret JP, Wolf SE, Desai MH, et al. Total burn wound excision of massive paedi-atric burns in the first 24 hours post-injury. Ann. Burns Fire Disasters 1999; XII(1):25–7.
43. Xiao-Wu W, Herndon DN, Spies M, et al. Effects of delayed wound excision and grafting in severely burned children. Arch Surg 2002;137(9):1049–54.
44. Hart DW, Wolf SE, Chinkes DL, et al. Effects of early excision and aggressive enteral feeding on hypermetabolism, catabolism, and sepsis after severe burn. J Trauma 2003;54(4):755–64.
45. Barret JP, Herndon DN. Modulation of inflammatory and catabolic responses in severely burned children by early burn wound excision in the first 24 hours. Arch Surg 2003;138(2):127–32.
46. Barret JP, Herndon DN. Effects of burn wound excision on bacterial colonization and invasion. Plast Reconstr Surg 2003;111(2):744–52.
47. Naoum JJ, Roehl KR, Wolf SE, et al. The use of homograft compared to topical antimicrobial therapy in the treatment of second-degree burns of more than 40% total body surface area. Burns 2004;30(6):548–51.
48. Wainwright D, Madden M, Luterman A, et al. Clinical evaluation of an acellular allograft dermal matrix in full-thickness burns. J Burn Care Rehabil 1996;17(2): 124–36.
49. Herndon DN, Rose JK. Cadaver skin allograft and the transmission of human cytomegalovirus in burn patients: Benefits clearly outweigh risks. J Am Coll Surg 1996;182(3):263–4.
50. Herndon DN. Multiple piece use of dermagraft-tc. J Burn Care Rehabil 1997;18(1 Pt 2):S14–5.
51. Herndon DN. Perspectives in the use of allograft. J Burn Care Rehabil 1997;18(1 Pt 2):S6.
52. Purdue GF, Hunt JL, Still JM Jr, et al. A multicenter clinical trial of a biosynthetic skin replacement, dermagraft-tc, compared with cryopreserved human cadaver skin for temporary coverage of excised burn wounds. J Burn Care Rehabil 1997; 18(1 Pt 1):52–7.
53. Rose JK, Desai MH, Mlakar JM, et al. Allograft is superior to topical antimicrobial therapy in the treatment of partial-thickness scald burns in children. J Burn Care Rehabil 1997;18(4):338–41.
54. Branski LK, Herndon DN, Celis MM, et al. Amnion in the treatment of pediatric partial-thickness facial burns. Burns 2008;34(3):393–9.
55. Herndon DN, Branski LK. Contemporary methods allowing for safe and conve-nient use of amniotic membrane as a biologic wound dressing for burns. Ann Plast Surg 2017;78(2 Suppl 1):S9–10.
56. Barret JP, Dziewulski P, Ramzy PI, et al. Biobrane versus 1% silver sulfadiazine in second-degree pediatric burns. Plast Reconstr Surg 2000;105(1):62–5.
57. Lal S, Barrow RE, Wolf SE, et al. Biobrane improves wound healing in burned chil-dren without increased risk of infection. Shock 2000;14(3):314–9.
58. Branski LK, Herndon DN, Pereira C, et al. Longitudinal assessment of integra in primary burn management: a randomized pediatric clinical trial. Crit Care Med 2007;35(11):2615–23.
59. Herndon DN, Rutan RL. Comparison of cultured epidermal autograft and massive excision with serial autografting plus homograft overlay. J Burn Care Rehabil 1992;13(1):154–7.
60. Barret JP, Wolf SE, Desai MH, et al. Cost-efficacy of cultured epidermal autografts in massive pediatric burns. Ann Surg 2000;231(6):869–76.

61. Heggers JP, Robson MC, Herndon DN, et al. The efficacy of nystatin combined with topical microbial agents in the treatment of burn wound sepsis. J Burn Care Rehabil 1989;10(6):508–11.

62. Heggers JP, Carino ES, Sazy JA, et al. A topical antimicrobial test system (topitest); nathan's agar well diffusion revisited. Surg Res Comm 1990;8:109–16.

63. Fujioka K, Sugi K, Isago T, et al. Thromboxane synthase inhibition and cardiopulmonary function during endotoxemia in sheep. J Appl Physiol 1991;71(4): 1376–81.

64. Meyer J, Traber LD, Nelson S, et al. Reversal of hyperdynamic response to continuous endotoxin administration by inhibition of no synthesis. J Appl Physiol 1992;73(1):324–8.

65. Tokyay R, Zeigler ST, Traber DL, et al. Postburn gastrointestinal vasoconstriction increases bacterial and endotoxin translocation. J Appl Physiol 1993;74(4): 1521–7.

66. Iglesias G, Zeigler ST, Lentz CW, et al. Thromboxane synthetase inhibition and thromboxane receptor blockade preserve pulmonary and circulatory function in a porcine burn sepsis model. J Am Coll Surg 1994;179(2):187–92.

67. Wolf SE, Jeschke MG, Rose JK, et al. Enteral feeding intolerance: An indicator of sepsis-associated mortality in burned children. Arch Surg 1997;132(12):1310–3.

68. Herndon DN, Lal S. Is bacterial translocation a clinically relevant phenomenon in burns? Crit Care Med 2000;28(5):1682–3.

69. Enkhbaatar P, Joncam C, Traber L, et al. Novel ovine model of methicillin-resistant staphylococcus aureus-induced pneumonia and sepsis. Shock 2008;29(5): 642–9.

Outpatient and Minor Burn Treatment

Elizabeth Chipp, FRCS (Plast)*

KEYWORDS

- Burn • Outpatient • Dressings • Telemedicine • First aid • Toxic shock syndrome

KEY POINTS

- Most burn injuries are minor and do not require admission to hospital.
- Even small burns can lead to significant physical and psychological morbidities.
- Involvement of the whole multidisciplinary team is key for the best outcome.

INTRODUCTION

Burns are the fourth most common type of trauma worldwide with approximately 11 million people each year suffering a burn injury severe enough to warrant medical attention. Most of those injuries, and the vast majority of associated deaths, are in low and middle-income countries (LMIC).[1]

Fortunately, most burn injuries in the developed world are minor and can be safely managed as an outpatient, without requiring admission to hospital. Of the more than 480,000 patients injured in 2016 in the United States, only approximately 40,000 required hospitalization according to the American Burn Association National Burn Repository.[2] There are likely to be many more minor burns that are treated in community facilities, which are not reported to the repository.

Managing burns on an outpatient basis avoids the costs associated with inpatient treatment, and allows the patient to remain at home with as little disruption to their life as possible. With careful patient selection and clearly defined pathways, this can lead to the best possible results for this large group of patients.

Even minor burns can cause pain, distress, scarring, functional problems, and loss of normal work activities. Optimum management of such injuries reduces infection, time to healing, and time away from work and daily activities.

PATIENT SELECTION

Although it is possible to safely manage many minor burns on an outpatient or ambulatory basis, careful patient selection is crucial. First comes the definition of a "minor

Consultant Burns and Plastic Surgeon, University Hospital Birmingham, Birmingham, UK
* Queen Elizabeth Hospital, Mindelsohn Way, Birmingham, B15 2GW, UK
E-mail address: elizabeth.chipp@uhb.nhs.uk

Surg Clin N Am 103 (2023) 377–387
https://doi.org/10.1016/j.suc.2023.02.006
0039-6109/23/© 2023 Elsevier Inc. All rights reserved.

surgical.theclinics.com

burn." Minor burns are those which affect a relatively small surface area, certainly less than 15% total body surface area (TBSA) in adults, and which are usually superficial in nature (**Fig. 1**). Patients with burns to complex areas, such as hands, face, and perineum, are generally excluded; however, they may be suitable for outpatient management after an initial brief admission for wound care, dressing, and to establish analgesia and commence rehabilitation. Suspicion of inhalation injury or other associated injuries would mandate hospital admission for assessment and treatment.

Managing a burn as an outpatient requires the patient to have a safe and appropriate home environment, with suitable family support and consideration given to additional mobility needs until they recover fully. The patient, or their caregiver, must be able to report any concerns or complications, to comply with therapy and basic dressings or wound care, and to have the means and ability to attend follow-up appointments. Patients with physical or psychological comorbidities may be difficult to manage as an outpatient, and each patient should be assessed on an individual basis in case they require admission. Other indications for hospitalization include associated traumatic injuries, suspicion of abuse, or patient preference.

Avoiding hospital admission and managing burns on an ambulatory basis can be particularly beneficial for children who often find hospital admission and treatment upsetting. Outpatient wound care in children can be accomplished with a low rate of admission and complications, including infection.[3] Avoiding admission helps to

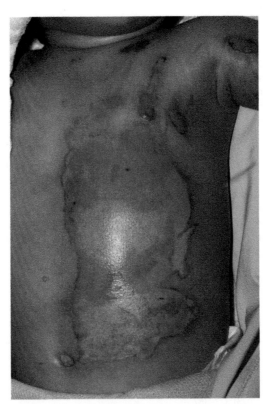

Fig. 1. A 4% TBSA scald in a 2-year-old child managed as an outpatient after an initial debridement and antimicrobial dressing.

minimize disruption to the entire family unit and may allow the child to continue attending school. Studies have shown that parents are able to change dressings at home to further reduce attendance at outpatient clinic appointments with a high level of parent satisfaction and low rate of complications.[4]

The coronavirus (COVID-19) global pandemic led to many burns services reevaluating the way they managed moderate-sized burns in an attempt to avoid admitting patients to hospital wherever possible. This was partly due to the overwhelming pressure on inpatient beds and partly due to the risk of hospital-acquired infection. Restructuring of minor-burn pathways can allow the vast majority of minor (<15% TBSA) burns to be managed nonoperatively as an outpatient with a high level of patient satisfaction.[5]

FIRST AID AND INITIAL WOUND MANAGEMENT

Adequate first aid, that is, stopping the burning process and cooling the burn wound, prevents burn-wound progression, improves outcome, and reduces pain. Cool running water applied to the burn wound for 20 minutes is effective within the first 3 hours postburn and has been shown to reduce the requirement for skin grafts.[6] Care should be taken to avoid hypothermia, especially in children who are more susceptible due to their larger surface-area: mass ratio. Ice should not be used because intense vasoconstriction can occur, which deepens the burn wound. Topical ointments should be avoided until the burn wound has been assessed because they can mask the appearance of the burn. Chemical burns should be treated with copious irrigation. In addition, Diphoterine is reportedly superior to water alone in normalizing pH after chemical injury.[7] This is an amphoteric, chelating, hypertonic washing agent designed to be used as a first-aid measure and effective against all chemicals but with limited efficacy on hydrofluoric acid.

Covering the burn with a simple nonadherent dressing will improve comfort and reduce contamination of the wound. Polyvinyl chloride film (cling wrap) is ideal and provides an inexpensive and readily available wound cover until definitive dressing is performed.[8]

Management of burns blisters remains controversial. Randomized controlled trials on this subject have not shown statistically significant differences in pain, healing time or wound colonisation.[9] Thin-walled blisters may spontaneously burst, leaving undebrided skin which is a potential nidus of infection. Blister fluid contains inflammatory mediators that may hinder wound healing. Blisters also prevent silver-based or other antimicrobial dressings from coming into direct contact with the wound bed, thus limiting their antimicrobial effect. For these reasons, fluid-filled blisters should be deroofed using an aseptic technique to aid patient comfort, allow proper wound assessment, and facilitate contact of antimicrobial dressings with the wound bed. Flat blisters, especially those on glabrous skin, may generally be left intact.

Burns are tetanus-prone wounds and tetanus immunoglobulin should be given to any patient with an uncertain or incomplete tetanus immunization history.

DEFINITIVE WOUND MANAGEMENT

The burn wound should first be cleansed using an antiseptic technique to remove dirt, debris, and loose blistered skin. This allows the assessment of the underlying burn wound to determine the size, depth, and healing potential. This assessment is vital in determining the ongoing patient management; superficial burns can be expected to heal with good wound care and appropriate dressings, whereas deeper burns (unless very small) are more likely to require surgical intervention.

Assessment of burn depth can be difficult, especially early after the burn or in patients with darker skin pigmentation. There are various adjuncts available to help the experienced burn-care provider assess the wound depth and healing potential, including laser Doppler imaging (LDI), infrared (IR) thermography, and hyperspectral imaging. Of these techniques, LDI is the most commonly used and has been shown to be more accurate than visual assessment alone.[10,11] LDI is a noninvasive method, which involves using a red diode laser to determine the dermal blood flow. This is used to produce a color map of the wound, in which each color correlates to predicted healing time. It is recommended by the National Institute for Health and Care Excellence in the United Kingdom to be used to "guide treatment decisions for patients in whom there is uncertainty about the depth and healing potential of burn wounds."[12] One drawback of this technique is the size of the machine and time taken to perform a scan, which can be particularly troublesome in pediatric patients. Handheld devices to perform IR thermography or hyperspectral imaging are likely to be more user friendly but LDI remains the superior technique.[13] (**Fig. 2**) shows images obtained from LDI and IR thermography.

Once a decision has been made that a burn should be managed nonoperatively, the most appropriate dressing needs to be selected in order to optimize wound healing conditions and minimize the time to healing. There are dozens of suitable dressings on the market and each burns service will undoubtedly have their own preferences.

The ideal dressing unfortunately does not exist, and a decision should be made considering multiple factors including availability, antimicrobial activity, cost, ease of use, patient comfort, exudate management, and storage. It is beyond the scope of this article to describe all of the available dressings but they can be broadly summarized into the following categories.[14]

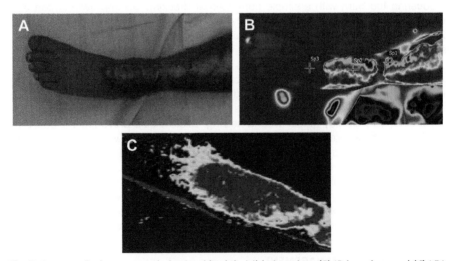

Fig. 2. Images of a burn wound obtained by (*A*) visible imaging, (*B*) IR imaging, and (*C*) LDI. The foot is on the left side of the 3 images. The LDI is a more close-up image of the burn on the dorsum of the ankle. All images suggest a burn, which is suitable to be managed conservatively. The visible-light photograph shows a relatively superficial burn. This is confirmed by the LDI (in this system, *red* indicates good blood flow and predicts a time to healing of less than 7 days). The IR image shows that the burn is cooler (depicted in this system as *light blue* and *green*) than the unburned skin on the foot (depicted as *red*) but it still has good blood flow.

- *Hydrocolloid dressings*, for example, Duoderm (ConvaTec, Reading, UK). These dressings form a gel when they are exposed to exudate, and this aids autolytic debridement of the wound.
- *Polyurethane film dressing*, for example, Tegaderm (3M, Saint Paul, Minnesota, USA), Opsite (Smith and Nephew, Watford, UK). These are transparent, adhesive film dressings, suitable for lightly exuding wounds.
- *Hydrogel dressings*, for example, Intrasite (Smith & Nephew). These dressings are able to deal with higher levels of exudate and to donate fluid to maintain a moist wound-healing environment.
- *Silicon-coated dressings*, for example, Mepitel (Mölnlycke, Gothenburg, Sweden). These dressings act as a nonadhesive wound contact layer to reduce trauma during dressing changes.
- *Antimicrobial (silver-containing or iodine-containing) dressings*, for example, Acticoat (Smith & Nephew), Aquacel Ag (ConvaTec), Silverlon (Argentum Medical, Geneva, IL, USA). These dressings aim to reduce the risk of invasive infection by minimizing bacterial colonization of the wound.
- *Fiber dressings*, for example, Kaltostat (ConvaTec). Absorbent dressings that can be used for moderately to heavily exuding wounds.
- *Topical antimicrobial burn creams*, for example, silver sulfadiazine (Silvadene; Flamazine), mafenide acetate (Sulfamylon, Mylan Pharmaceuticals, Canonsburg, Pennsylvania, USA). These are used in conjunction with a secondary dressing, except for when used to dress facial wounds. These are commonly used for more extensive burns (inpatients). They may be more challenging for outpatients to manage at home.
- *Biosynthetic skin substitutes*, for example, PermeaDerm (Milliken, Spartanburg, South Carolina, USA), Biobrane (Smith & Nephew), and Epiprotect (Regen Medical, Wiltshire, UK). These materials are designed to mimic the function of the skin and allow reepithelialization to occur, before separating spontaneously once wound healing has occurred.

In a Cochrane review of dressings for superficial and partial thickness burns, silver sulfadiazine was consistently associated with poorer healing outcomes than biosynthetic dressings, silver-containing dressings, and silicon-coated dressings,[14] which is thought to be due to a toxic effect on keratinocytes. It is widely available and relatively inexpensive and thus remains one of the most commonly used treatments for superficial burns. (In patients with larger and/or deeper burns that are assessed as requiring excision and grafting, the antimicrobial efficacy of silver sulfadiazine and mafenide acetate burn creams argues in favor of their use, despite any adverse effect on spontaneous wound healing.)

Superficial facial burns can be safely managed on an outpatient basis as long as inhalation and ocular injuries have been excluded. As with other areas of the body, the aim is to promote a moist burn-wound environment in order to speed reepithelialization, which in turn will reduce scarring and preserve function. Various topical agents may be used on the face such as bacitracin, or bacitracin and polymyxin B (Polysporin). Paraffin-based products may be used for facial burns but paraffin is highly flammable and patients must be strictly instructed not to smoke while using it because severe and even fatal injuries have been reported.[15]

When the dressing is applied, consideration should be given to frequency of dressing changes and whether these will be performed at home by the patient or in the health-care facility. In the latter scenario, the patient needs a reliable way of returning to the clinic for dressing changes as well as a reliable method of contacting the clinic if there are unexpected problems. In general, it is better to use a dressing, which can be left in place for several days before needing to be changed because this avoids traumatizing the healing wound and also avoids frequent potentially painful dressing changes. Frequency of dressing changes will be determined, in part, by the amount of exudate from the wound. Although antimicrobial dressings are more expensive than more traditional dressings, they require less frequent changes and, therefore, may actually represent an overall cost saving.

Dressing changes may be performed in the burn-care facility or by the patient or caregiver at home. Outreach nursing teams can be invaluable in managing outpatient cases, especially if the patient lives a long distance from the burn-care facility or finds it difficult to travel.

PAIN MANAGEMENT

Burns can be very painful. Adequate analgesia is important for successful outpatient management—at the time of initial debridement, during ongoing dressing changes, and as background analgesia in between dressings. Utilizing the pain ladder is an appropriate method for both adults and children, that is, starting with simple analgesics such as acetaminophen and ibuprofen and then escalating to opioids if required. Adjuncts such as pregabalin may be added for neuropathic pain if this is troublesome.

Dressing changes should be performed in a facility with the ability to deliver opioid analgesia if required and to monitor the patient for any adverse effects. Oral agents may be supplemented by patient-controlled inhalational agents such as nitrous oxide and oxygen mix (Entonox) or methoxyflurane (Penthrox) where these are available.

Nonpharmacological analgesia such as hypnosis and distraction techniques can be very helpful, particularly in managing associated anxiety. There is evidence that the use of virtual reality during burns dressing changes not only reduces pain and anxiety[16] but is also associated with reduced time to healing.[17] Studies have shown that even relatively low-fidelity solutions using a smart phone lead to a decrease in pain scores while being easy to use in a clinic setting.[18] Many patients will require multiple dressing changes during a period of weeks, and any techniques that reduce pain and anxiety during this time will lead to a more positive experience overall.

THE MULTIDISCIPLINARY TEAM

Patients treated on an outpatient basis should still be able to access the full burns multidisciplinary team, just as if they had been admitted. For example, even patients with minor burns can suffer significant psychological distress, which is unrelated to extent and visibility of the burn, circumstances of the injury, or the degree of disfigurement. This is described as "small burn, big problem"[19] and leads to significant psychological morbidity, which may require input from a psychologist.

Patients also require access to physiotherapy, occupational therapy, dietetics, and other support staff depending on the nature of their injuries. Outpatient care should not preclude access to patient support groups or burn camps, which may be as valuable for patients with "minor" burns as those who have been admitted with a more extensive injury.

MANAGEMENT OF COMPLICATIONS

Complications may develop at any time before the burn wound has healed, and it is important that the patient be able to communicate with the treating medical team in case of any concerns. The team may advise urgent review at a local medical facility, for example, in case of suspected infection or sepsis, or a planned review by the burn-care provider, for example, in case of problems with the dressing or poorly controlled pain.

BURN-WOUND INFECTION

All burn wounds are prone to infection due to the breach in the protective skin barrier, and a degree of immunosuppression is seen in even minor burns. Patients should be counselled about signs, which may indicate infection, and what steps to take if they are concerned. The incidence of burn-wound infection may be reduced by thorough wound debridement at the initial presentation and the use of antimicrobial dressings. Routine use of prophylactic antibiotics is best avoided due to the risk of resistant organisms and potential side effects. Burn wounds are frequently colonized with microorganisms, and a positive wound swab does not necessarily indicate a burn-wound infection. Clinical signs such as warmth, redness, discharge, increasing pain, or systemic upset should all prompt consideration of antibiotic therapy. Typical microorganisms are gram positive in the early stage of burn wound healing with gram-negative organisms becoming more prevalent after the first 7 to 10 days.

In cases of suspected burn-wound infection, broad-spectrum antibiotics should be commenced and then rationalized when microbiology results are available to guide antibiotic sensitivities. Depending on the clinical state of the patient and other factors such as comorbidities, treatment of early or minor burn-wound infection may be continued on an outpatient basis with oral antibiotics. Regular patient review is vital, and signs of systemic upset or deteriorating infection despite oral antibiotics warrants escalation to intravenous antibiotics. Although systemic antibiotics can be delivered in the community in some settings, admission is usually required at this point until the infection begins to respond to treatment.

TOXIC SHOCK SYNDROME

Parents of children with burn injuries should be carefully counselled about the symptoms of toxic shock syndrome (TSS) and the importance of seeking urgent medical attention if they develop. TSS is a rare but potentially fatal toxin-mediated disease usually caused by *Staphylococcus aureus* that can occur after seemingly trivial burns in children. Typical cases present within 2 days of injury in a child aged younger than 2 years with a burn smaller than 10% TBSA.[20] Clinical signs include pyrexia, rash, diarrhea, vomiting, and lethargy or irritability. Children with TSS can deteriorate very quickly without treatment and mortality of up to 50% is reported. Emergency departments should be educated that an unwell child with a burn has TSS until proven otherwise and should know how to commence urgent treatment. Parents should be advised to seek urgent attention at their closest medical facility rather than return to the burn-care provider because unnecessary delay may lead to worse outcomes. Symptoms can be vague and may be confused with other childhood illnesses but treatment should be commenced if suspicious and deescalated when appropriate. Treatment consists of fluid resuscitation, antibiotics, and consideration of fresh frozen plasma to provide passive immunity with preformed antibodies against the circulating toxin. Further treatment is supportive depending on the degree of organ dysfunction.

INADEQUATE BURN-WOUND HEALING

Careful follow-up is required for burns managed as an outpatient. If it becomes clear that the wound is not healing as expected or that healing is prolonged, then review by a burn-care provider is required to assess whether surgical intervention is indicated to expedite wound closure. Longer healing times are associated with higher rates of hypertrophic scarring, which can be unsightly, uncomfortable, and require prolonged periods of scar therapy.

Although traditionally 3 weeks has been used as a "safe" cutoff for wound healing (without the need for excision and grafting), hypertrophic scars can occur in burns that heal sooner than this, particularly in non-White skin types and in high-risk anatomical locations. Every additional day to healing carries a 1.138 relative risk of hypertrophic scarring and "every day counts" when considering healing time.[21]

Wounds that are failing to progress or that are expected to lead to adverse scarring should be considered for surgical management. This is not necessarily a failure of outpatient management; in burns of indeterminate depth, it is very reasonable to trial a period of conservative management providing there is the possibility of changing to a surgical approach if indicated. All management decisions should be made in conjunction with the patient wherever possible. Many patients are understandably reluctant to consider surgery and are keen to manage burns with dressings alone initially. They may become more keen on surgical intervention if wound healing is protracted and the burden of regular dressing changes becomes apparent.

TELEMEDICINE AND BURNS

Telemedicine is the term given to the practice of medicine using technology to deliver care at a distance. The use of telemedicine is already well established in burns and has been shown to be safe and accurate.[22] Its use was expanded across many specialties during the COVID-19 pandemic when steps were taken to reduce the number of face-to-face consultations. Increasing familiarity with video conferencing and remote working during the pandemic now means that telemedicine is more acceptable to patients than ever before. Telemedicine allows patients or referring services to send photographs of a burn wound to a specialist burns service. This can be used to assess the burn wound, make initial plans for management, and monitor ongoing progress without the need to see the patient face-to-face. Consultations may be carried out by telephone or by video, allowing real-time evaluation of the wound as well as assessment of range of movement, demonstration of dressing techniques, and so forth. This can be continued once the burn wound has healed for ongoing follow-up by phone or video according to patient preference and local services.

Telemedicine is particularly useful for patients who are geographically remote from a specialist burns service or those who have difficulties with mobility or transport. As well as being more convenient for patients, there are associated economic and environmental benefits in reducing unnecessary travel. The potential negatives of remote consultation include the inability to palpate scars, perform physical therapy, or to perform procedures such as intralesional steroid injections for scars.[23] Burn patients often have psychological morbidity and the loss of face-to-face interaction may be particularly harmful for this group of patients.

EDUCATION AND PREVENTION

Patient education and prevention are key aspects of burn care and can be delivered in the outpatient setting. Health-care providers should take the opportunity to provide basic health-promotion and burn-prevention information, which may prevent future, more serious injuries. Information should cover home safety topics such as keeping hot drinks away from children, safe use of kitchen appliances, use of smoke detectors in the home, and electrical safety. It should also cover appropriate first aid, which should include advice to apply cool running water for 20 minutes and to avoid applying substances such as creams, egg, butter, or turmeric to the wound.

LONG-TERM MANAGEMENT

Treatment does not end when the burn wound is healed. Patients managed as outpatients should have access to ongoing follow-up from the multidisciplinary team to monitor their progress. Burns that heal in less than 2 weeks do not generally heal with scarring but may result in dyspigmentation of the area, which can be very distressing. Patients should be advised to keep healed areas protected from direct ultraviolet light for up to 2 years. Areas that have healed with a scar should be regularly massaged with a bland emollient 2 to 3 times daily to help scars soften and fade. Newly healed skin may develop fragility blisters during massage, which generally resolve spontaneously and will settle as the healed skin matures.

Hypertrophic scars may develop, especially in those with delayed wound healing and non-White skin. Management of hypertrophic scars is multimodal and includes scar massage, topical silicone, and the use of pressure garments along with intralesional steroid injections and laser. Occasionally surgical revision of hypertrophic or contracted scars may be necessary. The impact of even small scars on a patient may be significant, and these can be assessed using a range of administered questionnaires such as the Patient and Observer Scar Assessment Scale.[24]

SUMMARY

Burn injuries are common and most may be considered minor and are suitable for outpatient management. Steps should be taken to ensure that patients managed in this way still retain access to the full burns multidisciplinary team and that admission remains an option if complications develop or according to patient preference. Modern antimicrobial dressings, outreach nursing teams, and the use of telemedicine means that the number of patients that can be safely managed without hospital admission is likely to increase further.

CLINICS CARE POINTS

- Most burn injuries are relatively minor and can be safely managed as an outpatient
- Appropriate first aid and wound management leads to superior outcomes
- A wide range of dressings is available, and selection should be tailored to the patient and the wound
- TSS is a rare but potentially fatal complication, which is typically seen in young children with small burns
- Hypertrophic scars may be seen even in burns, which heal sooner than 3 weeks; surgical management should be considered in patients at high risk of adverse scarring
- Patients with healed burns may require long-term follow-up by the whole multidisciplinary burns team in order to optimize their outcome and return to preinjury condition

DECLARATION OF INTERESTS

The author has no conflicts of interest to declare. The author has nothing to disclose.

REFERENCES

1. Peck MD. Epidemiology of burns throughout the world. Part I: distribution and risk factors. Burns 2011;37(7):1087–100.
2. American burn association: burn incidence fact sheet. Available at: https://ameriburn.org/who-we-are/media/burn-incidence-fact-sheet/. Accessed 28.09.2022.
3. Brown M, Coffee T, Adenuga P, et al. Outcomes of outpatient management of pediatric burns. J Burn Care Res 2014;35(5):388–94.
4. Thompson DM, Thomas C, Hyde L, et al. At home parent-administered dressing changes in paediatric burns aftercare: a survey of burns centres?" practice. Burns 2022;48(2):365–71.
5. Farid M, Al Omran Y, Lewis D, et al. Management of minor burns during the COVID-19 pandemic: a patient-centred approach. Scars Burn Heal 2021;7. 20595131211020566.
6. Griffin B, Cabilan CJ, Ayoub B, et al. The effect of 20 minutes of running water first aid within three hours of thermal burn injury on patient outcomes: A systematic review and meta-analysis. Australas Emerg Care 2022;25(4):367–76.
7. Zack-Williams SD, Ahmad Z, Moiemen NS. The clinical efficacy of Diphoterine® in the management of cutaneous chemical burns: a 2-year evaluation study. Ann Burns Fire Disasters 2015;28(1):9–12.
8. Wilson G, French G. Plasticised polyvinylchloride as a temporary dressing for burns. Br Med J 1987;294:556–7.
9. Ro HS, Shin JY, Sabbagh MD, et al. Effectiveness of aspiration or deroofing for blister management in patients with burns: a prospective randomized controlled trial. Medicine (Baltim) 2018;97(17):e0563.
10. Pape SA, Skouras CA, Byrne PO. An audit of the use of laser Doppler imaging (LDI) in the assessment of burns of intermediate depth. Burns 2001;27(3):233–9.
11. Jan SN, Khan FA, Bashir MM, et al. Comparison of laser doppler imaging (LDI) and clinical assessment in differentiating between superficial and deep partial thickness burn wounds. Burns 2018;44(2):405–8.
12. moorLDI2-BI: a laser Doppler blood flow imager for burn wound assessment. Medical technologies guidance. Available at: https://www.nice.org.uk/guidance/mtg2/resources/moorldi2bi-a-laser-doppler-blood-flow-imager-for-burn-wound-assessment-pdf-1788109070533. Accessed 27.9.22.
13. Wearn C, Lee KC, Hardwicke J, et al. Prospective comparative evaluation study of Laser Doppler Imaging and thermal imaging in the assessment of burn depth. Burns 2018;44(1):124–33.
14. Wasiak J, Cleland H, Campbell F, et al. Dressings for superficial and partial thickness burns. Cochrane Database Syst Rev 2013;2013(3):CD002106.
15. Ridd MJ, Hall S, Lane ME, et al. Burns with emollients. BMJ 2022;376:e066102.
16. Czech O, Wrzeciono A, Batalík L, et al. Virtual reality intervention as a support method during wound care and rehabilitation after burns: A systematic review and meta-analysis. Complement Ther Med 2022;68:102837.
17. Brown NJ, Kimble RM, Rodger S, et al. Play and heal: randomized controlled trial of Ditto™ intervention efficacy on improving re-epithelialization in pediatric burns. Burns 2014;40(2):204–13.
18. Xiang H, Shen J, Wheeler K, et al. Efficacy of smartphone active and passive virtual reality distraction vs standard care on burn pain among pediatric patients: a randomized clinical trial. JAMA Netw Open 2021;4(6):e2112082.

19. Blumenfield M, Reddish PM. Identification of psychologic impairment in patients with mild-moderate thermal injury: small burn, big problem. Gen Hosp Psychiatry 1987;9(2):142–6.
20. White M, Thornton K, Young A. Early diagnosis and treatment of toxic shock syndrome in paediatric burns. Burns 2005;31(2):193–7.
21. Chipp E, Charles L, Thomas C, et al. A prospective study of time to healing and hypertrophic scarring in paediatric burns: every day counts. Burns Trauma 2017; 5:3, eCollection 2017.
22. Saffle JR, Edelman L, Theurer L, et al. Telemedicine evaluation of acute burns is accurate and cost-effective. J Trauma 2009;67(2):358–65.
23. Brady C, Burke-Smith A, Williams A. COVID virtual burns clinics - Logistical advantages and the patient perspective. Burns 2021;47(4):961–2.
24. Draaijers LJ, Tempelman FR, Botman YA, et al. The patient and observer scar assessment scale: a reliable and feasible tool for scar evaluation. Plast Reconstr Surg 2004;113:1960–5.

Prehospital and Emergency Management

Jasmine M. Williams, MD[a],*, Chelsea L. Ingle, DO[a], Steven G. Schauer, DO, MS[a,b,c], Joseph K. Maddry, MD[a,b,c,d]

KEYWORDS

- Burn • Emergency • Fluid • Prehospital

KEY POINTS

- Patient's airway, breathing, and circulation are evaluated in the primary survey of any burn injury.
- Burns should be carefully assessed for their depth and extent.
- Accurate fluid resuscitation is a key feature in early care.
- Carbon monoxide and cyanide toxicity should be considered in patients with smoke inhalation.
- The American Burn Association criteria for burn center referral should be considered for all patients; disposition and need for escalation of care should be individualized.

EPIDEMIOLOGY/INTRODUCTION

Burns are a common presenting chief complaint in United States Emergency Departments (EDs). In 2018, more than 400,000 patients presented to an ED with some form of burn injury. The American Burn Association (ABA) repository of 2019 lists thermal burns as the leading cause of burn injuries in the United States, making up 41% of presentations. This is followed by scalds (31%), electrical burns (3.6%), and chemical burns (3.5%).[1] Presentation can range from small, superficial wounds, all the way to extensive deep-tissue injury with multisystem involvement requiring aggressive resuscitation. Emergency medicine and emergency medical services staff need to possess a proper understanding of how to triage, evaluate, and manage burn patients.

[a] Brooke Army Medical Center, JBSA Fort Sam Houston, TX, USA; [b] US Army Institute of Surgical Research, 3698 Chambers Pass, JBSA Fort Sam Houston, TX 78234, USA; [c] Uniformed Services University of the Health Sciences, Bethesda, MD, USA; [d] 59th Medical Wing, JBSA Lackland, TX, USA
* Corresponding author. 3551 Roger Brooke Drive, JBSA Fort Sam Houston, Texas, USA.
E-mail address: jasmine.willmd@gmail.com

Surg Clin N Am 103 (2023) 389–401
https://doi.org/10.1016/j.suc.2023.02.001
0039-6109/23/© 2023 Elsevier Inc. All rights reserved.
surgical.theclinics.com

PREHOSPITAL MANAGEMENT

In the prehospital environment, a rapid assessment of the scene safety should be conducted, and the patient should be removed from any potential hazards that could result in further injury. The initial assessment and triage of burn patients then begins with a primary survey encompassing airway, breathing, circulation, disability, and exposure similar to other trauma assessments. The primary survey can be completed in the following stepwise approach.[2] Repeat evaluations are often needed because changes can rapidly occur during the early phase.

Airway

Primary assessment begins by evaluating the patient's ability to maintain their own airway. In the awake and alert patient, this is achieved by assessing their ability to speak, taking special note of any changes in pitch or tone that would indicate an inhalation injury that could progress to airway compromise.[3] The status of the airway may evolve over time as edema develops, so the initial evaluation should be repeated throughout the course of care. The ABA has developed the following criteria for intubation in patients with suspected inhalation injury.[4]

1. Full-thickness burns of the face
2. Stridor
3. Respiratory distress
4. Airway swelling on laryngoscopy
5. Airway trauma
6. Altered mental status
7. Hypoxia/hypercarbia
8. Hemodynamic instability

Additional findings such as soot within the nose and mouth, carbonaceous sputum, and burn size greater than 30% total body surface area (TBSA) also raise the likelihood of underlying inhalation injury and/or impending airway edema.[5] However, these are frequently referred to as "soft" signs for intubation and should prompt further investigation or frequent reevaluation. If the decision is made to intubate a patient, an 8.0 endotracheal tube should be used, if possible, in order to facilitate future bronchoscopy.[6]

Breathing

Assessment of breathing is performed as a standard part of Advanced Trauma Life Support protocols. Bilateral lung fields are auscultated for equal breath sounds, making note of any wheezing that could indicate inhalation injury. Initial and continuous pulse oximetry may be used to monitor for hypoxemia. Patients with decreased oxygen saturation or increased work of breathing should be placed on supplemental oxygen as needed.

Circulation

Assessment of circulation includes palpating for pulses and measuring heart rate and blood pressure. As patients with significant burns require fluid resuscitation (eg, all patients with burn size ≥20% TBSA), it is crucial to establish either intravenous or interosseous access. Although it is acceptable to obtain intravenous access through burned skin, it is also associated with an increased risk of infection as well as a decreased rate of success due to loss of landmarks and difficulties with securing the line to the skin.[7] For this reason, we recommend that initial attempts be through undamaged skin (if available). Intraosseous access maybe used as an alternative when difficulty with IV access occurs.

Disability

The standard assessment of mental status in the trauma patient is through the Glasgow Coma scale. However, burns alone are not likely to cause changes in mental status. A change in mental status should prompt a search for other derangements.

Exposure

As burns encompass a wide range of causes to include thermal, electrical, and chemical, it is important to remove clothing that could possibly produce further heat or caustic damage to the tissue. Additionally, the clothing may become adherent to the wounds, which will make disrobing more challenging. An additional aspect of prehospital care includes consideration of body temperature. Burn injuries are associated with compromise of the body's normal ability to regulate temperature. Hypothermia has been associated with worse outcomes in trauma patients; this finding is similar in burn patients because it has been associated with a decreased time to mortality.[8,9] Although exposure is a part of the primary survey, there should be adequate external warming methods available. Passive warming methods may be used in a normothermic patient but those with hypothermia should undergo active warming methods such as warmed fluids.

EVALUATION IN THE EMERGENCY DEPARTMENT

Upon presentation to the ED, there is reassessment of the primary survey and evaluation of all interventions implemented in the field. It is important to note that all other injuries should be noted, addressed, and prioritized in order of their immediate risk to the patient. The injury that poses the greatest immediate threat to life, whether burn or trauma, should be prioritized.

Initial evaluation of burns includes classification based on depth of injury, as follows (**Table 1**).[1,6]

1. Superficial thickness (first degree): Burns to the epidermis (**Fig. 1**).
2. Partial thickness (second degree): Burns to the epidermis and a portion of the dermis. This category is further broken down into superficial partial and deep partial based on depth of extension into the dermis (**Fig. 2**).
3. Full thickness (third degree): Burns through the entirety of both the epidermis and dermis (**Fig. 3**).

Table 1
Burn depth classification

Classification	Skin Layer Involved	Physical Examination Findings
Superficial	Epidermis	Dry, red, blanches with pressure, painful
Superficial partial thickness	Epidermis and portion of dermis	Red, weeping, blisters, blanch with pressure, painful
Deep partial thickness	Epidermis and portion of dermis	Red, white patches, blisters, does not blanch with pressure, typically less painful
Full thickness	Epidermis, dermis, possibly deeper	Variable appearance. Can be charred or white. Usually dry, does not blanch with pressure, usually not painful

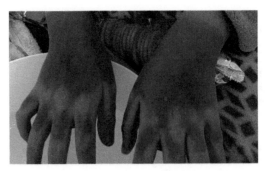

Fig. 1. Superficial burn: Burn to the epidermis layer only.

TBSA burned is the single most important metric for clinical decision-making. It is used to estimate fluid resuscitation needs, as well as in predicting overall prognosis. Although there are multiple tools to estimate TBSA, one method is the Rule of Nines. With this method, the body is broken into different sections, each of which has an allocated percentage. Burns are evaluated by their proportion of involved tissue in each region, and these values are summed to produce TBSA.[10] An alternative method is to use the patient's hand to estimate TBSA, with the palm (minus the fingers) being roughly equivalent to 0.5% and the entire hand (with the fingers) close to 1%. This is especially useful in children, in whom the use of traditional Rule of Nines could result in overestimation and overresuscitation.[11] It is important to note that TBSA excludes superficial wounds (first-degree burns) and only incorporates areas of partial-thickness and full-thickness burns (second-degree and third-degree burns). Once TBSA is calculated, the fluid infusion rate should then be revised using a burn resuscitation formula (see later discussion).

Evaluation apart from thorough physical examination may also include laboratory tests, which should be tailored to the patient's presentation and mechanism of injury. Laboratories such as a venous blood gas and lactate are trended to assess adequacy of resuscitation. In cases of moderate-to-severe injury, continued cardiac monitoring, end-tidal carbon dioxide monitoring, and pulse oximetry help to assess for any acute changes in oxygenation, ventilation, and hemodynamic stability that would require additional intervention.

EARLY MANAGEMENT
Fluid Resuscitation

Fluid resuscitation for the treatment of burn shock is one of the most important early interventions necessary in adults with 20% or greater TBSA and children with 15% or greater TBSA; some patients with preexisting medical illnesses require resuscitation for burn size 10% or greater. Burn patients experience increased microvascular permeability, with fluid shifts out of the intravascular compartment in damaged tissue. In patients with larger burns (≥25%), massive release of inflammatory mediators causes increased microvascular permeability in unburned tissue as well. Patients in burn shock also experience a varying degree of decreased cardiac contractility, and intense peripheral vasoconstriction. Replacing the ongoing volume losses and gradually restoring intravascular volume maintains vital-organ perfusion. After the first 24 hours, microvascular permeability improves, allowing titration to maintenance fluids to occur during the next 24 hours.[12,13]

There are multiple formulas to help guide initial fluid resuscitation during the first 24 hours. The 2 most common formulas are the Parkland or Baxter formula and the

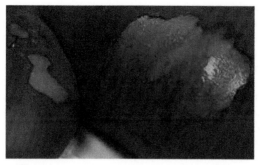

Fig. 2. Partial thickness burn: Burn to the epidermis and parts of the dermis.

modified Brooke formula. The ABA's Advanced Burn Life Support course now recommends the modified Brooke formula. The Institute of Surgical Research (ISR) Rule of Tens is a simplified formula that will typically put initial fluid rates between Parkland and modified Brooke recommendations and is the method recommended in the US Joint Trauma System guidelines for use in adults.[14] The ISR Rule of Tens is the simplest method for calculating fluid needs[15] but is not applicable to the pediatric population; for children (<40 kg) a weight-based formula such as the modified Brooke formula for children must be used.

- Parkland: The volume to be given during the first 24 hours is 4 mL/kg × TBSA%, with one-half of this volume given in the first 8 hours
- Modified Brooke (children): The volume to be given during the first 24 hours is 3 mL/kg × TBSA%, with one-half of this volume given in the first 8 hours
- Modified Brooke (adults): The volume to be given during the first 24 hours is 2 mL/kg × TBSA%, with one-half of this volume given in the first 8 hours
- Institute of Surgical Research Rule of Tens (adults): The starting rate is 10 mL/h × %TBSA, with an additional 100 mL/h for every 10 kg above 80 kg

Physiologic crystalloids, such as lactated Ringer's (LR) or Plasma-Lyte, are the recommended fluids in the first 24 hours, with LR being the most widely used. Excessive normal saline is associated with hyperchloremic acidosis.[12,16] It is for this reason that

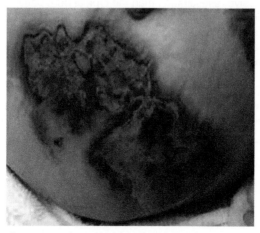

Fig. 3. Full thickness burn: Burn through the entire layer of both the epidermis and dermis.

we recommend the use of more balanced solutions. A 5% albumin infusion should be considered if the patient's response to initial resuscitation is such that they are predicted to receive greater than 250 mL/kg total fluid volume during the first 24 hours, or if the patient requires a sustained hourly infusion rate greater than 1500 mL/h.[14]

A common question is what to do about fluids given in the prehospital setting by EMS, or during transfer from an outside hospital. Although some authors have recommended adjusting the total volume to be infused based on these data, we recommend against this practice because it is mathematically more complex and because it risks underresuscitating patients who may have initially received too much. Rather, this volume should be noted, but the resuscitation continued based on the rate predicated by the formula, as if the patient was newly injured.

The above-mentioned formulas provide only a starting point. The fluid rate must be adjusted hourly, up or down, based on physiologic response. Urine output is the primary variable used to monitor fluid resuscitation and organ perfusion. A Foley catheter should be placed and urine output checked hourly once resuscitation has started. The goal urine output is 30 to 50 mL/h in adults and 0.5 to 1 mL/kg/h in children, as shown in **Table 2**. If a patient is oliguric despite several hours of resuscitation, reevaluate the patient from head to toe; check the lactate level; and consider inserting a central line to monitor central venous pressure. Other resuscitation endpoints can be found in **Box 1**.[17] Fluid boluses are not recommended (except in the presence of significant hypotension). This is because boluses, in the presence of increased microvascular permeability during burn shock, yield no lasting benefit and drive increased edema formation. Overresuscitation must be avoided because it results in numerous complications, such as pulmonary edema, compartment syndromes, and increased mortality.[12,13]

In addition to fluid resuscitation, pediatric burn patients, especially less than 20 kg, need fluids with glucose to prevent hypoglycemia. Use dextrose 5% in lactated Ringer's at a maintenance rate, in addition to the resuscitation LR. Use the pediatric 4-2-1 rule to calculate the maintenance rate (4 mL/kg for the first 10 kg + 2 mL/kg for the second 10 kg + 1 mL/kg for the third 10 kg and above). This infusion is not titrated.[13,14] Early nasogastric tube placement with enteral feeding in those who cannot continue bottle feeding is important for long-term outcomes.

Patients with gross myoglobinuria—most commonly caused by high-voltage electric injury—represent a special problem in burn-shock resuscitation.[18] These patients require more aggressive resuscitation than the typical burn patient. The fluid infusion rate should be rapidly increased to achieve a urine output of 70 to 100 mL/h in adults, in order to reduce myoglobin precipitation in the renal tubules. Failure to clear myoglobin on visual inspection of the urine over several hours may indicate ongoing myonecrosis and a need for surgery.

Pain Control

IV opioids are most often used to treat the severe pain caused by burns. Multimodal analgesia is appropriate, to include acetaminophen, selective Cox-2 inhibitors,

Table 2 Titrating burn resuscitation in adults	
Urine Output	**Action**
<30 mL/h	Increase fluid rate by 20%
30–50 mL/h	Maintain fluid rate
>50 mL/h	Decrease fluid rate by 20%

Box 1
Goals of burn resuscitation

Goals of burn resuscitation (Adults)

Urine output 30 to 50 mL/h

Heart rate less than 130

Systolic blood pressure greater than 90 mm Hg or mean arterial pressure greater than 60 mm Hg

Strong equal peripheral pulses

Base deficit less than 2 mEq/L

Lactate less than 2 mmol/L

---

gabapentin, and/or benzodiazepines.[1,18] Ketamine is the best option for conscious sedation because it causes a dissociative state with little effect on blood pressure and airway.[19] Ketamine has been shown to decrease the overall opioid requirements and decrease secondary hyperalgesia.[20] It can safely be used for patient-controlled analgesia with boluses for breakthrough pain.[21]

Wound Management/Infection Prophylaxis

All care should be performed in as warm an environment as possible, and active measures should be used to maintain core temperature.[9] As soon as possible (but certainly within the first 24 hours postburn), the patient should be completely cleansed with warm water and chlorhexidine to remove all nonviable skin and debris without causing further damage.[22] Afterward, a topical antimicrobial agent should be applied to help prevent infection and keep the tissue moist to promote healing. There are multiple topical agents applicable (**Table 3**). For deep burns with eschar formation, excision and debridement needs to occur but typically is performed after the first 24 hours.

Chemical Injuries

Chemical burns are managed with immediate and copious irrigation with water, as the major determinant of chemical burn severity is the duration of contact with the skin.[23] Exceptions include the following.[24]

- Phenols: Water insoluble; wipe with 50% polyethylene glycol first
- Dry lime: Exposure to water forms a strong base; substance should be brushed off the skin before irrigation
- Muriatic acid, concentrated sulfuric acid: Produce heat when mixed with water; consider neutralization with soap and water or lime water

Another special circumstance is hydrofluoric acid (HF), which may cause life-threatening hypocalcemia. These injuries should be treated with calcium gluconate, either as a topical gel, by intradermal injection, or by intra-arterial infusion.[24] Cutaneous exposure of a large area (>10%) or any ingestion of HF may necessitate intravenous calcium. Given the extremely dangerous nature of HF exposure, a medical toxicologist or Poison Control Center (1–800–222–1222) should be consulted immediately.

Escharotomy

The aim of burn resuscitation is to maintain vital-organ function while gradually restoring intravascular volume and avoiding the complications caused by edema.

Table 3
Topical agents for emergency department burn care

Topical Agent	Advantages	Disadvantages
Silver sulfadiazine	• Well-tolerated • Affordable • Broad-spectrum antimicrobial activity, including yeast	• Does not penetrate eschar • May cause transient neutropenia
Sulfamylon (mafenide acetate)	• Penetrates eschar and cartilage • Excellent antibacterial coverage, for example, *Pseudomonas*	• Painful application • Metabolic acidosis • No antifungal activity
Silver-containing dressings (eg, Acticoat, Aquacel Ag, Silverlon)	• May be used on clean wounds for up to 7 d	• Does not penetrate eschar • Prolonged use may result in inattention to wound status
Mupirocin	• Effective against Methacillin-Resistant Staphlococcus Aureus • Can use with other agents if needed	• Requires frequent dressing changes • No efficacy against gram-negative or fungal organisms
Combination antibiotic ointment, Bacitracin	• Well-tolerated • Inexpensive	• Limited antibacterial efficacy

Data from Sheridan, R.L., Critical care of the burn patient. 7th ed. Current Concepts in Adult Critical Care. 2016, Society of Critical Care Medicine; and Sheridan RL. Burns. Crit Care Med. 2002;30(11 Suppl):S500-S514.

Patients with full-thickness, circumferential burns to the extremities are at the highest risk of limb ischemia, or "eschar syndrome," caused by edema beneath the tight eschar. They should be monitored hourly with distal pulse checks by palpation or Doppler flowmetry. Delayed capillary refill, increasing pain in one extremity compared with the other, or paresthesia may be noted. If there is a concern with worsening examinations and pulses, escharotomy should not be delayed. Escharotomy can be performed at bedside with electrocautery (preferred) or a scalpel. An incision should be made in the midmedial and midlateral lines of the extremity, extending the entire length of the circumferential burn, and down to the level of the subcutaneous fat.[14] After completion of the escharotomy, distal pulses should be reexamined, and the extremity elevated above the heart. Escharotomy is not adequate to treat a true intramuscular compartment syndrome, which can also occur in burn patients, and which would require fasciotomy in the operating room. Chest escharotomies are discussed below.

Ventilation Management

Commonly used lung-protective strategies are appropriate for the early management of patients with burns and/or inhalation injury.[25] Lung-protective strategies consist of low tidal volumes (4–8 mL/kg of ideal body weight), maintaining plateau pressure less than 30 cm H_2O, and (if necessary) permissive hypercapnia. The head of the bed should be elevated.[25–28] Patients with circumferential full-thickness burns of the torso may develop a "thoracic eschar syndrome." Just as eschar and edema can cause limb ischemia in the extremities (see above), they can also cause hypoventilation in the chest. This may present as a life-threatening emergency requiring immediate bedside thoracic escharotomy to restore ventilation.

Carbon Monoxide Poisoning

Carbon monoxide (CO) poisoning is a serious complication that can occur in burn patients who suffered their injury indoors or in a confined space. CO toxicity is most common in those confined to an enclosed space with cooking stoves or engines.[14] CO has a higher affinity for hemoglobin than does oxygen, and shifts the oxyhemoglobin dissociation curve to the left, decreasing oxygen delivery to tissues. However, there are additional mechanisms to explain, for example, the delayed neurologic sequelae caused by CO. These include CO binding intracellular proteins such as myoglobin and cytochrome c oxidase, lipid peroxidation by neutrophils, and mitochondrial oxidative stress.[29] Common presenting symptoms include headache, dizziness, confusion, decreased or transient loss of consciousness, seizures, or cardiac ischemia. The classic teaching of cherry red skin is very rare late finding and usually only seen at lethal levels.[29]

The gold standard for diagnosis of CO poisoning is cooximetric measurement of carboxyhemoglobin (COHb) in arterial (preferred) or venous blood. A level greater than 3% to 4% in nonsmokers and greater than 10% in smokers is abnormal. A patient's peripheral saturation of oxygen by pulse oximetry may be normal despite elevated COHb. A newer method that may help screen for CO is a noninvasive pulse cooximeter, with values of SpCO greater than 6% in nonsmokers, and greater than 9% in smokers; however, we recommend that a confirmatory blood COHb be performed.[30] Due to the risk of cardiac injury, we also recommend a screening electrocardiogram be obtained when CO toxicity is probable.

Treatment of CO toxicity should begin as soon as there is any clinical suspicion, even before confirmatory testing results. The treatment consists of high flow 100% Fio_2 through face mask or endotracheal tube, which will shorten the half-life of COHb from 2.5 hours on room air to approximately 45 minutes. Oxygen supplementation should be continued until blood COHb is less than 3% to 5% and the patient's symptoms have resolved, typically around 6 hours.[18,29,31] Although studies evaluating the efficacy of hyperbaric oxygen have yielded conflicting results, it is recommended for special circumstances (**Box 2**) with the goal of decreasing delayed neurologic sequelae.[31] If considered, hyperbaric oxygen is recommended within 6 hours from injury but may be efficacious if initiated up to 24 hours after injury.

Cyanide Toxicity

Cyanide toxicity should be considered in structural or vehicular fires in which there is combustion of materials releasing hydrogen cyanide gas. These include certain synthetics (eg, polyurethane, vinyl), wool, and silk. Cyanide inhibits mitochondrial cytochrome c oxidase, causing inhibition of aerobic metabolism leading to anaerobic metabolism with cellular hypoxia. CN affects the nervous system first causing headaches, dizziness, confusion, and anxiety. In mild cases, hypertension and tachypnea are seen but in more severe toxicity, hypotension, bradypnea, pulmonary edema, seizures, and cardiac arrhythmias are more common.[32,33] CN toxicity is a clinical diagnosis due to the lack of blood cyanide testing capabilities in the ED. Burn patients with an appropriate mechanism of injury and neurologic symptoms (altered mental status, coma, seizure), hypotension, and lactic acidosis—in particular a lactate greater than 8 to 10 mmol/L—should be treated for a presumed cyanide toxicity.[34]

Hydroxocobalamin (a form of vitamin B_{12}) is the recommended antidote due to its rapid onset and safety. It works by binding to CN and forming cyanocobalamin and therefore does not affect hemodynamic stability or oxygen delivery. It is dosed at 5 g infused intravenously over 15 minutes with a repeat 5 g in severe cases.[32,33] If hydroxocobalamin is unavailable, sodium nitrite (300 mg) and sodium thiosulfate (12.5 g) are other options. Sodium nitrite is contraindicated if CO toxicity is a concern, due to it causing methemoglobinemia and worsening oxygen delivery.[27,34]

DISPOSITION

The ABA has recently revised its guidelines to help determine which patients merit referral to a burn center (**Table 4**).[35] Patients not meeting these criteria must be evaluated on an individualized basis, considering the extent of the burn, age of the patient, location of injuries, and comorbidities. Partial-thickness burns not meeting transfer criteria may still warrant admission, especially in young children and in the elderly. Typically, patients with superficial burns not requiring IV fluid resuscitation and with appropriate oral pain control can be discharged home with primary care follow-up. In cases where the disposition of the patient is unclear, the provider should consult burn specialists for further recommendations.[36]

Box 2
Indications for hyperbaric oxygen in carbon monoxide poisoning

Carboxyhemoglobin level greater than 25%

Carboxyhemoglobin level greater than 20% in pregnant patients

Loss of consciousness

Cardiac injury: EKG changes, elevated cardiac enzymes

End-organ damage: seizure, altered mental status

Severe metabolic acidosis (pH < 7.1)

Table 4 Guidelines for burn patient referral		
	Immediate Consultation with Consideration for Transfer	**Consultation Recommendation**
Thermal Burns	• Full thickness burns • Partial thickness ≥10% TBSA • Deep partial or full thickness burns involving face, hands, genitalia, feet, perineum, or over joints • Other comorbidities • Concomitant trauma • Poorly controlled pain	• Partial thickness burns <10% TBSA • Potentially deep burns of any size
Inhalation Injury	• Suspected inhalation injury	• Signs of potential inhalation such as facial flash burns, singed facial hairs, or smoke exposure
Pediatrics (≤14 y, or <30 kg)	• All pediatric burns may benefit from burn center referral due to pain, dressing change needs, rehabilitation, patient/caregiver needs, or nonaccidental trauma	
Chemical injuries	• All chemical injuries	
Electrical injuries	• All high voltage (≥1000 V) electrical injuries • Lightning injury	Low voltage (<1000 V) electrical injuries: consultation and consideration for follow-up in a burn center to screen for delayed symptoms, vision problems

Adapted from American Burn Association, "Guidelines for Burn Patient Referral" (2022 revision). Available at https://ameriburn.org/resources/burnreferral/; with permission.

CLINICS CARE POINTS

- Patient's airway, breathing, and circulation are evaluated in the primary survey of any burn injury
- Burns should be carefully assessed for their depth and extent
- Accurate fluid resuscitation is a key feature in early care
- CO and cyanide toxicity should be considered in patients with smoke inhalation
- The ABA criteria for burn center referral should be considered for all patients; disposition and need for escalation of care should be individualized

DECLARATION OF INTERESTS

The views expressed herein are those of the author(s) and do not reflect the official policy or position of Brooke Army Medical Center, the U.S. Army Medical Department, the U.S. Army Office of the Surgeon General, the Department of the Army, the Department of the Air Force, or the Department of Defense, or the U.S. Government.

REFERENCES

1. Jeschke MG, van Baar ME, Choudhry MA, et al. Burn injury. Nat Rev Dis Prim 2020;6(1):11.
2. Thim T, Krarup NH, Grove EL, et al. Initial assessment and treatment with the airway, breathing, circulation, disability, exposure (ABCDE) approach. Int J Gen Med 2012;5:117–21.
3. Witt CE, Stewart BT, Rivara FP, et al. Inpatient and Postdischarge Outcomes Following Inhalation Injury Among Critically Injured Burn Patients. J Burn Care Res 2021;42(6):1168–75.
4. Chotalia M, Pirrone C, Mangham T, et al. The predictive applicability of liberal vs restrictive intubation criteria in adult patients with suspected inhalation injury- a retrospective cohort Study. J Burn Care Res 2020;41(6):1290–6.
5. Kearns RD, Conlon KM, Matherly AF, et al. Guidelines for Burn Care Under Austere Conditions: Introduction to Burn Disaster, Airway and Ventilator Management, and Fluid Resuscitation. J Burn Care Res 2016;37(5):e427–39.
6. Newell CF, Edwards FJ, Winograd SM. A Review of Thermal Burns for Emergency Clinicians. Emergency Medicine Reports 2020;41(12).
7. Ciofi Silva CL, Rossi LA, Canini SR, et al. Site of catheter insertion in burn patients and infection: a systematic review. Burns 2014;40(3):365–73.
8. Lang TC, Zhao R, Kim A, et al. A critical update of the assessment and acute management of patients with severe burns. Adv Wound Care 2019;8(12):607–33.
9. Schauer SG, April MD, Fisher AD, et al. Hypothermia in the combat trauma population. Prehosp Emerg Care 2022;1–7.
10. Moore RA, Waheed A, Burns B. Rule of nines. In: *StatPearls*. StatPearls Publishing; 2022.
11. Nagel TR, Schunk JE. Using the hand to estimate the surface area of a burn in children. Pediatr Emerg Care 1997;13(4):254–5.
12. Rae L, Fidler P, Gibran N. The Physiologic Basis of Burn Shock and the Need for Aggressive Fluid Resuscitation. Crit Care Clin 2016;32(4):491–505.
13. Regan A, Hotwagner DT. Burn fluid management. In: *StatPearls*. StatPearls Publishing; 2022.
14. Driscoll IR, Mann-Salinas EA, Boyer NL, et al. Burn casualty care in the deployed setting. Mil Med 2018;183(suppl_2):161–7.
15. Chung KK, Salinas J, Renz EM, et al. Simple derivation of the initial fluid rate for the resuscitation of severely burned adult combat casualties: in silico validation of the rule of 10. J Trauma 2010;69(Suppl 1):S49–54.
16. Chan J, Ghosh S. Fluid resuscitation in burns: An update. Hong Kong J Emerg Med 2009;16(1):51–62.
17. Sheridan RL. Burns. Crit Care Med 2002;30(11 Suppl):S500–14.
18. Sheridan, R.L., Critical care of the burn patient. 7th edition Current concepts in adult critical care. 2016, Society of Critical Care Medicine.
19. Montgomery RK. Pain management in burn injury. Crit Care Nurs Clin 2004;16(1):39–49.
20. McGuinness SK, Wasiak J, Cleland H, et al. A systematic review of ketamine as an analgesic agent in adult burn injuries. Pain Med 2011;12(10):1551–8.
21. Schauer SG, April MD, Aden JK 3rd, et al. Impact of continuous ketamine infusion versus alternative regimens on mortality among burn intensive care unit patients: Implications for Prolonged Field Care. J Spec Oper Med 2019;19(2):77–80.
22. Rowan MP, Cancio LC, Elster EA, et al. Burn wound healing and treatment: review and advancements. Crit Care 2015;19:243–2015.

23. Brent J. Water-based solutions are the best decontaminating fluids for dermal corrosive exposures: A mini review. Clin Toxicol 2013;51(8):731–6.

24. Palao R, Monge I, Ruiz M, et al. Chemical burns: Pathophysiology and treatment. Burns 2010;36(3):295–304.

25. Palazzo S, James-Veldsman E, Wall C, et al. Ventilation strategies in burn intensive care: A retrospective observational study. Burns Trauma 2014;2(1):29–35.

26. Latenser BA. Critical care of the burn patient: the first 48 hours. Crit Care Med 2009;37(10):2819–26.

27. Dries DJ, Endorf FW. Inhalation injury: epidemiology, pathology, treatment strategies. Scand J Trauma Resuscitation Emerg Med 2013;21:31–2013.

28. Acute Respiratory Distress Syndrome Network, Brower RG, Matthay MA, et al. Ventilation with lower tidal volumes as compared with traditional tidal volumes for acute lung injury and the acute respiratory distress syndrome. N Engl J Med 2000;342(18):1301–8.

29. Hampson NB, Piantadosi CA, Thom SR, et al. Practice recommendations in the diagnosis, management, and prevention of carbon monoxide poisoning. Am J Respir Crit Care Med 2012;186(11):1095–101.

30. Sebbane M, Claret PG, Mercier G, et al. Emergency department management of suspected carbon monoxide poisoning: role of pulse CO-oximetry. Respir Care 2013;58(10):1614–20.

31. Wolf SJ, Maloney GE, Shih RD, et al, American College of Emergency Physicians Clinical Policies Subcommittee on Carbon Monoxide Poisoning. Clinical Policy: Critical issues in the evaluation and management of adult patients presenting to the emergency department with acute carbon monoxide poisoning. Ann Emerg Med 2017;69(1):98–107.e6.

32. Saeed O, Boyer NL, Pamplin JC, et al. Inhalation injury and toxic industrial chemical exposure. Mil Med 2018;183(suppl_2):130–2.

33. Lawson-Smith P, Jansen EC, Hyldegaard O. Cyanide intoxication as part of smoke inhalation–a review on diagnosis and treatment from the emergency perspective. Scand J Trauma Resuscitation Emerg Med 2011;19:14.

34. Baud FJ. Cyanide: critical issues in diagnosis and treatment. Hum Exp Toxicol 2007;26(3):191–201.

35. American Burn Association. Guidelines for Burn Patient Referral. Available at. https://ameriburn.org/resources/burnreferral/. Accessed 9 December 2022.

36. Warner PM, Coffee TL, Yowler CJ. Outpatient burn management. Surg Clin 2014; 94(4):879–92.

The First 24 Hours
Burn Shock Resuscitation and Early Complications

Shawn Tejiram, MD[a,b], Stephen P. Tranchina, BA[c],
Taryn E. Travis, MD[a,b,d], Jeffrey W. Shupp, MD[a,b,d,e,*]

KEYWORDS

- Burn • Resuscitation • Colloid • Fluid creep • Compartment syndrome

KEY POINTS

- The pathophysiologic response to burn injury drives fluid resuscitation requirements in burn shock.
- Formulas to predict fluid requirements in burn resuscitation have evolved over the past century in part due to significant historical events.
- Modern fluid resuscitation practices are augmented by colloid-based adjuncts and are titrated based on individualized physiologic response.
- Large-volume fluid resuscitation is associated with potential complications affecting several organ systems.

INTRODUCTION

Patients sustaining a thermal injury of 20% or greater of their total body surface area (TBSA) will require fluid resuscitation to treat shock.[1] Those patients with TBSA injury less than 20% may also require fluid resuscitation in cases of extremes of age, inhalation injury, or if a large proportion of TBSA is full thickness or deeper (such as in high-voltage electrical injury). The early pathophysiologic response to injury is termed burn shock in which increased microvascular permeability leads to intravascular hypovolemia requiring large volumes of fluid administration to maintain end-organ perfusion.[2]

[a] The Burn Center, MedStar Washington Hospital Center, 110 Irving Street, Northwest Suite 3B-55, Washington, DC 20010, USA; [b] Department of Surgery, Georgetown University School of Medicine, 3900 Reservoir Road NW, Washington, DC 20007, USA; [c] Georgetown University School, 3900 Reservoir Road NW, Washington, DC 20007, USA; [d] Department of Plastic and Reconstructive Surgery, Georgetown University School of Medicine, 3900 Reservoir Road NW, Washington, DC 20007, USA; [e] Department of Biochemistry and Molecular & Cellular Biology, Georgetown University Medical Center, 37th and O Street, Northwest, Washington, DC 20057, USA
* Corresponding author. The Burn Center, MedStar Washington Hospital Center, 110 Irving Street, Northwest Suite 3B-55, Washington, DC 20010.
E-mail address: Jeffrey.W.Shupp@medstar.net

Surg Clin N Am 103 (2023) 403–413
https://doi.org/10.1016/j.suc.2023.02.002
0039-6109/23/© 2023 Elsevier Inc. All rights reserved.

The treatment of burn shock using crystalloid infusions has been the mainstay of resuscitation for decades. Consensus on burn resuscitation has yet to be achieved and is an active area of research.

BURN PATHOPHYSIOLOGY

Burn shock is driven by a derangement of oncotic and hydrostatic pressures and damage to the barrier function of the microvasculature.[3] A surge in mediators such as histamine, serotonin, bradykinin, nitric oxide, oxygen-derived free radicals, tumor necrosis factor (TNF), interleukins (IL), prostaglandin, and thromboxane factor into this response. Histamine causes the formation of large endothelial gaps in response to the contraction of venular endothelial cells. Further interaction with oxygen-derived free radicals and xanthine oxidase plays a role in edema formation.[4,5] The helper T cell (Th1) response promotes release of TNF-alpha and IL-6, and promotes release of IL-10, a Th2 cytokine. The subsequent up-regulation of Th2 cells suppresses cytotoxic T cells and inhibits macrophage activation and T cell proliferation, altering the patient's ability to mount an effective immune response.[6,7]

Both local and systemic responses are evident following burn injury.[8] In injuries with smaller TBSA, the inflammatory response is typically localized and of relatively low intensity. As the burn size increases, a cytokine surge expands into systemic circulation affecting multiple organ systems.[9] Stress hormone production is redirected by the hypothalamus whereas the adrenal gland increases catecholamine and glucocorticoid release.[10] Cell–cell adhesions in capillaries weaken. This causes fluid leak from the intravascular to the interstitial space, and endothelial exposure that potentiates consumptive coagulopathy.[11–14] Recent research suggests that the endothelium (acting as its system) may be primarily injured and the degree to which this injury occurs can be measured by the breakdown products from its glycocalyx[15,16] (**Fig. 1**).

The response to burn injury is proportional to the size of the injury.[10] Injury mechanism, size, depth, concomitant inhalation or traumatic injury, and patient-specific factors all contribute to the degree of inflammatory response. Physiologic derangements following burn represent a dysregulation of homeostatic mechanisms. Increased microvascular permeability causes fluid and protein to shift into the extravascular

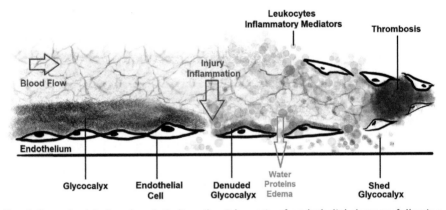

Fig. 1. Burn-shock-induced endotheliopathy. Schematic of endothelial damage following injury and inflammation resulting in increased vascular permeability, denuded glycocalyx, and migration of water, proteins, shed glycocalyx, and inflammatory mediators.

space, worsening hypovolemia, reducing cardiac output, and increasing systemic vascular resistance.[17] Myocardial dysfunction may be evident in some patients. Immediate and sustained release of catecholamines and increased adrenergic activity are key features of burn shock.[17,18] Nitric oxide released from hypoxic cells worsens hypotension, hypovolemia, and end-organ damage.[13] Hepatic injury and dysfunction may result, accompanied by transaminitis and hyperbilirubinemia.[19,20] Acute tubular necrosis may develop as a consequence of decreased cardiac output, and the effects of mediators such as aldosterone, angiotensin, and catecholamines.[17,21] Even in the absence of inhalation injury, extensive burns may cause acute respiratory distress syndrome (ARDS) (see below).[18,22]

RESUSCITATION FORMULAS

Early descriptions recognizing the need for fluid administration in burn patients date as far back as 1905 when Haldor Sneve provided oral and rectal delivery of salt solutions after burn injury.[23] In 1919, Archibald M. Fauntleroy added sodium bicarbonate to normal salt solutions via rectal infusion in the treatment of burn injury.[24] Literature suggesting fluid loss as a contributor to the physiologic response to burn injury was first described in 1930 when scientist Frank P. Underhill published his examination of the 1921 Rialto Theater Fire in New Haven, CT. Underhill studied patients involved in this fire and concluded that edema and death were related to fluid losses judged to be a filtrate of blood plasma.[25]

Current and historical formulas are summarized in **Table 1**. The modified Brooke formula recommends 2 mL/kg/%TBSA in adults and 3 mL/kg/%TBSA in children, with half administered in the first 8 hours following injury. It is the burn fluid resuscitation formula endorsed by the American Burn Association in its Advanced Burn Life

Table 1
Formulas for burn shock resuscitation (first 24 hours)

Formula	Description
Brooke	Lactated Ringer's (LR) 1.5 mL/kg/%TBSA burn + colloid 0.5 mL/kg/%TBSA burn
Burn Budget	LR 1000–4000 mL + 0.5 NS 1200 mL + 7.5% of body weight colloid + 1500–5000 mL 5% dextrose in water
Demling	*1st 8 h:* Dextran in normal saline at 2 mL/kg/h *After:* Fresh frozen plasma at 0.5 mL/kg/h starting at 8 h. Adjust LR based on urine output
Evans	Normal saline 1 mL/kg/%TBSA burn + colloids 1 mL/kg/% burn + 2000 mL glucose in water
Haifa	Plasma at 1.5 mL/kg/%TBSA burn + LR at 1 mL/kg/%TBSA burn. Adjust based on urine output
Harkins	1000 mL per 10% TBSA burned
Modified Brooke	LR at 2 mL/kg/% TBSA; half in first 8 h, remaining over next 16 h
Parkland	LR at 4 mL/kg/% TBSA; half in first 8 h, remaining over next 16 h
Monafo	Hypertonic saline (250 mEq/L Na$^+$, 150 mEq lactate, 100 mEq Cl$^-$)
Slater	LR 2000 mL + FFP at 75 mL/kg/24 h. Adjust based on urine output
Warden	*1st 8 h:* LR + 50 mEq/L NaHCO$_3$ at 4 mL/kg/% TBSA; half in first 8 h *After:* Switch to LR when pH normalizes or at 8 h. Adjust based on urine output

Support course. It should be noted that formulas are guides rather than guarantees. Titration of the fluid resuscitation rate is based on physiologic response. The principal indicator of the adequacy of resuscitation is the urine output. Fluid rates are generally increased or decreased to maintain a urine output of 30 to 50 mL/hour (0.5 mL/kg/hour) in adults, and 1 mL/kg/hour in children. The use of other endpoints remains debated; however, current literature suggests the use of base deficit and lactate to help guide resuscitation.[26,27] Early recognition of a difficult or failing resuscitation is critical to preventing refractory shock. Three specific periods have been suggested as critical in this regard: the initial 8 hours, hours 8 to 24, and after 24 hours.[28] Variables such as oliguria, anuria, fluid rates beyond predicted needs, worsening metabolic acidosis, abdominal distension, difficulty ventilating, and vasopressor use during resuscitation may suggest impending failure.[28] Software-based clinical decision-support tools have been employed to monitor fluid trends and predict fluid needs. Early use of these tools has been associated with lower delivered fluid volumes and decreased incidence of abdominal compartment syndrome (ACS).[29]

Modern resuscitative strategies have focused on better understanding the physiologic response to injury, use of adjuncts to resuscitation, and close frequent monitoring to optimize delivery of fluids. Extensive work has been done on understanding the contribution of burn injury to vasoplegia and the degree of vascular leakage that follows injury.[15] The provision of colloid-based solutions such as albumin is thought to help avoid excessive delivery of fluids.[30,31] More recently, the glycocalyx and its associated shedding from the endothelium have been identified as a contributor to improved microvascular permeability. It has been shown that fresh frozen plasma (FFP) compared to albumin better-restored glycocalyx function and may be a better adjunct to abating the vascular inflammatory response seen in large burn injuries.[15,16] Preliminary clinical work on the effect of plasma on resuscitation remains ongoing but suggests that plasma administration may alter required fluid rates during resuscitation. Other studies, such as the PROP-OLIS (plasma resuscitation without lung injury) seek to further explore the effect of FFP on 24-hour fluid requirements, any incidence of lung injury, and if there is an effect on the inflammatory response.[32]

COMPLICATIONS AND MANAGEMENT

Although goal-directed resuscitation formulas like the Parkland or modified Brooke are now widely used, they are not without complications. Recent evidence suggests the Parkland formula may not accurately predict necessary fluid requirements.[33] In one study, a cohort of burn patients from the 1970s was compared with matched counterparts from the year 2000. More recent patients received more than double the predicted resuscitation volume.[34] Engrav and colleagues[35] reported that 58% of patients with large burns received more than 4.3 mL/kg/% TBSA. A review of the modified Brooke formula demonstrated that patients actually received 4.9 mL/kg/% TBSA instead of the predicted 2 mL/kg/%TBSA.[36] A similar study found that patients resuscitated with the Parkland formula received 6.3 mL/kg/%TBSA compared with the predicted 4 mL/kg/%TBSA.[37]

The trend toward over-resuscitation was coined "fluid creep" by Basil Pruitt.[38] Fluid creep is reported to occur in up to 90% of patients with a 10% TBSA burn or greater, and is defined by an administered intravenous fluid volume in excess of formula-predicted needs.[39] Factors contributing to fluid creep include over-estimation of burn size, inexperience of clinical providers, inattention during resuscitation, delay in transport, and abandonment of colloid administration.[40] Fluid creep has been associated with adverse outcomes including compartment syndrome (CS), ARDS, pneumonia, infection, multiorgan failure, and death.[33] Awareness of these complications and prompt treatment are essential.

Orbital Compartment Syndrome

Orbital compartment syndrome (OCS) is a surgical emergency characterized by increased intraocular pressure (IOP) (>35 mm Hg), decreased visual acuity, fixed dilated pupil, ophthalmoplegia, and acute proptosis. Patients may report acute onset vision loss, decreased ocular mobility, double vision, and orbital pain.[41] In a manner analogous to other forms of CS, the increase in pressure leads to a decrease in ocular perfusion that compromises blood flow to the optic nerve and retina and may lead to ischemic or compressive optic neuropathy, nerve fiber layer loss, retinal vessel occlusion, and blindness.[42,43] Hayreh and colleagues[44] reported that as few as 60 minutes of increased IOP may result in permanent visual complications.

Factors associated with postburn OCS include resuscitation volumes in excess of Parkland formula prediction and large burn sizes.[45–48] In one retrospective chart review of severely burned patients, Singh and colleagues reported a positive relationship between fluid volume in the first 24 hours following injury and peak IOP in the first 48 hours. Patients who required orbital decompression were resuscitated with higher overall volumes than those who did not.[42] Lateral canthotomy and cantholysis decrease IOP and restore blood flow to the optic nerve and retina, and thus, remain the treatment of choice for OCS.[45,48]

There are no formalized criteria for ophthalmic evaluation or standardized timing of IOP checks in burn patients to assess the risk of developing OCS.[47] However, some recommend that patients receiving more than 5.5 mL/kg/%TBSA in the first 24 hours of resuscitation receive IOP checks once a day for at least 3 days following admission and more frequent monitoring when considering additional risk factors such as large TBSA burns, high predicted fluid volumes, volumes in excess of the Ivy index (>250 mL/kg in 24 hour), and the presence of deep periorbital burns.[42,46,47] Indeed, patients with deep periorbital burns can develop OCS within hours of injury, even before the administration of large volumes of fluid.

Extremity Compartment Syndrome

Extremity compartment syndrome (ECS) is defined as an increase in the osteofascial compartment pressure caused by the accumulation of blood or soft tissue edema within the investing fascia of an extremity. The fascia surrounding the muscles is unable to accommodate and stretch, resulting in a rise in compartment pressure, decreased capillary bed perfusion, cellular hypoxia, and eventually myonecrosis.[49,50] ECS takes only a few hours to develop. Patients may present with pain, paresthesia, paresis, tightness, cool temperature, or bruising in the affected limb.[49] ECS can occur in burn patients and is associated with over-resuscitation and may occur in burned or unburned limbs.[51–54] Investigators at the US Army Institute of Surgical Research (USAISR) established a link between ECS in unburned limbs of patients who received resuscitation volumes in excess of Parkland predictions.[55]

ECS is a surgical emergency, and if untreated, may lead to permanent dysesthesias, ischemic contractures, muscle dysfunction, loss of limb, and death. True intracompartmental ECS must be distinguished from limb ischemia caused by tight, circumferential burns of an extremity, or the extremity eschar syndrome. The treatment of the former is fasciotomy, and the treatment of the latter is escharotomy (**Figs. 2** and **3**). To be sure, inadequate or delayed escharotomy, by inciting an ischemia–reperfusion phenomenon, can cause true ECS and mandate fasciotomy.[56]

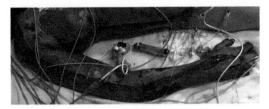

Fig. 2. Example of extremity escharotomy during burn resuscitation.

Abdominal Compartment Syndrome

ACS is characterized by the combination of intraabdominal hypertension (IAH), oliguria, and decreased pulmonary compliance.[57] Patients demonstrate IAH as measured by bladder pressure transduction, distended and tense abdomen, and related organ failure.[58,59] Mechanically ventilated patients with ACS may demonstrate decreased tidal volumes and increased inspiratory pressures.[60,61] IAH decreases perfusion due to impaired capillary and venous blood flow and risks multiorgan ischemia.[62,63]

Multiple studies have linked over-resuscitation to the development of ACS. Ivy and colleagues[57] reported that patients receiving more than 250 mL/kg in the first 24 hours (the "Ivy index") are at risk for developing ACS. In a group of 48 burn-injured patients, Oda and colleagues[64] identified eight patients with ACS and noted these patients had received more than 300 mL/kg of resuscitation fluid in the first 24 hours after burn injury. Markell and colleagues[65] found that the average fluid resuscitation volume administered to patients who developed ACS was 6.2 mL/kg/% TBSA, despite recommendations of 2 to 4 mL/kg/% TBSA. It should be noted that the Ivy index does not account for burn size, whereas modern burn resuscitation formulas deliver fluid volumes proportionally to burn size. Consequently, resuscitation of larger burns inherently increases the risk of exceeding the Ivy index, and therefore, the related risk of ACS. Evaluation of resuscitation strategies has been performed to reduce these complications.[66] O'Mara and colleagues compared crystalloid and colloid resuscitation and found that patients who received colloid required overall less fluid volume and were less likely to develop ACS.[67]

Decompression has been established as the treatment of choice for ACS. Decompressive laparotomy is a common treatment but carries significant associated morbidity and high mortality (**Fig. 4**).[68] Other studies have suggested percutaneous drainage (PD) as a viable treatment option if intraabdominal free fluid may be visualized on ultrasound. Reports by Corcos and colleagues[69] and Savino and colleagues[70] concluded that PD is a safe and effective method of decreasing IAH.

Acute Respiratory Distress Syndrome

ARDS may occur in burn patients as another consequence of massive systemic inflammation. Large-volume resuscitation, increased microvascular permeability, and direct injury from smoke inhalation can exacerbate this process.[71–74] One study

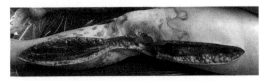

Fig. 3. Example of extremity fasciotomy during burn resuscitation.

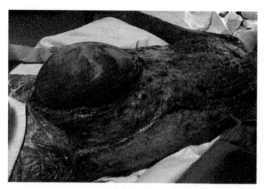

Fig. 4. Decompressive laparotomy after the development of ACS following burn resuscitation.

from the USAISR identified ARDS in one-third of mechanically ventilated burn patients. In an analysis of fluid resuscitation data from these 72 patients, increased volumes of fluid administration were shown to be independently associated with ARDS.[33,75] In a larger analysis of 330 patients, Mason and colleagues[76] classified patients by resuscitation volume as restrictive (<4 mL/kg/TBSA), standard (4–6 mL/kg/TBSA), or excessive (>6 mL/kg/TBSA) and demonstrated the presence of ARDS in 20% of the restrictive group, 35% of the standard group, and 42% of the excessive group. When ARDS develops in this patient population, management prioritizes lung-protective ventilation to minimize ventilator-induced lung injury,[77] utilizing volume-limited and pressure-limited ventilation with high positive end expiratory pressure (PEEP) and prone positioning in severe cases.[78] Later, pulmonary fibrosis and diffusion limitation may develop, complicating recovery from ARDS.[79]

SUMMARY

Advancements in burn resuscitation have occurred through clinical experience and scientific advancement. A better understanding of the physiologic response to burn injury has resulted in optimized fluid delivery practices and administration of colloid adjuncts. Early recognition of excess fluid-related complications is paramount to minimizing associated morbidity and mortality in burn-injured patients.

CLINICS CARE POINTS

- Severe burn injury requires resuscitation in the initial 24 hours following injury.
- A thorough understanding of burn pathophysiology is necessary to understand fluid needs following injury.
- Fluids are administered via consensus formulae and are titrated based on end points, primarily urine output, but also through other adjuncts such as blood gas analysis.
- Over resuscitation may result in major complications that require prompt recognition and management.

DISCLOSURE

The authors have nothing to disclose.

REFERENCES

1. Greenhalgh DG. Management of burns. N Engl J Med 2019;380(24):2349–59.
2. Tejiram S, Romanowski KS, Palmieri TL. Initial management of severe burn injury. Curr Opin Crit Care 2019;25(6):647–52.
3. Shirani KZ, Vaughan GM, Mason AD Jr, et al. Update on current therapeutic approaches in burns. Shock 1996;5(1):4–16.
4. Evers LH, Bhavsar D, Mailänder P. The biology of burn injury. Exp Dermatol 2010; 19(9):777–83.
5. Friedl HP, Till GO, Trentz O, et al. Roles of histamine, complement and xanthine oxidase in thermal injury of skin. Am J Pathol 1989;135(1):203–17.
6. Barrett LW, Fear VS, Waithman JC, et al. Understanding acute burn injury as a chronic disease. Burns Trauma 2019;7:23.
7. Hanschen M, Tajima G, O'Leary F, et al. Injury induces early activation of T-cell receptor signaling pathways in CD4+ regulatory T cells. Shock 2011;35(3):252–7.
8. Hettiaratchy S, Dziewulski P. ABC of burns: pathophysiology and types of burns. BMJ 2004;328(7453):1427–9.
9. Tejiram S, Shupp JW. Innovations in Infection Prevention and Treatment. Surg Infect 2021;22(1):12–9.
10. Jeschke MG, van Baar ME, Choudhry MA, et al. Burn injury. Nat Rev Dis Primers 2020;6(1):11.
11. Komarova YA, Kruse K, Mehta D, et al. Protein interactions at endothelial junctions and signaling mechanisms regulating endothelial permeability. Circ Res 2017;120(1):179–206.
12. Pober JS, Sessa WC. Evolving functions of endothelial cells in inflammation. Nat Rev Immunol 2007;7(10):803–15.
13. Greenhalgh DG. Sepsis in the burn patient: a different problem than sepsis in the general population. Burns Trauma 2017;5:5–23.
14. Du Clos TW. Function of C-reactive protein. Ann Med 2000;32(4):274–8.
15. Luker JN, Vigiola Cruz M, Carney BC, et al. Shedding of the endothelial glycocalyx is quantitatively proportional to burn injury severity. Ann Burns Fire Disasters 2018;31(1):17–22.
16. Keyloun JW, Le TD, Pusateri AE, et al. Circulating syndecan-1 and tissue factor pathway inhibitor, biomarkers of endothelial dysfunction, predict mortality in burn patients. Shock 2021;56(2):237–44.
17. Çakir B, Yegen B. Systemic responses to burn injury. Turk J Med Sci 2004;34(4): 215–26.
18. Schultz AM, Werba A, Wolrab C. Early cardiorespiratory patterns in severely burned patients with concomitant inhalation injury. Burns 1997;23(5):421–5.
19. Jeschke MG. Post-burn hypermetabolism: past, present and future. J Burn Care Res 2016;37(2):86–96.
20. Cota JM, FakhriRavari A, Rowan MP, et al. Intravenous antibiotic and antifungal agent pharmacokinetic-pharmacodynamic dosing in adults with severe burn injury. Clinical Therapeutics Clinical Therapeutics 2016;38(9):2016–31.
21. Kaddoura I, Abu-Sittah G, Ibrahim A, et al. Burn injury: review of pathophysiology and therapeutic modalities in major burns. Ann Burns Fire Disasters 2017;30(2): 95–102.
22. Nielson CB, Duethman NC, Howard JM, et al. Burns: pathophysiology of systemic complications and current management. J Burn Care Res 2017;38(1):e469–81.
23. Sneve H. The treatment of burns and skin grafting. JAMA 1905;47(1):1–8.

24. Fauntleroy AM, Hoagland AW. The treatment of burns: as exemplified in thirty-two cases. Ann Surg 1919 Jun;69(6):589–95.
25. Underhill FP. The significance of andydremia in extensive superficial burns. JAMA 1930;95(12):852–7.
26. Cancio LC, Galvez E Jr, Turner CE, et al. Base deficit and alveolar-arterial gradient during resuscitation contribute independently but modestly to the prediction of mortality after burn injury. J Burn Care Res 2006;27(3):289–96 [discussion: 296-287].
27. Muthukumar V, Arumugam PK, Narasimhan A, et al. Blood lactate and lactate clearance: refined biomarker and prognostic marker in burn resuscitation. Ann Burns Fire Disasters 2020;33(4):293–8.
28. Brownson EG, Pham TN, Chung KK. How to recognize a failed burn resuscitation. Crit Care Clin 2016;32(4):567–75.
29. Rizzo JA, Liu NT, Coates EC, et al. Initial results of the american burn association observational multicenter evaluation on the effectiveness of the burn navigator. J Burn Care Res 2022;43(3):728–34.
30. Lawrence A, Faraklas I, Watkins H, et al. Colloid administration normalizes resuscitation ratio and ameliorates "fluid creep". J Burn Care Res 2010;31(1):40–7.
31. Faraklas I, Lam U, Cochran A, et al. Colloid normalizes resuscitation ratio in pediatric burns. J Burn Care Res 2011;32(1):91–7.
32. Cancio L. Plasma resuscitation without lung injury (PROPOLIS), 2020. Available at: https://clinicaltrials.gov/ct2/show/NCT04681638. Accessed December 26, 2022.
33. Klein MB, Hayden D, Elson C, et al. The association between fluid administration and outcome following major burn: a multicenter study. Ann Surg 2007;245(4):622–8.
34. Friedrich JB, Sullivan SR, Engrav LH, et al. Is supra-Baxter resuscitation in burn patients a new phenomenon? Burns 2004;30(5):464–6.
35. Engrav LH, Colescott PL, Kemalyan N, et al. A biopsy of the use of the Baxter formula to resuscitate burns or do we do it like Charlie did it? J Burn Care Rehabil 2000;21(2):91–5.
36. Cancio LC, Chávez S, Alvarado-Ortega M, et al. Predicting increased fluid requirements during the resuscitation of thermally injured patients. J Trauma 2004;56(2):404–13 [discussion: 413-404].
37. Cartotto R, Zhou A. Fluid creep: the pendulum hasn't swung back yet. J Burn Care Res 2010;31(4):551–8.
38. Pruitt BA. Protection from excessive resuscitation: "pushing the pendulum back". J Trauma 2000;49(3):567–8.
39. Saffle JR. Fluid creep and over-resuscitation. Crit Care Clin 2016;32(4):587–98.
40. Atiyeh BS, Dibo SA, Ibrahim AE, et al. Acute burn resuscitation and fluid creep: it is time for colloid rehabilitation. Ann Burns Fire Disasters 2012;25(2):59–65.
41. Lima V, Burt B, Leibovitch I, et al. Orbital compartment syndrome: the ophthalmic surgical emergency. Surv Ophthalmol 2009;54(4):441–9.
42. Singh CN, Klein MB, Sullivan SR, et al. Orbital compartment syndrome in burn patients. Ophthal Plast Reconstr Surg 2008;24(2):102–6.
43. Vallejo A, Lorente JA, Bas ML, et al. Blindness due to anterior ischemic optic neuropathy in a burn patient. J Trauma 2002;53(1):139–41.
44. Hayreh SS, Kolder HE, Weingeist TA. Central retinal artery occlusion and retinal tolerance time. Ophthalmology 1980;87(1):75–8.
45. Sullivan SR, Ahmadi AJ, Singh CN, et al. Elevated orbital pressure: another untoward effect of massive resuscitation after burn injury. J Trauma 2006;60(1):72–6.

46. Vrouwe SQ, Zuo KJ, Grotski CH, et al. Orbital compartment syndrome following major burn resuscitation: a case series and survey of practice patterns. J Burn Care Res 2021;42(2):193–9.
47. Mai AP, Fortenbach CR, Wibbenmeyer LA, et al. Preserving vision: rethinking burn patient monitoring to prevent orbital compartment syndrome. J Burn Care Res 2020;41(5):1104–10.
48. Evans LS. Increased intraocular pressure in severely burned patients. Am J Ophthalmol 1991;111(1):56–8.
49. Olson SA, Glasgow RR. Acute compartment syndrome in lower extremity musculoskeletal trauma. J Am Acad Orthop Surg 2005;13(7):436–44.
50. von Keudell AG, Weaver MJ, Appleton PT, et al. Diagnosis and treatment of acute extremity compartment syndrome. Lancet 2015;386(10000):1299–310.
51. McQueen MM, Gaston P, Court-Brown CM. Acute compartment syndrome. Who is at risk? J Bone Joint Surg Br 2000;82(2):200–3.
52. Sheridan RL, Tompkins RG, McManus WF, et al. Intracompartmental sepsis in burn patients. J Trauma 1994;36(3):301–5.
53. Anjaria D, Deitich E. Burn injury, compartment syndromes. In: Vincent J-L, Hall JB, editors. Encyclopedia of intensive care medicine. Berlin, Heidelberg, Germany: Springer-Verlag Berlin Heidelberg; 2012. p. 408–12.
54. Boccara D, Lavocat R, Soussi S, et al. Pressure guided surgery of compartment syndrome of the limbs in burn patients. Ann Burns Fire Disasters 2017;30(3):193–7.
55. Beebe M, Cancio L, Goodwin C. Extremity compartment syndrome in thermally injured patients with unburned legs. J Burn Care Res 2000;21:S208.
56. Pruitt BA, Dowling JA, Moncrief JA. Escharotomy in early burn care. Arch Surg 1968;96(4):502–7.
57. Ivy ME, Atweh NA, Palmer J, et al. Intra-abdominal hypertension and abdominal compartment syndrome in burn patients. J Trauma 2000;49(3):387–91.
58. Newman R.K., Dayal N., Dominique E., Abdominal Compartment Syndrome. In: StatPearls [Internet]. Treasure Island (FL): StatPearls Publishing; 202. Available from: https://www.ncbi.nlm.nih.gov/books/NBK430932/. Accessed April 21, 2022.
59. Regli A, Pelosi P, Malbrain MLNG. Ventilation in patients with intra-abdominal hypertension: what every critical care physician needs to know. Ann Intensive Care 2019;9(1):52.
60. De Backer D. Abdominal compartment syndrom. Crit Care 1999;3:R103.
61. Maung AA, Kaplan LJ. Mechanical ventilation after injury. J Intensive Care Med 2014;29(3):128–37.
62. Maluso P, Olson J, Sarani B. Abdominal compartment hypertension and abdominal compartment syndrome. Crit Care Clin 2016;32(2):213–22.
63. Saffle JI. The phenomenon of "fluid creep" in acute burn resuscitation. J Burn Care Res 2007;28(3):382–95.
64. Oda J, Yamashita K, Inoue T, et al. Resuscitation fluid volume and abdominal compartment syndrome in patients with major burns. Burns 2006;32(2):151–4.
65. Markell KW, Renz EM, White CE, et al. Abdominal complications after severe burns. J Am Coll Surg 2009;208(5):940–7 [discussion: 947-949].
66. Azzopardi EA, McWilliams B, Iyer S, et al. Fluid resuscitation in adults with severe burns at risk of secondary abdominal compartment syndrome–an evidence based systematic review. Burns 2009;35(7):911–20.
67. O'Mara MS, Slater H, Goldfarb IW, et al. A prospective, randomized evaluation of intra-abdominal pressures with crystalloid and colloid resuscitation in burn patients. J Trauma 2005;58(5):1011–8.

68. De Waele JJ, Kimball E, Malbrain M, et al. Decompressive laparotomy for abdominal compartment syndrome. Br J Surg 2016;103(6):709–15.

69. Corcos AC, Sherman HF. Percutaneous treatment of secondary abdominal compartment syndrome. J Trauma 2001;51(6):1062–4.

70. Savino JA, Cerabona T, Agarwal N, et al. Manipulation of ascitic fluid pressure in cirrhotics to optimize hemodynamic and renal function. Ann Surg 1988;208(4):504–11.

71. Enkhbaatar P, Traber DL. Pathophysiology of acute lung injury in combined burn and smoke inhalation injury. Clin Sci (Lond) 2004;107(2):137–43.

72. Soejima K, Schmalstieg FC, Sakurai H, et al. Pathophysiological analysis of combined burn and smoke inhalation injuries in sheep. Am J Physiol Lung Cell Mol Physiol 2001;280(6):L1233–41.

73. Silva L, Garcia L, Oliveira B, et al. Acute respiratory distress syndrome in burn patients: incidence and risk factor analysis. Ann Burns Fire Disasters 2016;29(3):178–82.

74. Bhatia M, Moochhala S. Role of inflammatory mediators in the pathophysiology of acute respiratory distress syndrome. J Pathol 2004;202(2):145–56.

75. Sine CR, Belenkiy SM, Buel AR, et al. Acute respiratory distress syndrome in burn patients: a comparison of the berlin and american-european definitions. J Burn Care Res 2016;37(5):e461–9.

76. Mason SA, Nathens AB, Finnerty CC, et al. Hold the pendulum: rates of acute kidney injury are increased in patients who receive resuscitation volumes less than predicted by the parkland equation. Ann Surg 2016;264(6):1142–7.

77. Slutsky AS, Ranieri VM. Ventilator-induced lung injury. N Engl J Med 2013;369(22):2126–36.

78. Fan E, Brodie D, Slutsky AS. Acute respiratory distress syndrome: advances in diagnosis and treatment. JAMA 2018;319(7):698–710.

79. Ware LB, Matthay MA. The acute respiratory distress syndrome. N Engl J Med 2000;342(18):1334–49.

Critical Care of the Burn Patient

Garrett W. Britton, DO[a,b],*, Amanda R. Wiggins, MD[a], Barret J. Halgas, MD[a], Leopoldo C. Cancio, MD[a,b], Kevin K. Chung, MD[b]

KEYWORDS

- Burns • Inhalation injury • Teamwork • Critical-care medicine • Acute kidney injury

KEY POINTS

- Effective burn care must incorporate input from a multidisciplinary care team.
- A multimodal pain, agitation, and sedation regimen should be utilized to limit dose-dependent adverse effects as well as the incidence of delirium and should incorporate non-pharmacologic adjuncts.
- Application of traditional indicators of sepsis in the burn population is confounded by characteristic physiologic changes; several studies have demonstrated better-performing criteria.
- Management decisions for the critically ill burn patient should center around promoting wound closure and participation in rehabilitation.

PHASES OF BURN CARE

The continuum of care for burn patients consists of four overlapping phases: (1) initial assessment and triage, (2) acute burn-shock resuscitation, (3) wound closure, and (4) rehabilitation and reintegration. As they move through these phases, many patients will require intensive care, during which they will experience a continuous risk of infection, other complications, multisystem organ failure, and death. Severely burned patients will require intensive care unit (ICU) care for approximately one-half to 1 day per percent total body surface area burned (TBSA).[1,2]

Mortality associated with severe burns tends to occur in a bimodal distribution, either occurring during acute resuscitation or weeks later relating to complications and organ failure.[3] Sepsis and multisystem organ failure exceed burn shock as the leading causes of death, necessitating early identification and intervention for sepsis.[3,4] The critical-care management of these patients must complement their

[a] US Army Institute of Surgical Research, 3698 Chambers Pass Road, San Antonio, TX 78234, USA; [b] Uniformed Services University of Health Sciences, 4301 Jones Bridge Road, Bethesda, MD, USA
* Corresponding author.
E-mail address: Garrett.w.britton.mil@health.mil

surgical management to optimize wound closure and promote favorable long-term outcomes.[5]

TEAM-BASED AND SYSTEMS-BASED CARE

Burn ICU patients demonstrate complex and diverse issues, necessitating the integration of multidisciplinary services including intensivists, burn and reconstructive surgeons, physical and occupational therapists, respiratory therapists, pharmacists, dieticians, and behavioral health specialists.[6,7] With a team comprised of multiple health care providers of varying backgrounds, timely and effective communication is paramount. An effective team leader must be able to reconcile recommendations and goals from each service to best serve the patient, while managing the interpersonal and emotional dynamics relating to the delivery of care to the severely injured (**Box 1**).[7]

Because of the complexity of their injuries, burn patients should be managed methodically, utilizing a systems-based approach.[5]

NEUROLOGIC SYSTEM

Burns present a conundrum of balancing pain, agitation, anxiety, and delirium against the risks and side effects of agents used to treat them[8,9]; see Kim and colleagues[9] in this issue for a detailed discussion of the pharmacologic approach to these problems. Efforts to achieve adequate analgesia must avoid opiate-related complications, prevent delirium, and promote early mobilization. This requires a multimodal analgesia regimen incorporating both pharmacologic and non-pharmacologic strategies. Each component of the regimen should be assessed and escalated or de-escalated daily.[10] See **Box 2** for non-pharmacologic interventions.

Achieving adequate sedation is challenging as physiologic derangements and alterations to pharmacokinetics and pharmacodynamics affect how patients respond to usual therapies.[11,12] The sedation regimen should be protocol-driven to avoid oversedation, promote early mobility, and decrease delirium.[13] A multimodal sedation regimen is favorable to decrease dose-dependent side effects.[9]

Delirium increases length of stay and mortality.[13] In burn patients requiring mechanical ventilation, the prevalence of delirium is as high as 80%.[14] A protocolized approach must be implemented for delirium prevention including a measure such as the Confusion Assessment Method for the ICU and non-pharmacologic interventions.[14,15] Patients who develop delirium are at risk for removing life-sustaining devices and dressings, and while pharmacologic agents have generally not been shown to reduce the duration of delirium, sedatives and antipsychotic medications with sedating effects may prevent harm to the patients with hyperactive delirium.[15–18] Efforts to minimize delirium must be implemented and discussed daily by the team (**Box 3**).[13]

Box 1
Skills required of an effective multidisciplinary burn-team leader

- Understand the goals and perspectives of each team member
- Acknowledge and reinforce the value of each discipline/team member
- Respectfully reconcile conflicting recommendations or competing interests
- Guide the team to understanding and working toward the common goal in a timely and efficient manner

Box 2
Non-pharmacologic analgesic adjuncts

- Virtual reality
- Hypnosis
- Massage therapy
- Music therapy
- Aromatherapy

Alcohol and substance abuse are common among burn patients, with an incidence ranging from 8% to 27% for a single agent and up to 18% for at least two substances.[19] Intoxication seems to be associated with a need for higher level of care (ICU), increased length of stay, and increased injury recidivism.[19] Routine serum alcohol and urine drug screening for burn ICU patients are appropriate.

Psychological disability must be recognized as a threat to successful reintegration into society. Psychosocial care must begin immediately. Acute stress reaction, post-traumatic stress disorder, and major depression occur in up to one-third of patients with severe burns and must be addressed.[20]

PULMONARY

Approximately one-third of burn ICU patients will require mechanical ventilation relating to airway edema, inhalation injury, pulmonary edema, infection, or acute respiratory distress syndrome[21,22]; see Edward Bittner and Robert Sheridan's article, "ARDS, Mechanical Ventilation, and Inhalation Injury in Burn Patients," in this issue for a detailed discussion. These patients may have increased minute ventilation and oxygen consumption owing to hypermetabolism, resulting in challenges associated with lung-protective strategies.[23,24] Although strong evidence exists to support a low-tidal-volume strategy in the general ICU population, burn patients with TBSA greater than 20% were excluded from many trials.[25] Patients with inhalation injury benefit from high-frequency percussive ventilation (HFPV) using the volumetric diffusive respiration (VDR-4) ventilator.[26–29] In inhalation injury, this ventilator improves clearance of debris from the airways while facilitating lung-protective ventilation and improving gas exchange.[26] In one trial, burn patients with and without inhalation injury were randomized to either HFPV or low-tidal-volume ventilation. This study demonstrated a reduced need for rescue to another mode of ventilation in the HFPV group.[30]

A multidisciplinary program must be implemented to liberate patients from mechanical ventilation.[31] Daily sedation interruption and spontaneous breathing trials increase ventilator-free days in burn patients.[32] Achieving such trials may be challenging due to complex analgesia needs. Traditional measures to predict extubation success have demonstrated mixed utility in burn patients.[33,34]

Box 3
Risk factors for delirium

- Electrolyte abnormalities–hypernatremia, hyponatremia
- Uremia
- Alteration from normal sleep–wake cycle
- Use of deliriogenic medications including opiates, benzodiazepines, anticholinergics
- Sensory impairment: hearing deficits, decreased visual acuity

There is no consensus regarding indications or timing of tracheostomy in burn patients. Most undergo tracheostomy due to prolonged mechanical ventilation (after days 7–14).[35] Patients who undergo early tracheostomy (<7–14 days), do so typically because of full-thickness burns to the head and neck or for pulmonary toilet following inhalation injury.[35] Tracheostomy may decrease the need for sedatives and analgesics, enabling increased participation in rehabilitation.[36,37]

CARDIOVASCULAR SYSTEM

The goal of hemodynamic support in the burn patient is to maintain tissue perfusion, promote wound closure, and avoid end-organ injury.[5] The reduction in cardiac output and rise in systemic vascular resistance early postburn ("ebb phase") is supplanted by a persistent elevation in cardiac output and reduction in vascular tone ("flow phase") (**Fig. 1**).[38] Burn patients with prolonged critical illness and immobility demonstrate

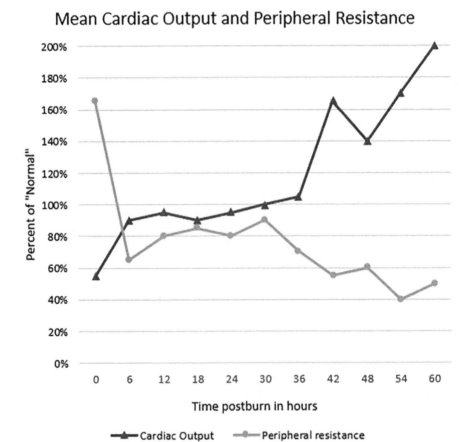

Fig. 1. Postburn changes in cardiac output and peripheral vascular resistance from Pruitt's study of seven patients with burn size of 64.5% TBSA, resuscitated with the Brooke formula. (Pruitt, Basil A. Jr. Ltc. Mc.; Mason, Arthur D. Jr. M.d.; Moncrief, John A. M.d.. Hemodynamic Changes In The Early Postburn Patient The Influence Of Fluid Administration And Of A Vasodilator (hydralazine). The Journal Of Trauma: Injury, Infection, And Critical Care 11(1):p 36-46, January 1971.)

decreased ability to defend against orthostatic stressors and abrupt alterations to sympathetic tone such as during induction of general anesthesia.

Generally, a single modality for assessing hemodynamic performance and volume status is insufficient; a composite of endpoints should be utilized.[5] When choosing between fluids and vasopressors in treating a hypotensive burn patient, careful consideration must be applied concerning wound status and risk of organ failure. Both intravenous fluids (by causing edema), and vasoconstrictive agents (by decreasing wound perfusion) may adversely affect wound healing.

In addition to baseline sinus tachycardia, up to 10% of burn patients experience new-onset atrial fibrillation (NOAF), which is associated with increased mortality.[39,40] Causes of postburn NOAF include increased catecholamines, inflammation, atrial pressure changes, and electrolyte abnormalities. Inciting events may include sepsis and multi-organ dysfunction.[41] The best treatment of postburn NOAF is not clear; rate and rhythm control remain mainstays.[3]

GASTROINTESTINAL SYSTEM

The incidence of postburn gastroduodenal stress ulcers (Curling's ulcers) has decreased significantly because of early enteral nutrition and the use of acid suppression.[42] The authors recommend stress-ulcer chemoprophylaxis for any patient with $\geq$ 20% TBSA injury, mechanical ventilation, prolonged vasopressor use, or inability to receive enteral nutrition.[43]

Decreased gut motility, manifested as nausea, vomiting, and tube feeding intolerance, should prompt an evaluation for sepsis, ischemia, mechanical obstruction, electrolyte derangements, and medication effects.[44]

One of the most catastrophic postburn complications is of full-thickness gut necrosis. Early gut infarction may be due to abdominal compartment syndrome; late gut infarction principally reflects non-occlusive mesenteric ischemia.[44]

Critically ill burn patients are also susceptible to acalculous cholecystitis, acute pancreatitis, and hepatic dysfunction.[45] Symptoms of these disease processes may be confounded or obscured by symptoms related to the patients' injuries.

RENAL SYSTEM

Approximately 20% to 46% of burn ICU patients develop renal dysfunction.[46,47] Patients with advanced-stage acute kidney injury (AKI) or those requiring renal replacement therapy experience a mortality of 62% to 100%.[48,49] Variability in reporting likely relates to the application of various staging criteria including the Risk, Injury, Failure, Loss, End-stage (RIFLE), Acute Kidney Injury Network (AKIN), and Kidney Disease Improving Global Outcomes (KDIGO) criteria.[50] AKIN and RIFLE criteria have been validated in burn patients whereas KDIGO criteria have not.[51] Changes in serum creatinine and urine output may be late findings[51]; work continues to identify better markers of AKI.

Postburn AKI can generally be divided into two cohorts based on timing and etiology. Early AKI (<3 days postburn) relates to burn shock, inflammation, rhabdomyolysis, and cardiac dysfunction; late AKI relates to sepsis, nephrotoxic agents, and fluid overload.[51]

When supportive care is not enough to limit AKI progression, renal replacement therapy (RRT) should be initiated. Timing, indications, and modalities vary. In many centers, continuous renal replacement therapy (CRRT) is employed and managed by the surgeon or intensivist, whereas in others, intermittent hemodialysis (iHD) or slow low-efficiency dialysis is used and managed by a nephrologist.[52] CRRT proponents cite gradual volume removal resulting in less hemodynamic change and precise titration of ultrafiltration (UF) and solute goals.[53,54]

The long-term risk conferred by postburn AKI is not clear. In a systematic review, no studies reported a prolonged need for dialysis (>6 months following discharge). In a multicenter observational study, 90% of RRT patients did not require dialysis at discharge or at 6-month follow-up.[53,54]

ELECTROLYTE DERANGEMENTS

Burn patients are likely to experience electrolyte derangements during hospitalization, which are associated with increased length of stay and mortality.[55]

Hypernatremia

Approximately 24% to 35% of patients will experience hypernatremia (serum sodium > 145 meq/L).[56,57] During burn shock, the renin-aldosterone system becomes upregulated resulting in sodium retention. Thereafter, hypernatremia is driven by evaporative water losses across open wounds. Postburn catabolism and uremia likely contribute to renal water losses.[55–58] Hypernatremia is managed with the administration of electrolyte-free water (enterally, or 5% dextrose in water intravenously).[59] Renal wasting of sodium can be promoted with thiazide diuretics.[60]

Hypophosphatemia

The hypermetabolic response to injury increases energy expenditure and rapidly depletes phosphate stores. Nadiring around postburn days 3 to 5, postburn hypophosphatemia may be life-threatening, precipitating weakness, encephalopathy, cardiac dysfunction, and respiratory failure.[61] The authors recommend frequent monitoring of serum phosphorus and repletion to maintain levels between 3.0 and 4.0 mg/dL.[61]

HEMATOLOGIC SYSTEM

The hematologic derangements experienced by burn patients may be varied and profound. Patients are likely to experience wide-ranging changes to cell lines through the course of their hospitalization owing to hemoconcentration during the resuscitative phase and then to consumption during the recovery phase due to recurring surgical insults. The coagulation cascade is also significantly altered during the course of management continuously tipping between hypercoagulable and hypocoagulable phases.[62,63]

Changes in the coagulation system are common postburn. In a study of patients with burns exceeding 15% TBSA, the majority (60%) had thromboelastography results consistent with a hypercoagulable state, whereas a minority (24%) had a hypocoagulable state.[64] In vivo studies show an increase in procoagulant markers within the first 48 hours, such as thrombin–antithrombin complex, and factors VIIa and VIII. Simultaneously, the levels of endogenous anticoagulants (antithrombin; proteins C and S) fall. The net direction of fibrinolysis is less defined with increases in both plasminogen activator and inhibitor. Tissue plasminogen activator is released locally in burned tissues and may play a role in burn-wound progression.[65]

The incidence of venous thromboembolic complications is uncertain, given variations in screening methodology.[66] Chemoprophylaxis should be started upon admission unless contraindicated. Growing evidence suggests that standard dosing of low-molecular-weight heparin is inadequate due to alterations in pharmacokinetics and pharmacodynamics.

Many patients experience leukocytosis and thrombocytosis during critical illness confounding sepsis diagnosis. Anemia is common after resuscitation and restoration of circulating plasma volume. Patients may require many units of blood products relating to intraoperative blood loss. A conservative transfusion strategy is appropriate for most.[67,68] Anemia does not impair wound healing.[5]

INFECTIOUS DISEASE

As improvements in the resuscitative management and resuscitative mortality are made, more patients are surviving the critical-care phase of severe injury and are exposed to recurring bouts of sepsis; for a detailed discussion, see John L. Kiley and David G. Greenhalgh's article, "Infections in Burn Patients," in this issue. Sepsis remains the leading cause of death in burn patients who survive the initial injury, highlighting the need for early detection, appropriate antimicrobial administration, and source control.[69] Owing to the hypermetabolic response, traditional diagnostic criteria for sepsis lack utility. Furthermore, burn patients with greater than 20% TBSA involvement are typically excluded from pivotal sepsis studies.[70]

In particular, a thorough wound evaluation must be performed in all burn patients suspected of having sepsis, and indwelling vascular devices should be changed.

NUTRITION AND METABOLISM

Optimizing postburn nutrition is paramount to wound healing and survival; see Shahriar Shahrokhi and Marc G. Jeschke's article, "Metabolic and Nutritional Support," in this issue for detailed discussion. Estimating caloric needs following burn injury is best accomplished using indirect calorimetry. The Carlson and Milner equations seem to correlate most closely to calorimetry.[71,72] Those with severe burn injuries (eg, >30% TBSA) will typically not be able to meet their needs without an enteral tube. The provision of early enteral nutrition has been shown to promote wound closure and decrease the risk of infection. We, therefore, aim to initiate nutrition within 24 hours of injury.[73] Formulations high in protein and carbohydrates and low in lipids are favored.[74]

PALLIATIVE AND COMFORT CARE

Death is a common occurrence in most burn centers; there are approximately 180,000 deaths due to burn injuries worldwide annually.[75] For survivors, we increasingly recognize the importance of quality of life for those with life-limiting injuries.[76] Historically, the role of palliative care in burns has been reserved for those with injuries understood to be non-survivable, traditionally referred to as comfort care. But many burn patients are faced with severe and life-altering disabilities or disfigurement and must come to terms with their new existence. Family members may experience difficulty as well. Palliative-care experts may serve as a resource to the patient, family, and care team.[76,77] There is no consensus on when to consult palliative-care services. Generally, patients with severe burns and inhalation injury or those at an advanced age and with severe comorbid illness should be considered for early palliative-care involvement.[78] When conducting care discussions with patients and families, a palliative-care specialist may provide additional perspective.

Three comfort-care pathways have been described for burns: Burn-Modified Liverpool Care Pathway, Comfort-Care Protocol, and the Do Not Resuscitate-Comfort Measures Only pathway. Generally, all pathways consist of similar components (**Box 4**).

Box 4
Components of a comfort-care pathway

- Symptom management
  ○ Nausea
  ○ Pain
  ○ Agitation
  ○ Dyspnea
- Spiritual aspects of care
- Enhancing patient–family communication, liberalizing visiting hours
- Removal of tubes, lines, and drains that do not serve a palliative purpose
- Discontinuing vasoactive medications
- Discontinuing antibiotics
- Discontinuing restorative wound care
- Post-bereavement care

DISPOSITION OF BURN PATIENTS

Determining when to transfer severely burned patients out of the ICU may be confounded by wound status, wound-care burden, rehabilitative needs, and nutritional needs. In other words, patients may be liberated from mechanical organ support but require continued intensive care due to wound and rehabilitation needs. The degree of insensible volume loss, wound-care duration and resource intensity, patient ability to indicate the need for assistance, ability to take nutrition, and need for high-dose or high-risk medications should be considered.

SUMMARY

Care for severely injured burn patients is complex and resource intensive. The provision of comprehensive burn care requires the integration of an experienced multidisciplinary care team to develop and effectively execute individualized care plans. It is important to recognize unique physiologic derangements of burn patients in contradistinction to non-burn critically ill patients.

CLINICS CARE POINTS

- Effective burn care must incorporate input from a multidisciplinary care team.
- A multimodal pain and sedation regimen should be utilized to limit dose-dependent adverse effects such as delirium and should incorporate non-pharmacologic adjuncts.
- Application of traditional indicators of sepsis in burn patients is confounded by the hypermetabolic, systemic inflammatory response to injury.
- Management decisions for the critically ill burn patient should center around promoting wound closure and participation in rehabilitation.

DISCLOSURE

The views expressed herein are those of the authors and do not reflect the official policy or position of the Department of the Army, the Department of Defense, or the US Government. No funding was received for this research.

REFERENCES

1. Jeschke MG, Chinkes DL, Finnerty CC, et al. Pathophysiologic response to severe burn injury. Ann Surg 2008;248(3):387–401.
2. Frugoni B, Gabriel RA, Rafaat K, et al. A predictive model for prolonged hospital length of stay in surgical burn patients. Burns 2020;46(7):1565–70.
3. Culnan DM, Sherman WC, et al. Critical care in the severely burned: organ support and management of complications. In: Herndon DN, editor. Total burn care. 5th edition. New York: Elsevier; 2018. p. 328–54.
4. Publications. American Burn Association. 2022. Available at: https://ameriburn.org/education/publications/. Accessed December 22, 2022.
5. Parrillo JE, Dellinger RP, Chung KK, et al. Critical care of the severely burned. In: Critical care medicine: principles of diagnosis and management in the adult. 5th ed. Philadelphia, PA: Elsevier; 2019.
6. Win TS, Nizamoglu M, Maharaj R, et al. Relationship between multidisciplinary critical care and burn patients survival: A propensity-matched national cohort analysis. Burns 2018;44(1):57–64.
7. Al-Mousawi AM, Mecott-Rivera GA, Jeschke MG, et al. Burn teams and burn centers: The importance of a comprehensive team approach to burn care. Clin Plast Surg 2009;36(4):547–54.
8. Bayuo J. Nurses' experiences of caring for severely burned patients. Collegian 2018;25(1):27–32.
9. Kim DE, Pruskowski KA, Ainsworth CR, et al. A review of adjunctive therapies for burn injury pain during the opioid crisis. J Burn Care Res 2019;40(6):983–95.
10. Herndon DN, Meyer WJ, Martyn JAJ, et al. Management of pain and other discomforts in burned patients. In: Total burn care. 5th ed. Edinburgh: Elsevier; 2018. p. 679–99.
11. Blanchet B, Jullien V, Vinsonneau C, et al. Influence of burns on pharmacokinetics and pharmacodynamics of drugs used in the care of burn patients. Clin Pharmacokinet 2008;47(10):635–54.
12. Steele AN, Grimsrud KN, Sen S, et al. Gap analysis of pharmacokinetics and pharmacodynamics in burn patients. J Burn Care Res 2015;36(3):194–211.
13. Devlin JW, Skrobik Y, Gélinas C, et al. Clinical practice guidelines for the prevention and management of pain, agitation/sedation, delirium, immobility, and sleep disruption in adult patients in the ICU. Crit Care Med 2018;46(9):825–73.
14. Agarwal V, O'Neill PJ, Cotton BA, et al. Prevalence and risk factors for development of delirium in burn intensive care unit patients. J Burn Care Res 2010;31(5):706–15.
15. Girard TD, Pandharipande PP, Ely EW. Delirium in the intensive care unit. Crit Care 2008;12(Suppl 3):S3.
16. Girard TD, Pandharipande PP, Carson SS, et al. Feasibility, efficacy, and safety of antipsychotics for Intensive Care Unit delirium: The mind randomized, placebo-controlled trial. Crit Care Med 2010;38(2):428–37.
17. Page VJ, Ely EW, Gates S, et al. Effect of intravenous haloperidol on the duration of delirium and coma in critically ill patients (hope-ICU): A randomised, double-blind, placebo-controlled trial. Lancet Respir Med 2013;1(7):515–23.
18. Devlin JW, Roberts RJ, Fong JJ, et al. Efficacy and safety of quetiapine in critically ill patients with delirium: A prospective, multicenter, randomized, double-blind, placebo-controlled pilot study. Crit Care Med 2010;38(2):419–27.
19. Williams FN, Chrisco L, Strassle PD, et al. Association Between Alcohol, Substance Use, and Inpatient Burn Outcomes. J Burn Care Res 2021;42(4):595–9.

20. Blakeney PE, Rosenberg L, Rosenberg M, et al. Psychosocial care of persons with severe burns. Burns 2008;34(4):433–40.
21. Belenkiy SM, Buel AR, Cannon JW, et al. Acute respiratory distress syndrome in wartime military burns: application of the Berlin criteria. J Trauma Acute Care Surg 2014;76(3):821–7.
22. Folwell JS, Basel AP, Britton GW, et al. Mechanical Ventilation Strategies in the Critically Ill Burn Patient: A Practical Review for Clinicians. EBJ 2021;2(3):140–51.
23. Childs C, Little RA. Acute changes in oxygen consumption and body temperature after burn injury. Arch Dis Child 1994;71(1):31–4.
24. Gore DC, Chinkes D, Sanford A, et al. Influence of fever on the hypermetabolic response in burn-injured children. Arch Surg 2003;138(2):169–74.
25. Acute Respiratory Distress Syndrome Network, Brower RG, Matthay MA, Schoenfeld D, et al. Ventilation with lower tidal volumes as compared with traditional tidal volumes for acute lung injury and the acute respiratory distress syndrome. N Engl J Med 2000;342(18):1301–8.
26. Cioffi WG Jr, Rue LW 3rd, Graves TA, et al. Prophylactic use of high-frequency percussive ventilation in patients with inhalation injury. Ann Surg 1991;213(6):575–82.
27. Rodeberg DA, Housinger TA, Greenhalgh DG, et al. Improved ventilatory function in burn patients using volumetric diffusive respiration. J Am Coll Surg 1994;179(5):518–22.
28. Reper P, Wibaux O, Van Laeke P, et al. High frequency percussive ventilation and conventional ventilation after smoke inhalation: a randomised study. Burns 2002;28(5):503–8.
29. Carman B, Cahill T, Warden G, et al. A prospective, randomized comparison of the Volume Diffusive Respirator vs conventional ventilation for ventilation of burned children. 2001 ABA paper. J Burn Care Rehabil 2002;23(6):444–8.
30. Chung KK, Wolf SE, Renz EM, et al. High-frequency percussive ventilation and low tidal volume ventilation in burns: a randomized controlled trial. Crit Care Med 2010;38(10):1970–7.
31. Morandi A, Piva S, Ely EW, et al. Worldwide Survey of the "Assessing Pain, Both Spontaneous Awakening and Breathing Trials, Choice of Drugs, Delirium Monitoring/Management, Early Exercise/Mobility, and Family Empowerment" (ABC-DEF) Bundle. Crit Care Med 2017;45(11):e1111–22.
32. Smailes ST, Martin RV, McVicar AJ. Evaluation of the spontaneous breathing trial in burn intensive care patients. Burns 2009;35(5):665–71.
33. Rizzo JA, Haq M, McMahon RA, et al. Extubation Failure in a Burn Intensive Care Unit: Examination of Contributing Factors. J Burn Care Res 2021;42(2):177–81.
34. Smailes ST, Martin RV, McVicar AJ. The incidence and outcome of extubation failure in burn intensive care patients. J Burn Care Res 2009;30(3):386–92.
35. Aggarwal S, Smailes S, Dziewulski P. Tracheostomy in burns patients revisited. Burns 2009;35(7):962–6.
36. Hosokawa K, Nishimura M, Egi M, et al. Timing of tracheotomy in ICU patients: a systematic review of randomized controlled trials. Crit Care 2015;19:424.
37. Delaney A, Bagshaw SM, Nalos M. Percutaneous dilatational tracheostomy versus surgical tracheostomy in critically ill patients: a systematic review and meta-analysis. Crit Care 2006;10(2):R55.
38. Pruitt BA Jr, Mason AD Jr, Moncrief JA. Hemodynamic changes in the early post-burn patient: the influence of fluid administration and of a vasodilator (hydralazine). J Trauma 1971;11(1):36–46.

39. Morsy M, Slomka T, Shukla A, et al. Clinical and echocardiographic predictors of new-onset atrial fibrillation in patients admitted with blunt trauma. Echocardiography 2018;35(10):1519–24.
40. Arrigo M, Ishihara S, Feliot E, et al. New-onset atrial fibrillation in critically ill patients and its association with mortality: A report from the FROG-ICU study. Int J Cardiol 2018;266:95–9.
41. O'Connor JM, Helmer SD, Khandelwal A. Atrial fibrillation in elderly burn patients. Am Surg 2014;80(6):623–4.
42. Raff T, Germann G, Hartmann B. The value of early enteral nutrition in the prophylaxis of stress ulceration in the severely burned patient. Burns 1997;23(4):313–8.
43. Choi YH, Lee JH, Shin JJ, et al. A revised risk analysis of stress ulcers in burn patients receiving ulcer prophylaxis. Clin Exp Emerg Med 2015;2(4):250–5.
44. Markell KW, Renz EM, White CE, et al. Abdominal complications after severe burns. J Am Coll Surg 2009;208(5):940–9.
45. Walsh K, Goutos I, Dheansa B. Acute Acalculous Cholecystitis in Burns: A Review. J Burn Care Res 2018;39(5):724–8.
46. Chung KK, Stewart IJ, Gisler C, et al. The Acute Kidney Injury Network (AKIN) criteria applied in burns. J Burn Care Res 2012;33(4):483–90.
47. Brusselaers N, Monstrey S, Colpaert K, et al. Outcome of acute kidney injury in severe burns: a systematic review and meta-analysis. Intensive Care Med 2010;36(6):915–25.
48. Stewart IJ, Tilley MA, Cotant CL, et al. Association of AKI with adverse outcomes in burned military casualties. Clin J Am Soc Nephrol 2012;7(2):199–206.
49. Mosier MJ, Pham TN, Klein MB, et al. Early acute kidney injury predicts progressive renal dysfunction and higher mortality in severely burned adults. J Burn Care Res 2010;31(1):83–92.
50. Basel AP, Britton GW, Chung KK. Acute kidney injury in burns patients, In: Koyner JL, Lerma EV, Topf JM, editors. Handbook of critical care nephrology, 2021, Wolters Kluwer; Netherlands, p. 520–525.
51. Niculae A, Peride I, Tiglis M, et al. Burn-Induced Acute Kidney Injury-Two-Lane Road: From Molecular to Clinical Aspects. Int J Mol Sci 2022;23(15):8712.
52. Folkestad T, Brurberg KG, Nordhuus KM, et al. Acute kidney injury in burn patients admitted to the intensive care unit: a systematic review and meta-analysis. Crit Care 2020;24(1):2.
53. Clark A, Neyra JA, Madni T, et al. Acute kidney injury after burn. Burns 2017;43(5):898–908.
54. Chung KK, Coates EC, Hickerson WL, et al. Renal Replacement Therapy in Severe Burns: A Multicenter Observational Study. J Burn Care Res 2018;39(6):1017–21.
55. Lam NN, Minh NTN. Risk factors and outcome of Hypernatremia amongst severe adult burn patients. Ann Burns Fire Disasters 2018;31(4):271–7.
56. Namdar T, Siemers F, Stollwerck PL, et al. Increased mortality in hypernatremic burned patients. Ger Med Sci 2010;8:Doc11.
57. Rugg C, Ströhle M, Schmid S, et al. The Link between Hypermetabolism and Hypernatremia in Severely Burned Patients. Nutrients 2020;12(3):774.
58. Chand R, Chand R, Goldfarb DS. Hypernatremia in the intensive care unit. Curr Opin Nephrol Hypertens 2022;31(2):199–204.
59. Chauhan K, Pattharanitima P, Patel N, et al. Rate of Correction of Hypernatremia and Health Outcomes in Critically Ill Patients. Clin J Am Soc Nephrol 2019;14(5):656–63.

60. Overgaard-Steensen C, Ring T. Clinical review: practical approach to hypona-traemia and hypernatraemia in critically ill patients. Crit Care 2013;17(1):206.
61. Herndon DN, Mozingo DW, Mason AD. Hypophosphatemia. In: Total burn care. 5th ed. Edinburgh: Elsevier; 2018. p. 280–6.
62. Geng K, Liu Y, Yang Y, et al. Incidence and Prognostic Value of Acute Coagulop-athy After Extensive Severe Burns. J Burn Care Res 2020;41(3):544–9.
63. Glas GJ, Levi M, Schultz MJ. Coagulopathy and its management in patients with severe burns. J Thromb Haemostasis 2016;14(5):865–74.
64. Huzar TF, Martinez E, Love J, et al. Admission Rapid Thrombelastography (rTEG®) Values Predict Resuscitation Volumes and Patient Outcomes After Ther-mal Injury. J Burn Care Res 2018;39(3):345–52.
65. Ball RL, Keyloun JW, Brummel-Ziedins K, et al. Burn-Induced Coagulopathies: a Comprehensive Review. Shock 2020;54(2):154–67.
66. Barret JP, Dziewulski PG. Complications of the hypercoagulable status in burn injury. Burns 2006;32(8):1005–8.
67. Palmieri TL, Holmes JH 4th, Arnoldo B, et al. Transfusion Requirement in Burn Care Evaluation (TRIBE): A Multicenter Randomized Prospective Trial of Blood Transfusion in Major Burn Injury. Ann Surg 2017;266(4):595–602.
68. Palmieri TL. Transfusion and Infections in the Burn Patient. Surg Infect 2021; 22(1):49–53.
69. Greenhalgh DG. Sepsis in the burn patient: a different problem than sepsis in the general population. Burns Trauma 2017;5:23.
70. Marik PE, Taeb AM. SIRS, qSOFA and new sepsis definition. J Thorac Dis 2017; 9(4):943–5.
71. Carlson DE, Cioffi WG Jr, Mason AD Jr, et al. Resting energy expenditure in pa-tients with thermal injuries. Surg Gynecol Obstet 1992;174(4):270–6.
72. Milner EA, Cioffi WG, Mason AD, et al. A longitudinal study of resting energy expenditure in thermally injured patients. J Trauma 1994;37(2):167–70.
73. Rodriguez NA, Jeschke MG, Williams FN, et al. Nutrition in burns: Galveston con-tributions. JPEN - J Parenter Enter Nutr 2011;35(6):704–14.
74. Herndon DN, Carson JS, Khosrozadeh H, et al. Nutritional needs and support for the burned patient. In: Total burn care. 5th ed. Edinburgh: Elsevier; 2018. p. 287–300.
75. World Health Organization. (n.d.). Burns. World Health Organization. Available at: https://www.who.int/news-room/fact-sheets/detail/burns. Accessed June 28, 2022.
76. Bayuo J, Bristowe K, Harding R, et al. The Role of Palliative Care in Burns: A Scoping Review. J Pain Symptom Manag 2020;59(5):1089–108.
77. Ray DE, Karlekar MB, Crouse DL, et al. Care of the Critically Ill Burn Patient. An Overview from the Perspective of Optimizing Palliative Care. Ann Am Thorac Soc 2017;14(7):1094–102 [published correction appears in Ann Am Thorac Soc. 2017 Dec;14(12):1866].
78. Bagley BA, Senthil-Kumar P, Pavlik LE, et al. Care of the Critically Injured Burn Patient. Ann Am Thorac Soc 2022;19(6):880–9.

Infections in Burn Patients

John L. Kiley, MD[a],*, David G. Greenhalgh, MD[b]

KEYWORDS

- Burn wound infections • Immunosuppression • Multidrug-resistant
- Gram-negative bacteria • Fungal wound infection

KEY POINTS

- Infections are the leading cause of mortality in burn patients who survive their initial resuscitation.
- Burn injury leads to immunosuppression and a dysregulated inflammatory response.
- Early surgical excision of burn wounds along with the support of the multidisciplinary team in burn intensive care units has had a profound impact on mortality from burns.
- The diagnosis and management of infections after burns can be challenging.

INTRODUCTION

Infections are the leading cause of mortality in burn patients who survive initial resuscitation[1,2] and present diagnostic and therapeutic challenges.[3] Here, the authors discuss the role of immunosuppression, the timing of infections, infecting syndromes, diagnostic challenges, and management strategies.

IMMUNOSUPPRESSION

One key effect of thermal injury is immunosuppression and a dysregulated inflammatory response.[4] Leukocyte populations in burned mice models, when transferred into healthy mice, are subsequently able to impact the recognition of pathogens in those healthy mice as well as adversely affect the ratio of suppressor T cells to helper T cells.[5–7] Studies in humans have yielded similar supporting evidence. Toll-like receptors are downregulated, resulting in the decreased production of interleukin (IL)-6 and IL-12. This results in a decreased antigen presentation and T-cell proliferation, two key

Disclaimer: The opinions or assertions contained herein are the private views of the authors, and are not to be construed as official or as reflecting the views of the Department of the Army or the Department of Defense.

[a] Infectious Disease, Brooke Army Medical Center, Uniformed Services University of the Health Sciences, 3551 Roger Brooke Drive, JBSA Fort Sam, Houston, TX 78341, USA; [b] Shriners Children's Northern California, University of California, Davis, 2425 Stockton Boulevard, Sacramento, CA 95817, USA
* Corresponding author.
E-mail address: john.l.kiley.mil@health.mil

Surg Clin N Am 103 (2023) 427–437
https://doi.org/10.1016/j.suc.2023.02.005
0039-6109/23/Published by Elsevier Inc.

processes in a regulated immune response.[8] Of note, these impacts can be prolonged, as shown by Fear and colleagues in the case of natural killer (NK) cell cytotoxicity as well as antibody-dependent cellular cytotoxicity.[9] In that paper, the investigators were able to demonstrate prolonged (weeks) dysregulation of NK T-cell response and CD8 cell response in a murine model. They also documented increased hazard ratios acute upper and lower respiratory infections in human patient up to 5 years after burn injury.

Burn immunosuppression is also thought to impact the ability to regulate changes to the gut that occur postburn, in particular increasing mucosal permeability. The increased gut mucosal permeability and resultant translocation of bacteria or their products are likely a result of converging factors: gut vasoconstriction in response to burn shock and downregulation of the innate immune system's response to bacterial invasion of the gut wall.[10,11] Animal models have provided supporting evidence for these changes, but further studies are needed in humans to identify effective interventions.[12]

DIAGNOSIS OF INFECTION IN BURNED PATIENTS

Diagnosis of sepsis is particularly challenging in burn patients.[13] Severe burns, that is, those involving greater than 20% of the patient's total body surface area (TBSA), cause a pronounced inflammatory response. Following the burn shock phase and resuscitation, a hypermetabolic phase ensues, marked by catabolic physiology, catecholamine production, peripheral insulin resistance, and multi-organ dysfunction.[14] This hypermetabolic phase can last for weeks, months, and in some cases years. During this phase, the traditional signs of sepsis including tachycardia, tachypnea, fever, and leukocytosis are often present, even in the absence of infection.

The American Burn Association published criteria from a consensus conference in 2007 that aimed to overcome the lack of specificity and sensitivity of non-burn sepsis scores (**Box 1**). Hogan and colleagues evaluated the correlation of these criteria with bacteremia in a 1-year retrospective study.[15] They found that the American Burn Association (ABA) criteria yielded an area under the receiver operating characteristic curve (AUC-ROC) of 0.638, sensitivity 78.2%, and specificity 49.5%. Mann-Salinas

---

Box 1
American burn association sepsis criteria for adults

Sepsis is defined as at least three of the following:
1. Temperature greater than 39 or less than 36.5°C
2. Progressive tachycardia (>110 beats/min)
3. Progressive tachypnea (>25 breaths/min or minute ventilation >12 L/min)
4. Thrombocytopenia (<100,000/μL at least 3 days after the burn)
5. Hyperglycemia (plasma glucose >200 mg/dL, or insulin resistance defined as >7 units of insulin/h IV drip or >25% increase in insulin requirements over 24 hours)
6. Inability to continue enteral feedings longer than 24 hours (abdominal distension, residual twice the feeding rate, or diarrhea >2.5 L/d)

In addition, a documented infection is required (culture-positive infection, pathologic tissue source identified, or clinical response to antimicrobials).

Adapted from American Burn Association Consensus Conference on Burn Sepsis and Infection Group, Greenhalgh DG, Saffle JR, Holmes IV JH, Gamelli RL, Palmieri TL, Horton JW, Tompkins RG, Traber DL, Mozingo DW, Deitch EA, et al. American Burn Association consensus conference to define sepsis and infection in burns. J Burn Care Res. 2007;28(6):776-90; with permission.

and colleagues developed six criteria that performed better than the ABA criteria in identifying bacteremic burn patients (AUC-ROC 0.755). These criteria include temperature, tachycardia, hypotension, use of vasopressors, acidosis, and hyperglycemia.[16] There have been efforts to identify molecular correlates of sepsis; Burmeister and colleagues identified a correlation between novel protein biomarkers (complement C5, metalloproteinases, syndecan-1, p-selectin, galectin-1) and clinical suspicion of sepsis.[17] Future research is needed to develop better predictors in the burn population.[18,19]

Timing of Infections and Microbiology After Burns

Given the challenges in diagnosing postburn sepsis, it can be helpful to recognize that there are well-described timelines for various infection syndromes. For example, Van-Duin and colleagues in a single-center study showed that skin and soft-tissue infections occur early in the hospital course, whereas pneumonia, bloodstream infections, and urinary tract infections occur later.[20] This also applies to the timing of emergence of specific organisms that may complicate the burn patient's recovery. In general, gram-positive organisms colonize burn wounds shortly after injury (first 48 hours), followed by gram-negative and fungal organisms (5–7 days postburn).[21] Certain gram-negative organisms, such as *Pseudomonas aeruginosa*, present in delayed fashion.

Bacterial Wound Infection

Burn wound infections have decreased in prevalence in large part due to the advancements in wound and surgical care.[21] Clinical suspicion and bedside examination of wounds are key in diagnosing burn wound infection. Changes in the eschar color, erythema at the wound margin, increased edema, and graft failure can all be the signs of wound infection. Histopathological examination of full-thickness wound biopsies is a gold-standard method of diagnosis. Pruitt and colleagues developed staging criteria that distinguish between colonization (the presence of microorganisms in nonviable tissue) and infection (the presence of microorganisms in viable tissue) **(Table 1)**. Another diagnostic option is the quantitative culture of wound biopsies, but the utility of this approach is uncertain.[22] The use of superficial swabs is hampered by issues with biofilm formation, particularly in the case of *Pseudomonas aeruginosa*.

As noted above, early bacterial wound infections feature gram-positive organisms (classically *Streptococcus*, but increasingly *Staphylococcus aureus*, including

Table 1
Histopathological criteria for staging the microbial status of burn wounds

Stage I: Colonization	
A. Superficial	Sparse microbial population on burn wound surface
B. Penetration	Microorganisms present in variable thickness of eschar
C. Proliferation	Dense population of microorganisms at nonviable/viable interface
Stage II: Invasion	
A. Microinvasion	Microscopic foci of microorganisms in viable tissue immediately below eschar
B. Generalized	Widespread penetration of microorganisms deep into viable tissues
C. Microvascular	Involvement of lymphatics and microvasculature

Adapted from Pruitt BA Jr, McManus AT. The changing epidemiology of infection in burn patients. World J Surg. 1992;16(1):57-67. https://doi.org/10.1007/BF02067116; with permission.

methicillin-resistant *S aureus* [MRSA]). Later in the hospital course gram-negative organisms will predominate (*Enterobacteriaceae* as well as *Pseudomonas aeruginosa*).[23,24] Investigations into the cutaneous microbiome might prove useful in understanding the evolution of the postburn microbiology.[25,26]

Fungal Wound Infection

Invasive fungal wound infections (FWI) often have devastating clinical consequences including increased mortality. Risk factors include prior fungal wound colonization (FWC), higher TBSA, broad-spectrum antimicrobials, and total parenteral nutrition. FWI but not FWC was associated with increased mortality in one series.[27] Histopathology and culture are both important in making FWI diagnosis. Histopathologic morphology cannot be used to identify fungal organisms to the species level, whereas culture cannot differentiate colonization from invasion.[28] A molecular marker,[1,3] β-D-glucan, has not been shown to be useful in the diagnosis of FWI in burn patients.[29–31] Fungal organisms that commonly cause FWI include *Candida*, *Aspergillus*, *Fusarium*, and the Mucorales.[32] FWI with molds impact mortality disproportionately when compared with yeasts such as *Candida*.

Bloodstream Infection

Multiple factors place burn patients at risk of bacteremia: intravascular catheters, mechanical ventilation, Foley catheters, and open wounds. Burn wound manipulation itself is associated with transient bacteremia; however, the significance thereof in the era of early excision and grafting is less clear. Burn patients can develop the complications of bacteremia to include endocarditis, with resultant very high mortality.[33–35]

Pneumonia

Pneumonia is an important infectious complication in burn patients which increases postburn mortality in many series.[36] The diagnosis can be challenging particularly when there is concomitant inhalation injury or pulmonary edema, as these can make interpreting infiltrates on chest imaging difficult.[37] Clinical, radiologic, and physiologic criteria should be used to make the diagnosis (eg, new or persistent infiltrate, sepsis, and change in sputum). Other authors have proposed confirmed, probable and possible as diagnostic categories: confirmed when a patient meets the clinical syndrome (two clinical criteria plus microbiologic confirmation), probable if only the clinical syndrome, and possible with only abnormal chest imaging.[38]

Viral Infections

Viral infections in burns include asymptomatic shedding, wound involvement, and lower respiratory tract infections; the latter are associated with high mortality.[39] Latent virus reactivation, primary infection, and, rarely, nosocomial reinfection have been postulated as the three main mechanisms. Pathogens include the herpesvirus family (herpes simplex virus [HSV], cytomegalovirus [CMV], and VZV), hepatitis, human immunodeficiency virus (HIV), and severe acute respiratory syndrome - coronavirus -2 (SARS-CoV-2).[40,41] Studies on the epidemiology of cutaneous HSV infections in burn patients are typically limited by the number of subjects.[42] Cutaneous HSV infections classically occur 1 to 3 weeks postburn and involve areas of healing partial-thickness burns as opposed to full-thickness burns. Tzanck smears demonstrating multinucleated giant cells can be helpful for screening but are unable to differentiate among viruses and have largely been supplanted by polymerase chain reaction. CMV and VZV are notable in that most reports are in pediatric patients.[43,44] Similar to HSV, VZV is reported to occur more frequently in re-epithelializing skin.[45,46] CMV infection in burn patients can range from asymptomatic viral shedding to end-organ disease and hepatitis.[47–52]

The clinical significance of asymptomatic herpes viremia in burn patients is not well understood and is often extrapolated from other critically ill populations.[53] Multiple authors have suggested that this is a "bystander phenomenon" rather than clinical disease.[54–56] Ong and colleagues showed that in previously immunocompetent patients with septic shock, 70% developed viremia with at least one herpesvirus (CMV, epstein-barr virus [EBV], or human herpes virus [HHV]-6) and 30% developed viremia with more than one.[57] Although mortality was increased in those patients with both CMV and EBV viremia, it is unclear whether there is a role for antiviral use in these patients. Tuxen and colleagues studied prophylactic acyclovir administration in patients with acute respiratory distress syndrome (ARDS), although HSV disease was prevented, they were not able to show any significant impact on mortality.[58,59] Further research is needed in this area.[60,61]

MANAGEMENT
Antibacterials

Antimicrobial considerations in the burn patient largely revolve around two main questions: multidrug resistance and dosing.[62] The length of stay—often a function of TBSA and other markers of severity—is a risk factor for the acquisition of an infection with a multiple-drug-resistant (MDR) organism.[63] Widespread resistance to beta-lactams can make the selection of an empiric regimen and of targeted therapy, extremely challenging. This includes carbapenem resistance secondary to carbapenemase production, metallo-beta-lactamase production, combinations of porin mutations, efflux pumps, or target inhibition. In a 6-year review at the US Army Burn Center, the most prevalent organisms were *Acinetobacter baumannii, Pseudomonas aeruginosa*, and *Klebsiella pneumonia*. Over half of the *Acinetobacter* were MDR, and the *Pseudomonas* and *Klebsiella* isolates were MDR greater than 15% of the time. Drug resistance was more common 15 days versus less than 5 days post-admission. Drug-resistant gram-positive organisms such as MRSA are also common to include in wound infections.[64] Thus, some centers have adopted alternative preoperative antimicrobial prophylaxis regimens such as vancomycin and amikacin. Whether prophylactic antibiotics in general would improve burn patient outcomes was addressed in one meta-analysis with mixed results, and they are not recommended.[65,66] Advances in MDR gram-negative therapies include new combination beta-lactam/beta-lactamase inhibitors, new tetracyclines (omadacycline, eravacycline), new aminoglycosides (plazomicin), and siderophores (cefiderocol).

Dosing antimicrobials in burn patients is made challenging by the shift to a hypermetabolic state around 48 to 72 hours postburn.[14,67,68] This is marked by increased cardiac output, changes in gut function, and augmented hepatic and renal clearance.[69] Furthermore, the volume of distribution is often altered by large-volume fluid resuscitation. These facts may support higher or more frequent dosing of antimicrobials, but further work on dosing in burn patients is needed. Piperacillin–tazobactam can serve as a useful example. Either higher doses (8/1 g four times daily) or prolonged infusion times (4.5 g every 6 hours, infused over 3 hours) are more likely to achieve probability of target attainment (ie, the percentage time above minimum inhibitory concentration). Selig and colleagues recently showed that dosing decisions for burn patients based solely on TBSA does not impact probability of target attainment.[70] Multidisciplinary care that includes a clinical pharmacist and infectious-disease specialist can help confront these complex issues.

Topical antimicrobials were a revolutionary advance in the care of burned patients. Products used today include mafenide acetate (Sulfamylon), silver-based products, and honey.[71–73] The reader is directed to a review by Cancio.[71]

Antifungals

The cornerstone of management of FWI in these patients is aggressive surgical debridement. Having underscored that, antifungals often are empirically started in cases of suspected FWI. Empiric antifungal therapy often attempts to address the wide variety of noncandidal organisms that can cause FWI including *Aspergillus* and Mucorales. This typically results in combination therapy with liposomal amphotericin B and a broad-spectrum triazole (eg, voriconazole, posaconazole, or isavuconazole).

Questions about antifungals in burn patients include the following. How does hypermetabolism affect dosing strategies? What if any pharmacokinetic–pharmacodynamic parameters exist to help guide therapy? Are susceptibilities available, and if so are there any clinical breakpoints?[74] How does intrinsic resistance impact antifungal choice? (eg, *Aspergillus terreus* has intrinsic resistance to amphotericin B, but not to broad-spectrum triazoles.) How long should these patients be treated after surgical debridement? What is the role of newer antifungal agents like rezafungin, ibrexafungerp, olorofim, and fosmanogepix?[75] Last, whereas the development of topical antimicrobials by Pruitt and colleagues was a key step in preventing bacterial burn wound infections, the same is not true of topical antifungals. Compounds with some topical antifungal efficacy include honey, silver, and cerium nitrate. Nystatin has been used to treat established FWC or FWI. A combination of mafenide acetate (aqueous solution) and amphotericin B has been used, but in one study, the amphotericin component was undetectable after 2 days of exposure to high temperatures.[76] This is an area that requires further research.

Excision of the Burn Wound

Early surgical excision of the burn wound is generally considered to be the standard of care and decreases burn wound infection risk. The definition of early excision in the literature varies between a few days and 2 weeks; at many burn centers, the goal is excision of all full-thickness burns within 1 week of injury. Janzekovic published experience with tangential excision in 1972, overcoming concerns about excessive blood loss.[77,78] A meta-analysis in 2006 showed that early excision improved mortality and length of stay, but not blood transfusion requirements.[79] In patients who have already developed invasive burn wound infections, aggressive excision is even more critical to survival, as demonstrated by Spegar and colleagues for noncandidal FWIs.[80] Some investigators have unsuccessfully attempted to determine when to perform delayed excision in countries with limited resources.[81]

INFECTION PREVENTION AND CONTROL

Infection prevention and control (IPAC), along with antimicrobial stewardship, is vital in burn care[82] (**Box 2**). Burn units are often be threatened by routine outbreaks with gram-negative organisms such as *Pseudomonas aeruginosa* and *Acinetobacter baumannii*, in part because of the fastidious nature of the organisms, as well as their proclivity to form reservoirs in areas that are difficult to disinfect and form part of a units' infrastructure (eg, sinks, faucets, toilets, showers).[83–85] These two organisms are particularly challenging due to the risk they pose of transmitted resistance, and their risk of developing multidrug resistance including up to all classes of agents currently available.[86] Having a robust IPAC service with the ability to investigate outbreaks in

---

Box 2
Infection control and prevention in the burn center

- Universal precautions
- Additional barrier precautions
- Early removal of intravascular and urinary catheters
- Ventilator-associated pneumonia prevention bundles; early ventilator liberation
- Antibiotic stewardship
- Early excision and grafting of deep-partial-thickness and full-thickness burns

---

burn units is crucial. Previously, if phenotypic susceptibilities to antimicrobials raised clinical suspicion, pulse-field gel electrophoresis (PFGE) could be used to link organisms to outbreaks. As whole-genome sequencing becomes more ubiquitous, this is technology is likely to supplant PFGE because of its ability to detect small differences between organisms.[87,88] The outbreaks of atypical organisms in burn units can occasionally occur (eg, Orf virus; invasive fungal infections) highlighting the need for careful attention to IPAC practices in burn units.[89,90]

CLINICS CARE POINTS

- Early excision of burn wounds and support from a multidisciplinary burn team improves mortality from burns.
- Timing and microbiology of burn infections has been well described and can assist in gauging pre-test probability of disease.
- Infection prevention and control is vital in preventing and responding to outbreaks in burn units.

REFERENCES

1. Church D, Elsayed S, Reid O, et al. Burn wound infections. Clin Microbiol Rev 2006;19(2):403–34.
2. D'Avignon LC, Hogan BK, Murray CK, et al. Contribution of bacterial and viral infections to attributable mortality in patients with severe burns: an autopsy series. Burns 2010;36(6):773–9.
3. Norbury W, Herndon DN, Tanksley J, et al. Infection in Burns. Surg Infect 2016; 17(2):250–5.
4. Moore CB, Medina MA, van Deventer HW, et al. Downregulation of immune signaling genes in patients with large surface burn injury. J Burn Care Res 2007;28(6):879–87.
5. Hansbrough JF, Field TO Jr, Gadd MA, et al. Immune response modulation after burn injury: T cells and antibodies. J Burn Care Rehabil 1987;8(6):509–12.
6. Mistry S, Mistry NF, Antia NH, et al. Cellular immune mechanisms in thermally injured mice. Burns Incl Therm Inj 1986;12(3):188–92.
7. Mistry S, Mistry NP, Arora S, et al. Cellular immune response following thermal injury in human patients. Burns Incl Therm Inj 1986;12(5):318–24.
8. D'Arpa P, Leung KP. Toll-Like Receptor Signaling in Burn Wound Healing and Scarring. Adv Wound Care 2017;6(10):330–43.

9. Fear VS, Boyd JH, Rea S, et al. Burn Injury Leads to Increased Long-Term Susceptibility to Respiratory Infection in both Mouse Models and Population Studies. PLoS One 2017;12(1):e0169302.
10. Rendon JL, Li X, Akhtar S, et al. Interleukin-22 modulates gut epithelial and immune barrier functions following acute alcohol exposure and burn injury. Shock 2013;39(1):11–8.
11. Wang C, Li Q, Ren J. Microbiota-Immune Interaction in the Pathogenesis of Gut-Derived Infection. Front Immunol 2019;10:1873.
12. Adiliaghdam F, Cavallaro P, Mohad V, et al. Targeting the gut to prevent sepsis from a cutaneous burn. JCI Insight 2020;5(19).
13. Greenhalgh DG. Sepsis in the burn patient: a different problem than sepsis in the general population. Burns Trauma 2017;5:23.
14. Williams FN, Herndon DN. Metabolic and Endocrine Considerations After Burn Injury. Clin Plast Surg 2017;44(3):541–53.
15. Hogan BK, Wolf SE, Hospenthal DR, et al. Correlation of American Burn Association sepsis criteria with the presence of bacteremia in burned patients admitted to the intensive care unit. J Burn Care Res 2012;33(3):371–8.
16. Mann-Salinas EA, Baun MM, Meininger JC, et al. Novel predictors of sepsis outperform the American Burn Association sepsis criteria in the burn intensive care unit patient. J Burn Care Res 2013;34(1):31–43.
17. Burmeister DM, Heard TC, Chao T, et al. A Prospective Observational Study Comparing Clinical Sepsis Criteria to Protein Biomarkers Reveals a Role for Vascular Dysfunction in Burn Sepsis. Crit Care Explor 2022;4(1):e0610.
18. Mann EA, Wood GL, Wade CE. Use of procalcitonin for the detection of sepsis in the critically ill burn patient: a systematic review of the literature. Burns 2011;37(4):549–58.
19. Ruiz-Castilla M, Roca O, Masclans JR, et al. RECENT ADVANCES IN BIOMARKERS IN SEVERE BURNS. Shock 2016;45(2):117–25.
20. van Duin D, Strassle PD, DiBiase LM, et al. Timeline of health care-associated infections and pathogens after burn injuries. Am J Infect Control 2016;44(12):1511–6.
21. Mayhall CG. The epidemiology of burn wound infections: then and now. Clin Infect Dis 2003;37(4):543–50.
22. Halstead FD, Lee KC, Kwei J, et al. A systematic review of quantitative burn wound microbiology in the management of burns patients. Burns 2018;44(1):39–56.
23. Azzopardi EA, Azzopardi E, Camilleri L, et al. Gram negative wound infection in hospitalised adult burn patients–systematic review and metanalysis. PLoS One 2014;9(4):e95042.
24. Park HS, Pham C, Paul E, et al. Early pathogenic colonisers of acute burn wounds: A retrospective review. Burns 2017;43(8):1757–65.
25. Johnson TR, Gómez BI, McIntyre MK, et al. The Cutaneous Microbiome and Wounds: New Molecular Targets to Promote Wound Healing. Int J Mol Sci 2018;19(9).
26. Kelly DC, Rizzo J, Yun HC, et al. Microbiology and clinical characteristics of industrial oil burns. Burns 2020;46(3):711–7.
27. Horvath EE, Murray CK, Vaughan GM, et al. Fungal wound infection (not colonization) is independently associated with mortality in burn patients. Ann Surg 2007;245(6):978–85.
28. Schofield CM, Murray CK, Horvath EE, et al. Correlation of culture with histopathology in fungal burn wound colonization and infection. Burns 2007;33(3):341–6.

29. Kaita Y, Tarui T, Otsu A, et al. The Clinical Significance of Serum 1,3-β-D-Glucan For the Diagnosis of Candidemia in Severe Burn Patients. J Burn Care Res 2019; 40(1):104–6.

30. Shupp JW, Petraitiene R, Jaskille AD, et al. Early serum (1→3)-β-D-glucan levels in patients with burn injury. Mycoses 2012;55(3):224–7.

31. Blyth DM, Chung KK, Cancio LC, et al. Clinical utility of fungal screening assays in adults with severe burns. Burns 2013;39(3):413–9.

32. Ballard J, Edelman L, Saffle J, et al. Positive fungal cultures in burn patients: a multicenter review. J Burn Care Res 2008;29(1):213–21.

33. Aurora A, Le TD, Akers KS, et al. Recurrent bacteremia: A 10-year retrospective study in combat-related burn casualties. Burns 2019;45(3):579–88.

34. Lago K, Decker CF, Chung KK, et al. Difficult to Treat Infections in the Burn Patient. Surg Infect 2021;22(1):95–102.

35. Regules JA, Glasser JS, Wolf SE, et al. Endocarditis in burn patients: clinical and diagnostic considerations. Burns 2008;34(5):610–6.

36. Liodaki E, Kalousis K, Mauss KL, et al. Epidemiology of pneumonia in a burn care unit: the influence of inhalation trauma on pneumonia and of pneumonia on burn mortality. Ann Burns Fire Disasters 2015;28(2):128–33.

37. Edelman DA, Khan N, Kempf K, et al. Pneumonia after inhalation injury. J Burn Care Res 2007;28(2):241–6.

38. Mosier MJ, Pham TN. American Burn Association Practice guidelines for prevention, diagnosis, and treatment of ventilator-associated pneumonia (VAP) in burn patients. J Burn Care Res 2009;30(6):910–28.

39. Graham BS, Snell JD Jr. Herpes simplex virus infection of the adult lower respiratory tract. Medicine (Baltim) 1983;62(6):384–93.

40. Edge JM, Van der Merwe AE, Pieper CH, et al. Clinical outcome of HIV positive patients with moderate to severe burns. Burns 2001;27(2):111–4.

41. Lachance P, Chen J, Featherstone R, et al. Association Between Cytomegalovirus Reactivation and Clinical Outcomes in Immunocompetent Critically Ill Patients: A Systematic Review and Meta-Analysis. Open Forum Infect Dis 2017;4(2):ofx029.

42. Bourdarias B, Perro G, Cutillas M, et al. Herpes simplex virus infection in burned patients: epidemiology of 11 cases. Burns 1996;22(4):287–90.

43. Kagan RJ, Naraqi S, Matsuda T, et al. Herpes simplex virus and cytomegalovirus infections in burned patients. J Trauma 1985;25(1):40–5.

44. Sheridan RL, Weber JM, Pasternak MM, et al. A 15-year experience with varicella infections in a pediatric burn unit. Burns 1999;25(4):353–6.

45. Kubota Y, Kosaka K, Hokazono T, et al. Disseminated zoster in an adult patient with extensive burns: a case report. Virol J 2019;16(1):68.

46. Sheridan RL, Schulz JT, Weber JM, et al. Cutaneous herpetic infections complicating burns. Burns 2000;26(7):621–4.

47. Bordes J, Maslin J, Prunet B, et al. Cytomegalovirus infection in severe burn patients monitoring by real-time polymerase chain reaction: A prospective study. Burns 2011;37(3):434–9.

48. Deepe GS Jr, MacMillan BG, Linnemann CC Jr. Unexplained fever in burn patients due to cytomegalovirus infection. JAMA 1982;248(18):2299–301.

49. Jain M, Duggal S, Chugh TD. Cytomegalovirus infection in non-immunosuppressed critically ill patients. J Infect Dev Ctries 2011;5(8):571–9.

50. Lodding IP, Schultz HH, Jensen JU, et al. Cytomegalovirus Viral Load in Bronchoalveolar Lavage to Diagnose Lung Transplant Associated CMV Pneumonia. Transplantation 2018;102(2):326–32.

51. Moran KT, Thupari JN, O'Reilly TJ, et al. Effect of immunoglobulin G therapy on serum antibody titers to cytomegalovirus in burn patients. Am J Surg 1988; 155(2):294–7.

52. Osawa R, Singh N. Cytomegalovirus infection in critically ill patients: a systematic review. Crit Care 2009;13(3):R68.

53. Dreyfus DH. Herpesviruses and the microbiome. J Allergy Clin Immunol 2013; 132(6):1278–86.

54. Agut H, Bonnafous P, Gautheret-Dejean A. Laboratory and clinical aspects of human herpesvirus 6 infections. Clin Microbiol Rev 2015;28(2):313–35.

55. Limaye AP, Boeckh M. CMV in critically ill patients: pathogen or bystander? Rev Med Virol 2010;20(6):372–9.

56. Limaye AP, Kirby KA, Rubenfeld GD, et al. Cytomegalovirus reactivation in critically ill immunocompetent patients. JAMA 2008;300(4):413–22.

57. Ong DS, Bonten MJM, Spitoni C, et al. Epidemiology of Multiple Herpes Viremia in Previously Immunocompetent Patients With Septic Shock. Clin Infect Dis 2017; 64(9):1204–10.

58. Luyt CE, Combes A, Deback C, et al. Herpes simplex virus lung infection in patients undergoing prolonged mechanical ventilation. Am J Respir Crit Care Med 2007;175(9):935–42.

59. Luyt CE, Forel JM, Hajage D, et al. Acyclovir for Mechanically Ventilated Patients With Herpes Simplex Virus Oropharyngeal Reactivation: A Randomized Clinical Trial. JAMA Intern Med 2020;180(2):263–72.

60. Kiley JL, Chung KK, Blyth DM. Viral Infections in Burns. Surg Infect 2021;22(1): 88–94.

61. Sen S, Szoka N, Phan H, et al. Herpes simplex activation prolongs recovery from severe burn injury and increases bacterial infection risk. J Burn Care Res 2012; 33(3):393–7.

62. Keen EF 3rd, Robinson BJ, Hospenthal DR, et al. Prevalence of multidrug-resistant organisms recovered at a military burn center. Burns 2010;36(6): 819–25.

63. Lachiewicz AM, Hauck CG, Weber DJ, et al. Bacterial Infections After Burn Injuries: Impact of Multidrug Resistance. Clin Infect Dis 2017;65(12):2130–6.

64. Singh NP, Rani M, Gupta K, et al. Changing trends in antimicrobial susceptibility pattern of bacterial isolates in a burn unit. Burns 2017;43(5):1083–7.

65. Avni T, Levcovich A, Ad-El DD, et al. Prophylactic antibiotics for burns patients: systematic review and meta-analysis. BMJ 2010;340:c241.

66. Putra ON, Saputro ID, Hidayatullah AYN. A retrospective surveillance of the prophylactic antibiotics for debridement surgery in burn patients. Int J Burns Trauma 2021;11(2):96–104.

67. Cota JM, FakhriRavari A, Rowan MP, et al. Intravenous Antibiotic and Antifungal Agent Pharmacokinetic-Pharmacodynamic Dosing in Adults with Severe Burn Injury. Clin Ther 2016;38(9):2016–31.

68. Pruskowski KA. Pharmacokinetics and Pharmacodynamics of Antimicrobial Agents in Burn Patients. Surg Infect 2021;22(1):77–82.

69. Selig DJ, Akers KS, Chung KK, et al. Meropenem pharmacokinetics in critically ill patients with or without burn treated with or without continuous veno-venous haemofiltration. Br J Clin Pharmacol 2022;88(5):2156–68.

70. Selig DJ, Akers KS, Chung KK, et al. Comparison of Piperacillin and Tazobactam Pharmacokinetics in Critically Ill Patients with Trauma or with Burn. Antibiotics (Basel) 2022;11(5).

71. Cancio LC. Topical Antimicrobial Agents for Burn Wound Care: History and Current Status. Surg Infect 2021;22(1):3–11.
72. Dai T, Huang YY, Sharma SK, et al. Topical antimicrobials for burn wound infections. Recent Pat Anti-Infect Drug Discov 2010;5(2):124–51.
73. Lewandowski L, Purcell R, Fleming M, et al. The use of dilute Dakin's solution for the treatment of angioinvasive fungal infection in the combat wounded: a case series. Mil Med 2013;178(4):e503–7.
74. Wiederhold NP. Antifungal Susceptibility Testing: A Primer for Clinicians. Open Forum Infect Dis 2021;8(11):ofab444.
75. Lamoth F, Lewis RE, Kontoyiannis DP. Investigational Antifungal Agents for Invasive Mycoses: A Clinical Perspective. Clin Infect Dis 2022;75(3):534–44.
76. Rizzo JA, Martini AK, Pruskowski KA, et al. Thermal stability of mafenide and amphotericin B topical solution. Burns 2018;44(2):475–80.
77. Jackson D. Excision and closure of the wound as applied to burns. Proc R Soc Med 1972;65(1):23–4.
78. Janzekovic Z. A new concept in the early excision and immediate grafting of burns. J Trauma 1970;10(12):1103–8.
79. Ong YS, Samuel M, Song C. Meta-analysis of early excision of burns. Burns 2006; 32(2):145–50.
80. Spebar MJ, Walters MJ, Pruitt BA Jr. Improved survival with aggressive surgical management of noncandidal fungal infections of the burn wound. J Trauma 1982; 22(10):867–8.
81. Wong L, Rajandram R, Allorto N. Systematic review of excision and grafting in burns: Comparing outcomes of early and late surgery in low and high-income countries. Burns 2021;47(8):1705–13.
82. Rafla K, Tredget EE. Infection control in the burn unit. Burns 2011;37(1):5–15.
83. Kanamori H, Parobek CM, Juliano JJ, et al. A Prolonged Outbreak of KPC-3-Producing Enterobacter cloacae and Klebsiella pneumoniae Driven by Multiple Mechanisms of Resistance Transmission at a Large Academic Burn Center. Antimicrob Agents Chemother 2017;61(2).
84. Mabrouk A, Chebbi Y, Raddaoui A, et al. Clonal spread of PER-1 and OXA-23 producing extensively drug resistant Acinetobacter baumannii during an outbreak in a burn intensive care unit in Tunisia. Acta Microbiol Immunol Hung 2020;67(4):222–7.
85. Yagnik KJ, Kalyatanda G, Cannella AP, et al. Outbreak of Acinetobacter baumannii associated with extrinsic contamination of ultrasound gel in a tertiary centre burn unit. Infect Prev Pract 2019;1(2):100009.
86. Smoke SM, Brophy A, Reveron S, et al. Evolution and transmission of cefiderocol-resistant Acinetobacter baumannii during an outbreak in the burn intensive care unit. Clin Infect Dis 2023;76(3):e1261-e1265.
87. Be NA, Allen JE, Brown TS, et al. Microbial profiling of combat wound infection through detection microarray and next-generation sequencing. J Clin Microbiol 2014;52(7):2583–94.
88. Yun HC, Tully CC, Mende K, et al. A single-center, six-year evaluation of the role of pulsed-field gel electrophoresis in suspected burn center outbreaks. Burns 2016;42(6):1323–30.
89. Midilli K, Erkiliç A, Kuşkucu M, et al. Nosocomial outbreak of disseminated orf infection in a burn unit, Gaziantep, Turkey, October to December 2012. Euro Surveill 2013;18(11):20425.
90. Struck MF. Infection control in burn patients: are fungal infections underestimated? Scand J Trauma Resusc Emerg Med 2009;17:51.

Acute Respiratory Distress Syndrome, Mechanical Ventilation, and Inhalation Injury in Burn Patients

Edward Bittner, MD[a,b], Robert Sheridan, MD[c],*

KEYWORDS

- ARDS • Burn injury • Inhalation injury • Mechanical ventilation
- Protective ventilation • Ventilator-induced lung injury

KEY POINTS

- Acute respiratory distress syndrome (ARDS) is common in seriously burned patients, driven by a combination of inflammatory and infection factors.
- Inhalation injury contributes to respiratory failure in some burn patients.
- In burn patients, ARDS with or without inhalation injury is effectively managed using principles evolved for non–burn patients.

ACUTE RESPIRATORY DISTRESS SYNDROME
Epidemiology and Pathophysiology

Burn patients are at risk of developing acute respiratory distress syndrome (ARDS) as a result of systemic inflammation, fluid resuscitation, protein loss, prolonged mechanical ventilation (MV), and multiorgan dysfunction (MODS) (**Fig. 1**). Inhalation injury—via direct cellular damage, disruption of mucociliary clearance, airway obstruction, and proinflammatory cytokines—further increases the risk.[1] Between 20% and 50% of mechanically ventilated burn patients will develop ARDS. Onset is most commonly during the first week postburn, although it may be delayed.[2,3] Pathologically, ARDS is acutely characterized by inflammation-mediated injury resulting in increased alveolar-capillary permeability, edema, alveolar collapse/derecruitment, reduced lung compliance, increased pulmonary vascular resistance, ventilation-perfusion (VQ) mismatch and shunting, and impaired gas exchange.[4] Chronic changes are

[a] Department of Anesthesia, Critical Care, and Pain Medicine, Massachusetts General Hospital and Shriners Hospital for Children, 51 Blossom Street, Boston, MA 02114, USA; [b] Department of Anesthesia, Massachusetts General Hospital, 55 Fruit Street, Boston, MA 02114, USA; [c] Department of Surgery, Massachusetts General Hospital and Shriners Hospital for Children, 51 Blossom Street, Boston, MA 02114, USA
* Corresponding author.
E-mail address: rsheridan@mgh.harvard.edu

Surg Clin N Am 103 (2023) 439–451
https://doi.org/10.1016/j.suc.2023.01.006
0039-6109/23/© 2023 Elsevier Inc. All rights reserved.

surgical.theclinics.com

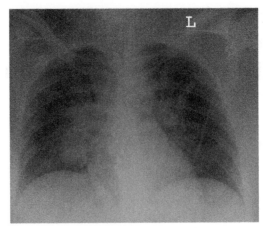

Fig. 1. Postburn ARDS are often nonspecific, showing inhomogeneous consolidation and perihilar fullness.

characterized by fibrosis, vascular smooth muscle hypertrophy, and capillary obliteration.[4] ARDS contributes to mortality and morbidity in burn patients.[5] Mortality in ARDS is caused primarily by the development of MODS.[6]

The management of ARDS is largely supportive, and most approaches in burn patients have been translated from the non–burn population. Although MV is often essential, the process itself can inflict further damage to the lungs, referred to as ventilator-induced lung injury (VILI).[7] Mechanisms of VILI include high inspiratory pressures (barotrauma), high tidal volumes (TV; volutrauma), repeated opening and closing of alveoli (atelectrauma), oxygen toxicity, and inflammatory cytokine release (biotrauma).[8,9] Recently, additional mechanisms of injury have been implicated, including high mechanical power (ergotrauma), stress frequency, respiratory muscle overuse/underuse (myotrauma), and pulmonary capillary stress failure.[10–12]

Protective Ventilation

The standard approach to protective mechanical ventilation (PMV) includes small TVs to limit volutrauma, setting positive end-expiratory pressure (PEEP) to minimize atelectrauma, and recruitment maneuvers (RMs) to open collapsed regions of the lung. An individualized approach to MV based on lung pathophysiology and morphology, ARDS cause, and lung imaging and monitoring has been suggested to improve ventilation practice and outcome.[13] In addition, PMV has been expanded beyond the lung itself to include right-heart-protective ventilation, diaphragmatic-protective ventilation, minimization of repetitive-stress injury, capillary-stress reduction, and consideration of patient self-inflicted lung injury (P-SILI).[11]

Tidal Volumes

A TV of 4 to 6 mL/kg predicted body weight is commonly used to maintain a plateau pressure (Pplat) < 30 cm H_2O.[14] Minimizing airway driving pressure (DP), calculated as Pplat minus PEEP, is another suggested strategy for selecting TV.[15] Importantly, Pplat and DP are indirect measures for peak lung stress. When functional residual capacity is markedly reduced in severe ARDS, overdistention can occur in nondependent regions despite achieving target levels. Real-time bedside monitoring with pressure and imaging techniques, such as esophageal manometry, electrical impedance tomography, and lung ultrasound, are increasingly used to select TV to minimize overdistention.[16–18]

Unique characteristics of burn patients may affect the successful application of a low-TV approach. For example, low TV in a burn patient with poor chest compliance and/or inhalation injury with obstruction of the conducting airways can result in lung underinflation. A retrospective study in pediatric burn patients with inhalation injury found that a low-TV approach was associated with more atelectasis, longer duration of MV, and a higher incidence of ARDS than a higher-TV approach.[19] A recent international cohort study found that low-TV ventilation was used in most burn patients, but was not associated with a reduction in days ventilator-free and alive at day 28.[20] Strict application of low-TV ventilation in the setting of increased CO_2 production from burn-associated hypermetabolism can result in "air hunger," patient-ventilator dyssynchrony, and hypercapnia. Although hypercapnia may be tolerated to an extent ("permissive hypercapnia"), adjustments to the ventilator mode and increases in sedation are often needed.

POSITIVE END-EXPIRATORY PRESSURE

PEEP is used in ARDS to minimize atelectasis and reduce lung heterogeneity, thereby increasing the amount of aerated lung available for ventilation. PEEP may also shift edema fluid from the flooded alveoli into the interstitial space, decreasing shunt fraction and promoting more uniform alveolar mechanics.[8] However, PEEP will only have benefit when alveolar recruitment surpasses overexpansion of patent alveoli. There is no simple method to assess the risk-to-benefit ratio of different PEEP levels. In ARDS, derecruitment is a continuous process in which the rate of collapse increases as PEEP decreases. With decreasing levels of PEEP, derecruitment ceases in the sternal lung zones at PEEP of 10 cm H_2O, whereas it continues in dorsal regions down to 0 cm H_2O.[21] Consequently, a minimum PEEP of 10 to 12 cm H_2O might reduce derecruitment during the acute phase of ARDS, and higher levels may be necessary in severe cases. Approaches to select an optimal PEEP level in ARDS include the use of tables that assign PEEP based on Fio_2, use of the highest PEEP that optimizes oxygenation while allowing an acceptable TV and Pplat, and bedside PEEP titration based on lung compliance and recruitability.[22]

Recruitment Maneuvers

Computed tomographic (CT) scans have indicated that tissue consolidation can account for up to 50% of the lung in ARDS.[23] RMs apply a higher-than-normal inflation pressure (usually ≥35 cm H_2O) to the lungs for 20 to 40 seconds to "open the lung" by recruiting atelectatic regions.[24] Evidence to support their routine use in ARDS is lacking.[25] However, RMs may be beneficial for improving oxygenation in patients with hypoxemia.[25] The improvement in oxygenation from an RM is often greatest when followed by an increase in the level of PEEP.[25] Repeated RMs during lung-protective ventilation can improve pulmonary compliance and oxygenation and do not appear to worsen lung injury in severe ARDS.[26] Most alveolar recruitment occurs during the first 10 seconds of an RM; extended durations (eg, minutes) may be associated with worse outcomes.[27] RMs appear to be most effective in improving oxygenation during early ARDS rather than during the fibroproliferative phase.[28]

Right-Heart-Protective Ventilation

Pulmonary hypertension (PH) in ARDS results from pulmonary vasoconstriction (caused by hypoxia or hypercarbia), microthrombosis, and ventilation with high

DPs.[29] Right-ventricular (RV) dysfunction develops with sustained elevations in PH, as the RV has no adaptive mechanism other than dilatation when its afterload is increased.[30] In ARDS, RV dysfunction can lead to RV failure (acute cor pulmonale), and if left untreated, cardiogenic shock can develop. Elevated right-heart pressure can also worsen hypoxemia by right-to-left intracardiac shunting of deoxygenated blood through a patent foramen ovale. RV PMV has been suggested to reduce RV afterload to include the following: (1) minimizing lung stress by limiting Pplat and DP, (2) reducing pulmonary vasoconstriction by improving oxygenation and control of CO_2, and (3) prone positioning (PP) to unload the RV.[31] Optimization of RV-protective PEEP must balance alveolar recruitment and overdistention. If RV-protective measures are insufficient (or unfeasible), ancillary therapies, such as inhaled vasodilators or extracorporeal membrane oxygenation (ECMO), may be required.

Diaphragm

Respiratory-muscle weakness rapidly develops in critically ill, mechanically ventilated patients and carries a poorer prognosis.[32,33] Exposure to excessive workloads even for brief periods can result in diaphragmatic inflammation referred to as use atrophy.[11] Failing to allow full rest following the onset of acute respiratory failure or after a failed weaning trial can induce this injury and prolong MV.[11] Furthermore, sepsis can incite and exacerbate diaphragmatic injury, through the effects of proinflammatory cytokines.[34] Disuse atrophy can result from prolonged periods of MV and loss of electro-myographic stimulation.[35] Diaphragmatic PMV uses the following dual approach[12]: (1) early after the onset of acute respiratory failure, avoiding prolonged periods of high work of breathing (WOB) by providing adequate ventilatory support and sedation; (2) during recovery, limiting passive ventilation and targeting an inspiratory effort level similar to that of healthy subjects at rest to accelerate liberation from ventilation.[33]

Self-Induced Lung Injury

Increased respiratory drive and vigorous inspiratory efforts are often attempts to compensate for impairments in respiratory mechanics and gas exchange. These vigorous spontaneous breathing efforts may have injurious physiologic effects mediated by swings in transpulmonary pressure (TPP), increases in transvascular pressure resulting in edema, intratidal shift of gas between different lung zones (pendelluft), and diaphragmatic injury. This is referred to as P-SILI.[36] In patients receiving MV, vigorous respiratory efforts may also result in patient-ventilator dyssynchrony and increased mechanical lung injury owing to high TPPs and/or cyclic atelectasis.[37,38] Preventing P-SILI in clinical practice requires assessment of a patient's inspiratory effort and the detection of potentially harmful patient-ventilator interactions. For some patients with vigorous spontaneous breathing and/or patient-ventilator dyssynchrony, sedation or paralysis may be protective treatment.

Stress Frequency and Permissive Hypercapnia

Higher ventilatory frequencies are often used with low-TV ventilation to reduce hypercapnia, but this may have detrimental effects on respiratory mechanics, gas exchange, and cumulative lung trauma.[39,40] Higher ventilatory frequencies shorten inspiratory time, resulting in the need for higher peak-flow rates, which may augment parenchymal shear stress, worsen oxygenation, and contribute to greater pressure-related cyclic lung stress and strain. Shortened expiration times may have detrimental effects, including dynamic hyperinflation, reduced compliance, increased TPP, and diaphragmatic dysfunction. A reduction of the frequency of ventilation with resulting hypercapnia may be beneficial in ARDS by facilitating a reduction of the cumulative intensity of cyclic stress and strain. Hypercapnia itself may also have beneficial physiologic benefits, including improved VQ matching from pulmonary vasoconstriction, increased local alveolar ventilation from inhibition of airway tone, increased oxygen delivery from an increase in cardiac output, increased unloading of oxygen in the tissues, microvascular vasodilation, and anti-inflammatory effects.[41] Some studies have reported benefit from permissive hypercapnia in ARDS, although they are confounded by the inability to dissect the effects of permissive hypercapnia from the effects of low TV.[42] Because hypercapnia increases respiratory drive, deep sedation or neuromuscular blockade may be required.

Fluid Overload and Capillary Stress Reduction

Fluid-conservative approaches have been associated with improved outcomes in non–burn ARDS, but have the potential to compromise burn resuscitation.[43] Consequently, application of a fluid-conservative approach in a burn patient with ARDS should be considered carefully, with close attention to administering the least amount of fluid that still achieves adequate organ perfusion.

Unconventional Mechanical Ventilation

A variety of unconventional modes of MV, including high-frequency percussive ventilation (HFPV), high-frequency oscillatory ventilation (HFOV), or airway-pressure-release ventilation (APRV), are used in some burn centers for patients with ARDS.[44]

HFPV delivers very small, high-frequency tidal breaths superimposed on a conventional pressure-controlled breath.[45] HFPV improves oxygenation, improves ventilation, and lowers airway pressures compared with other modes of MV. HFPV also produces intrabronchial percussion, airway turbulence, and higher airflow, all of which enhance mobilization and clearance of airway debris and secretions. HFPV, although shown not to be superior to conventional ventilation in the general ARDS population, has a suggested role in inhalation injuries and burn-related ARDS.[46] HFPV is routinely used in some burn centers, particularly in patients with inhalation injury or in those who fail conventional MV.

HFOV delivers small, sub-dead-space TVs at high frequency to maximize lung recruitment and avoid cyclic alveolar collapse.[47] HFOV in burn-related ARDS has not been extensively studied. HFOV is sometimes used as a rescue approach for burn patients with refractory hypoxemia but is generally unsuccessful in improving oxygenation in inhalation injury, probably because effective lung recruitment is impaired by obstruction of the conducting airways.[48]

APRV is a mode of pressure-controlled ventilation that allows spontaneous breathing at regularly fluctuating high and low levels of continuous positive airway pressure.[49] Proposed benefits include alveolar recruitment and stabilization, improved VQ matching, increased mean airway pressure, and minimization peak and Pplats.[50] Spontaneous breathing in APRV reduces sedation requirements, thereby preserving airway reflexes and facilitating cough and pulmonary toilet. There is limited literature supporting the benefit of APRV for ARDS. Specific evidence in the burn population is lacking.

Noninvasive Ventilation

For patients with mild ARDS, noninvasive ventilation (NIV) may be beneficial, as it allows patients to communicate more easily, requires less sedation, allows more effective cough and expectoration of secretions, and avoids intubation-related complications. NIV appears safe and effective in mild to moderate hypoxemia, but it may delay intubation and increase mortality in more severe hypoxemia.[51] In patients with inhalation injury or that have received large-volume fluid resuscitation, NIV may mask evidence of progressive airway obstruction.[52] There is currently limited literature examining the impact of NIV in the burn population.[53]

High-Flow Nasal Cannula

High-flow nasal cannula (HFNC) is increasingly used in the management of respiratory failure, including mild ARDS.[54] HFNC is capable of delivering up to 100% heated and humidified oxygen at flow rates of up to 60 L per minute. The benefits include a reduction in WOB, reduction of the anatomic dead space, generation of a small amount of PEEP, and improvement of mucociliary clearance.[55] There are limited reports of HFNC use in patients with burns and/or inhalation injury.[56]

STRATEGIES FOR REFRACTORY HYPOXEMIA
Prone Positioning

When a patient with ARDS is turned from supine to prone, the atelectatic dorsal lung regions are freed from the weight of the more ventral lung, the heart, and the mediastinum, favoring expansion of dorsal regions. The net effect is more homogeneous aeration with a more uniform strain distribution leading to an improvement of gas exchange and a decreased risk of VILI.[57] A systematic review of 9 randomized controlled trials (RCTs) concluded that patients with ARDS most likely to derive a survival benefit from PP were those with severe hypoxemia and in whom it was used more than 16 hours per day.[58] Data on PP of burn patients are limited; it presents logistical and safety challenges.[59] A case series reports improvements in oxygenation and a low rate of complications in patients with burn-related ARDS undergoing PP.[60] PMV should continue to be used during PP, and reassessment of ventilatory parameters should be performed, as respiratory mechanics may change with proning.[61,62] Increased sedation and neuromuscular blockade may be required.

Neuromuscular Blockade

Neuromuscular blocking agents (NMBAs) are sometimes used in patients with severe ARDS to enhance gas exchange and reduce Pplats, ventilator dyssynchrony, and VILI. A meta-analysis of 5 RCTs in moderate to severe ARDS concluded that early initiation (within 36–48 hours of ARDS diagnosis) of a 48-hour infusion of cisatracurium improved oxygenation and lowered barotrauma risk without increasing intensive care unit weakness.[63] There is no specific evidence to guide the use of NMBAs in burn-injured patients with ARDS. It is reasonable to consider them in burn patients with severe ARDS.[64]

Inhaled Pulmonary Vasodilators

Inhaled pulmonary vasodilators, including nitric oxide (NO) and epoprostenol, selectively increase blood flow to ventilated lung regions, thereby improving VQ matching and improving oxygenation.[65] They can also benefit ARDS patients with right-heart failure. A meta-analysis of 14 RCTs in adults with ARDS found that inhaled NO increased oxygenation but did not affect duration of MV or survival.[66] Improvement in oxygenation with inhaled NO has been demonstrated in burn-injured patients with ARDS.[67] Inhaled epoprostenol is a less-expensive agent that has similar effects.[68]

Extracorporeal Life Support

If other rescue strategies used in ARDS management fail to improve oxygenation, ECMO may be beneficial. A recent report concluded that mortality for burn-injured patients receiving ECMO was comparable that for non–burn ECMO patients.[69] Considerations include the risks of anticoagulation, need for further operative care, and consideration of the goals or futility of care.[70] Patients most likely to benefit from ECMO are those with severe ARDS within the first week of MV and without multiple organ failure.[71] ECMO for burn patients should be provided only in centers experienced in both burn care and in the use of extracorporeal support for ARDS.

INHALATION INJURY

Usually sustained in structural or vehicular fires, inhalation injury occurs in about 5% of burn-unit admissions.[72,73] Survival has improved with the evolution of supportive respiratory care, but inhalation injury remains a significant source of morbidity and mortality in burn patients. It increases mortality in patients with large cutaneous burns.[74]

Pathophysiology

The smoke generated during structural fires contains many incomplete combustion products, chemicals, and fine debris with varied particle size and weight. Gas temperatures can rise above floor level to several hundred degrees Fahrenheit. Exposure to such temperatures in inhaled gas can cause direct thermal damage to the supraglottic airway. Rarely, particularly with steam inhalation injury in enclosed spaces, thermal injury below the glottis can occur. Aerosolized irritants can cause inflammation, bronchospasm, increased bronchial blood flow, surfactant depletion, and mucosal slough. The local response to inhaled irritants attracts inflammatory cells, generates reactive oxygen species, and causes local release of proinflammatory molecules.[75] These can induce variable degrees of alveolar flooding and bronchial exudate with secondary VQ mismatching. These inflammatory changes are thought to explain the significant resuscitation fluid volume required by burn patients with inhalation injury.[76–78] Inhalation injury may be accompanied and complicated by carbon monoxide and/or cyanide poisoning.

Inhalation injury carries a strong risk of ARDS, and of pneumonia secondary to sloughing of the respiratory epithelium with resulting loss of ciliary clearance and accrual of obstructive endobronchial debris. This results in small-airway occlusion, atelectasis, and infection. Deaths owing to inhalation injury are often related to secondary ARDS and infection, with a classic report suggesting up to a 60% increase in expected burn mortality in the setting of coincident inhalation injury and pneumonia.[79]

Diagnosis

Tools to evaluate the presence and severity of inhalation injury include clinical evaluation, bronchoscopy, and radiography. Unfortunately, none of these tools reliably predict clinical course.[80] Severity grading schemes have been proposed,[81] but have not proven to be reliably useful for clinical care. History and clinical presentation are the most reliable methods of evaluation. Burns occurring in a closed space, burns around the nose and mouth, singed nasal hair, soot in the airway, carbonaceous sputum, hoarseness, wheezing, and stridor all suggest inhalation injury. Bronchoscopic examination will often reveal carbonaceous debris, ulceration, pallor, and mucosal slough, although patients inhaling fine-particle smoke or burning hydrocarbons may have deceptively unremarkable bronchoscopy. Those with overt bronchoscopic signs on initial evaluation seem to have more challenging clinical courses.[82] Serial bronchoscopy for pulmonary toilet may have value later in the hospital course, but there is no demonstrated role for early bronchoscopic removal of visible soot. Early chest radiographs are usually normal. Radionuclide ventilation scanning with xenon-133, technetium-99 DTPA, or macroaggregated albumin may show inhomogeneous tracer clearance suggestive of small airway obstruction.[83] CT scanning has been proposed for early diagnosis.[84–88]

Management

During initial evaluation, intubation is indicated for usual reasons of obtunded mental state or respiratory distress. Inhalation injury alone does not mandate intubation unless airway patency is threatened, particularly if cutaneous burns are small. In patients with severe facial edema or stridor, rapid assessment is critical, and intubation is often required. Evolving upper airway edema may complicate reintubation, so tube security is essential. Routine use of prophylactic antibiotics or empiric steroids is not supported.

Inhalation injury is associated with mucosal slough and loss of ciliary clearance with compromised pulmonary toilet. Chest physiotherapy and suctioning or stimulated cough is front-line therapy. Uncommonly, repeated bronchoscopy for pulmonary toilet may be needed.[89] Tracheobronchitis and pneumonia may occur and are addressed with targeted antibiotics and pulmonary toilet. Additional proposed therapies have included HFPV,[90] high-volume ventilation,[91] and nebulized heparin and N-acetylcysteine.[92] Tracheostomy, weaning, and extubation follow standard critical-care indications. Rarely, patients will suffer tracheal injury requiring reconstruction[93]; most survivors have no long-term pulmonary sequalae.[94]

SUMMARY

ARDS is common in patients with burn injury, and the need for large-volume fluid resuscitation, frequent surgery, presence of inhalation injury, superimposed sepsis, and burn-associated hypermetabolism all contribute to ventilation challenges.

CLINICS CARE POINTS

- Respiratory distress and failure are common occurences in burn patients driven by direct respiratory system injury, pulmonary and systemic infection, and systemic inflammation
- Inhalalation injury is caused by inhaled irritants and can result in multi-level iinvolvement of the respiratory system

DISCLOSURE

The authors have nothing to disclose.

REFERENCES

1. Lam NN, Hung TD. ARDS among cutaneous burn patients combined with inhalation injury: early onset and bad outcome. Ann Burns Fire Disasters 2019;32:37–42.
2. Lam NN, Hung TD, Hung DK. Acute respiratory distress syndrome among severe burn patients in a developing country: application result of the berlin definition. Ann Burns Fire Disasters 2018;31:9–12.
3. Cartotto R, Li Z, Hanna S, et al. The acute respiratory distress syndrome (ARDS) in mechanically ventilated burn patients: an analysis of risk factors, clinical features, and outcomes using the Berlin ARDS definition. Burns 2016;42:1423–43.

4. Matthay MA, Zemans RL, Zimmerman GA, et al. Acute respiratory distress syndrome. Nat Rev Dis Primers 2019;5:18.
5. Zavlin D, Chegireddy V, Boukovalas S, et al. Multi-institutional analysis of independent predictors for burn mortality in the United States. Burns Trauma 2018; 6:24.
6. Del Sorbo L, Slutsky AS. Acute respiratory distress syndrome and multiple organ failure. Curr Opin Crit Care 2011;17:1–6.
7. Beitler JR, Malhotra A, Thompson BT. Ventilator-induced Lung Injury. Clin Chest Med 2016;37:633–46.
8. Ohshimo S. Oxygen administration for patients with ARDS. J Intensive Care 2021; 9:17.
9. Slutsky AS, Ranieri VM. Ventilator-induced lung injury. N Engl J Med 2013;369: 2126–36.
10. Kallet RH. Mechanical Ventilation in ARDS: Quo Vadis? Respir Care 2022;67: 730–49.
11. Marini JJ. Evolving concepts for safer ventilation. Crit Care 2019;23:114.
12. Bertoni M, Spadaro S, Goligher EC. Monitoring patient respiratory effort during mechanical ventilation: lung and diaphragm-protective ventilation. Crit Care 2020;24:106.
13. Pelosi P, Ball L, Barbas CSV, et al. Personalized mechanical ventilation in acute respiratory distress syndrome. Crit Care 2021;25:250.
14. Papazian L, Aubron C, Brochard L, et al. Formal guidelines: management of acute respiratory distress syndrome. Ann Intensive Care 2019;9:69.
15. Pereira Romano ML, Maia IS, Laranjeira LN, et al. Driving Pressure-limited Strategy for Patients with Acute Respiratory Distress Syndrome. A Pilot Randomized Clinical Trial. Ann Am Thorac Soc 2020;17:596–604.
16. Pham T, Telias I, Beitler JR. Esophageal Manometry. Respir Care 2020;65: 772–92.
17. Rubin J, Berra L. Electrical impedance tomography in the adult intensive care unit: clinical applications and future directions. Curr Opin Crit Care 2022;28: 292–301.
18. Cylwik J, Buda N. Lung Ultrasonography in the Monitoring of Intraoperative Recruitment Maneuvers. Diagnostics 2021;11:276.
19. Sousse LE, Herndon DN, Andersen CR, et al. High tidal volume decreases adult respiratory distress syndrome, atelectasis, and ventilator days compared with low tidal volume in pediatric burned patients with inhalation injury. J Am Coll Surg 2015;220:570–8.
20. Schultz MJ, Horn J, Hollmann MW, et al. LAMiNAR investigators. Ventilation practices in burn patients-an international prospective observational cohort study. Burns Trauma 2021;9. tkab034.
21. Crotti S, Mascheroni D, Caironi P, et al. Recruitment and derecruitment during acute respiratory failure: a clinical study. Am J Resp Crit Care Med 2001 Jul 1; 164(1):131–40.
22. Gattinoni L, Collino F, Maiolo G, et al. Positive end-expiratory pressure: how to set it at the individual level. Ann Transl Med 2017;5:288.
23. Gattinoni L, Caironi P, Cressoni M, et al. Lung recruitment in patients with the acute respiratory distress syndrome. N Engl J Med 2006;354:1775–86.
24. Hess DR. Recruitment Maneuvers and PEEP Titration. Respir Care 2015;60: 1688–704.
25. Pensier J, de Jong A, Hajjej Z, et al. Effect of lung recruitment maneuver on oxygenation, physiological parameters and mortality in acute respiratory distress

syndrome patients: a systematic review and meta-analysis. Intensive Care Med 2019;45:1691–702.

26. Li MQ, Han GJ, Li JQ, et al. Effect of Repeated Recruitment Manoeuvres on Patients with Severe Acute Respiratory Distress Syndrome. West Indian Med J 2015;64:362–6.

27. Arnal JM, Paquet J, Wysocki M, et al. Optimal duration of a sustained inflation recruitment maneuver in ARDS patients. Intensive Care Med 2011;37:1588–94.

28. Spieth PM, Gama de Abreu M. Lung recruitment in ARDS: we are still confused, but on a higher PEEP level. Crit Care 2012;16:108.

29. Revercomb L, Hanmandlu A, Wareing N, et al. Mechanisms of Pulmonary Hypertension in Acute Respiratory Distress Syndrome (ARDS). Front Mol Biosci 2021 Jan 18;7:624093.

30. Zochios V, Parhar K, Tunnicliffe W, et al. The Right Ventricle in ARDS. Chest 2017; 152:181–93.

31. Paternot A, Repesse X, Vieillard-Baron A. Rationale and description of right ventricle-protective ventilation in ARDS. Respir Care 2016;61:1391–6.

32. Jaber S, Petrof BJ, Jung B, et al. Rapidly progressive diaphragmatic weakness and injury during mechanical ventilation in humans. Am J Respir Crit Care Med 2011;183:364–71.

33. Goligher EC, Dres M, Fan E, et al. Mechanical Ventilation-induced Diaphragm Atrophy Strongly Impacts Clinical Outcomes. Am J Respir Crit Care Med 2018;197: 204–13.

34. Hussain SN, Simkus G, Roussos C. Respiratory muscle fatigue: a cause of ventilatory failure in septic shock. J Appl Physiol 1985;58:2033–40.

35. Levine S, Nguyen T, Taylor N, et al. Rapid disuse atrophy of diaphragm fibers in mechanically ventilated humans. N Engl J Med 2008;358:1327–35.

36. Carteaux G, Parfait M, Combet M, et al. Patient-Self Inflicted Lung Injury: A Practical Review. J Clin Med 2021;10:2738.

37. Yoshida T, Uchiyama A, Matsuura N, et al. Spontaneous breathing during lung-protective ventilation in an experimental acute lung injury model: high transpulmonary pressure associated with strong spontaneous breathing effort may worsen lung injury. Crit Care Med 2012;40:1578–85.

38. Yoshida T, Torsani V, Gomes S, et al. Spontaneous effort causes occult pendelluft during mechanical ventilation. Am J Respir Crit Care Med 2013;188:1420–7.

39. Tonetti T, Vasques F, Rapetti F, et al. Driving pressure and mechanical power: new targets for VILI prevention. Ann Transl Med 2017;5:286.

40. Akoumianaki E, Vaporidi K, Georgopoulos D. The Injurious Effects of Elevated or Nonelevated Respiratory Rate during Mechanical Ventilation. Am J Respir Crit Care Med 2019;199:149–57.

41. Curley GF, Laffey JG, Kavanagh BP. CrossTalk proposal: there is added benefit to providing permissive hypercapnia in the treatment of ARDS. J Physiol 2013;591: 2763–5.

42. Barnes T, Zochios V, Parhar K. Re-examining Permissive Hypercapnia in ARDS: A Narrative Review. Chest 2018 Jul;154(1):185–95.

43. Guilabert P, Usúa G, Martín N, et al. Fluid resuscitation management in patients with burns: update. Br J Anaesth 2016;117:284–96.

44. Folwell JS, Basel AP, Britton GW, et al. Mechanical Ventilation Strategies in the Critically Ill Burn Patient: A Practical Review for Clinicians. Eur. Burn J 2021;2: 140–51.

45. Miller AG, Bartle RM, Feldman A, et al. A narrative review of advanced ventilator modes in the pediatric intensive care unit. Transl Pediatr 2021;10:2700–19.

46. Chung KK, Rhie RY, Lundy JB, et al. A Survey of Mechanical Ventilator Practices Across Burn Centers in North America. J Burn Care Res 2016;37:e131–9.
47. Sklar MC, Fan E, Goligher EC. High-Frequency Oscillatory Ventilation in Adults With ARDS: Past, Present, and Future. Chest 2017;152:1306–17.
48. Cartotto R, Walia G, Ellis S, et al. Oscillation after inhalation: high frequency oscillatory ventilation in burn patients with the acute respiratory distress syndrome and co-existing smoke inhalation injury. J Burn Care Res 2009;30:119–27.
49. Swindin J, Sampson C, Howatson A. Airway pressure release ventilation. BJA Educ 2020;20:80–8.
50. Fredericks AS, Bunker MP, Gliga LA, et al. Airway Pressure Release Ventilation: A Review of the Evidence, Theoretical Benefits, and Alternative Titration Strategies. Clin Med Insights Circ Respir Pulm Med 2020;14:1179548420903297.
51. Non-invasive ventilatory support and high-flow nasal oxygen as first-line treatment of acute hypoxemic respiratory failure and ARDS. Intensive Care Med 2021;47:851–66.
52. Goh CT, Jacobe S. Ventilation strategies in paediatric inhalation injury. Paediatr Respir Rev 2016;20:3–9.
53. Endorf FW, Dries DJ. Noninvasive ventilation in the burned patient. J Burn Care Res 2010;31:217–28.
54. Helviz Y, Einav S. A Systematic Review of the High-flow Nasal Cannula for Adult Patients. Crit Care 2018;22:71.
55. Nishimura M. High-flow nasal cannula oxygen therapy in adults. J Intensive Care 2015;3:15.
56. Byerly FL, Haithcock JA, Buchanan IB, et al. Use of high flow nasal cannula on a pediatric burn patient with inhalation injury and post-extubation stridor. Burns 2006;32:121–5.
57. Guérin C, Albert RK, Beitler J, et al. Prone position in ARDS patients: why, when, how and for whom. Intensive Care Med 2020;46:2385–96.
58. Bloomfield R, Noble DW, Sudlow A. Prone position for acute respiratory failure in adults. Cochrane Database Syst Rev 2015;11:CD008095.
59. Oto B, Orosco RI, Panter E, et al. Prone Positioning of the Burn Patient With Acute Respiratory Distress Syndrome: A Review of the Evidence and Practical Considerations. J Burn Care Res 2018;39:471–5.
60. Hale DF, Cannon JW, Batchinsky AI, et al. Prone positioning improves oxygenation in adult burn patients with severe acute respiratory distress syndrome. J Trauma Acute Care Surg 2012;72:1634–9.
61. Park SY, Kim HJ, Yoo KH, et al. The efficacy and safety of prone positioning in adults patients with acute respiratory distress syndrome: a meta-analysis of randomized controlled trials. J Thorac Dis 2015;7:356–67.
62. Papazian L, Munshi L, Guérin C. Prone position in mechanically ventilated patients. Intensive Care Med 2022;48:1062–5.
63. Ho ATN, Patolia S, Guervilly C. Neuromuscular blockade in acute respiratory distress syndrome: a systematic review and meta-analysis of randomized controlled trials. J Intensive Care 2020;8:12.
64. Martyn JAJ, Sparling JL, Bittner EA. Molecular mechanisms of muscular and non-muscular actions of neuromuscular blocking agents in critical illness. Br J Anaesth 2022;S0007-0912(22):00451–2.
65. Torbic H, Szumita PM, Anger KE, et al. Inhaled epoprostenol vs inhaled nitric oxide for refractory hypoxemia in critically ill patients. J Crit Care 2013;28:844–8.

66. Gebistorf F, Karam O, Wetterslev J, et al. Inhaled nitric oxide for acute respiratory distress syndrome (ARDS) in children and adults. Cochrane Database Syst Rev 2016;2016:CD002787.
67. Sheridan RL, Hurford WE, Kacmarek RM, et al. Inhaled nitric oxide in burn patients with respiratory failure. J Trauma 1997;42:629–34.
68. Fuller BM, Mohr NM, Skrupky L, et al. The use of inhaled prostaglandins in patients with ARDS: a systematic review and meta-analysis. Chest 2015;147: 1510–22.
69. Nosanov LB, McLawhorn MM, Vigiola Cruz M, et al. A National Perspective on ECMO Utilization in Patients with Burn Injury. J Burn Care Res 2017;39:10–4.
70. Kennedy JD, Thayer W, Beuno R, et al. ECMO in major burn patients: feasibility and considerations when multiple modes of mechanical ventilation fail. Burns Trauma 2017;5:20.
71. Combes A, Peek GJ, Hajage D, et al. ECMO for severe ARDS: systematic review and individual patient data meta-analysis. Intensive Care Med 2020;46:2048–57.
72. Veeravagu A, Yoon BC, Jiang B, et al. National trends in burn and inhalation injury in burn patients: results of analysis of the nationwide inpatient sample database. J Burn Care Res 2015;36(2):258–65.
73. Aub JC, Pittman H, Brues AM. The pulmonary complications: a clinical description. Ann Surg 1943 Jun;117(6):834–40.
74. Ryan C, Schoenfeld R, Thorpe W, et al. Objective estimates of the probability of death from burn injuries. NEJM 1998;338:362–6.
75. Albright JM, Davis CS, Bird MD, et al. The acute pulmonary inflammatory response to the graded severity of smoke inhalation injury. Crit Care Med 2012 Apr;40(4):1113–21.
76. Endorf FW, Gamelli RL. Inhalation injury, pulmonary perturbations, and fluid resuscitation. J Burn Care Res 2007 Jan-Feb;28(1):80–3.
77. Barillo DJ, Goode R, Esch V. Cyanide poisoning in victims of fire: analysis of 364 cases and review of the literature. J Burn Care Rehabil 1994;15(1):46–57.
78. Cumpston KL, Rodriguez V, Nguyen T, et al. Evaluation of prehospital hydroxocobalamin use in the setting of smoke inhalation. Am J Emerg Med 2021 Dec;50: 365–8.
79. Shirani KZ, Pruitt BA Jr, Mason AD Jr. The influence of inhalation injury and pneumonia on burn mortality. Ann Surg 1987 Jan;205(1):82–7.
80. Hassan Z, Wong JK, Bush J, et al. Assessing the severity of inhalation injuries in adults. Burns 2010 Mar;36(2):212–6.
81. Ryan CM, Fagan SP, Goverman J, et al. Grading inhalation injury by admission bronchoscopy. Crit Care Med 2012 Apr;40(4):1345–6.
82. Spano S, Hanna S, Li Z, et al. Does Bronchoscopic Evaluation of Inhalation Injury Severity Predict Outcome? J Burn Care Res 2016;37(1):1–11.
83. Shiau YC, Liu FY, Tsai JJ, et al. Usefulness of technetium-99m hexamethylpropylene amine oxime lung scan to detect inhalation lung injury of patients with pulmonary symptoms/signs but negative chest radiograph and pulmonary function test findings after a fire accident–a preliminary report. Ann Nucl Med 2003;17(6):435–8.
84. Yamamura H, Morioka T, Hagawa N, et al. Computed tomographic assessment of airflow obstruction in smoke inhalation injury: Relationship with the development of pneumonia and injury severity. Burns 2015;41(7):1428–34.
85. Roderique JD, Josef CS, Feldman MJ, et al. A modern literature review of carbon monoxide poisoning theories, therapies, and potential targets for therapy advancement. Toxicology 2015;334:45–58.

86. Buckley NA, Juurlink DN, Isbister G, et al. Hyperbaric oxygen for carbon monoxide poisoning. Cochrane Database Syst Rev 2011;4:CD002041.
87. Dumestre D, Nickerson D. Use of cyanide antidotes in burn patients with suspected inhalation injuries in North America: a cross-sectional survey. J Burn Care Res 2014;35(2):e112-7.
88. Anseeuw K, Delvau N, Burillo-Putze G, et al. Cyanide poisoning by fire smoke inhalation: a European expert consensus. Eur J Emerg Med 2013;20(1):2–9.
89. Carr JA, Crowley N. Prophylactic sequential bronchoscopy after inhalation injury: results from a three-year prospective randomized trial. Eur J Trauma Emerg Surg 2013;39(2):177–83.
90. Ashry HS, Mansour G, Kalil AC, et al. Incidence of ventilator associated pneumonia in burn patients with inhalation injury treated with high frequency percussive ventilation versus volume control ventilation: A systematic review. Burns 2016;S0305–4179.
91. Sousse LE, Herndon DN, Andersen CR, et al. High tidal volume decreases adult respiratory distress syndrome, atelectasis, and ventilator days compared with low tidal volume in pediatric burned patients with inhalation injury. J Am Coll Surg 2015;220(4):570–8.
92. Miller AC, Elamin EM, Suffredini AF. Inhaled anticoagulation regimens for the treatment of smoke inhalation-associated acute lung injury: a systematic review. Crit Care Med 2014;42(2):413–9.
93. Gaissert HA, Lofgren RH, Grillo HC. Upper airway compromise after inhalation. Complex strictures of the larynx and trachea and their management. Ann Surg 1993;218(5):672–8.
94. Palmieri TL. Long term outcomes after inhalation injury. J Burn Care Res 2009; 30(1):201–3.

The Burn Wound

Nikhil R. Shah, MD[a], Alen Palackic, MD[a], Kimberley C. Brondeel, BS[b],
Elliot T. Walters, MD[a], Steven E. Wolf, MD[a],*

KEYWORDS

- Burn • Wound • Debridement • Epithelialization • Wound healing • Scar

KEY POINTS

- The skin is a versatile organ system that plays a crucial role in physiologic homeostasis, including thermoregulation, maintenance of fluid balance, and protection against pathogens.
- Burn injury induces severe damage to the structural components of the integumentary system, leading to activation of various regional and systemic proinflammatory cascades.
- Awareness of vulnerable wound zones and phases of healing is pivotal to facilitate targeted therapies, including adequate resuscitation, early excision and grafting, integrative wound care, and nutritional and endocrinologic support.

PATHOPHYSIOLOGY OF THE BURN WOUND

The epidermis consists of five distinct layers, listed deepest to most superficial: stratum basale, stratum spinosum, stratum granulosum, stratum lucidum, and stratum corneum.[1] Predominantly composed of keratinocytes, these strata proliferate longitudinally from the innermost layer, eventually leading to sloughing of the stratum corneum in 2 to 4 weeks.[2] Conversely in the axial plane, epithelialization progresses from wound edges inward as keratinocyte division occurs. Other cell types within the epidermis include melanocytes, which are responsible for melanin production and protect against ultraviolet radiation; Merkel cells, which conduct sensorineural feedback functions; and Langerhans cells, which act as the primary phagocytic and immunologic response against presented antigens.[3]

Both tensile and elastic strength are provided by the dermis, anchored below the epidermis by interdigitating papillae.[4] Its versatile extracellular matrix, composed of collagen, elastin, and glycosaminoglycans, facilitates structural resilience from mechanical forces and ample absorptive capacity.[5] The dermis also houses the origins of epidermal appendages, such as hair follicles, sudoriferous glands, and sebaceous glands. Perhaps most importantly, angiogenesis and neural proliferation occur in the

[a] Department of Surgery, University of Texas Medical Branch, 301 University Boulevard, Galveston, TX 77555, USA; [b] John Sealy School of Medicine, University of Texas Medical Branch, 301 University Boulevard, Galveston, TX 77555, USA
* Corresponding author. 815 Market Street, Galveston, TX 77550.
E-mail address: swolf@utmb.edu

Surg Clin N Am 103 (2023) 453–462
https://doi.org/10.1016/j.suc.2023.01.007
0039-6109/23/© 2023 Elsevier Inc. All rights reserved.

dermal-subcutaneous junction, thus making it a crucial determinant of wound healing. A thorough comprehension of these anatomic layers facilitates accurate evaluation of the burn wound, because its classification and subsequent therapy is predicated on depth of injury.

Prolonged increased thermal contact induces protein denaturation and cell membrane breakdown, with higher temperature of the insult and length of contact relating directly to the extent of damage.[6,7] Identifying the cause by which energy transfer occurs allows better understanding of wound formation because the pathogenesis of tissue injury varies greatly between various thermal insults. Flame burns notably involve prolonged contact with the heat source, particularly if clothes or coverings are present because these articles potentiate flammability. Conversely, clothing may act as a protective agent in flash burns, which are precipitated by rapid explosions of natural gas, propane, or gasoline. Flash burns preferentially affect exposed skin, with the most severe injury in the region facing the source. However, it is important to consider that flash burns may become flame burns should clothing or hair ignite after initial explosion.

Damage exerted by scald burns depends on the temperature and specific heat of the liquid, duration of contact, and viscosity of the heated substance.[8,9] For example, soups or sauces are inherently thicker than water and thus are more difficult to evacuate from the skin surface. Similarly to flame burns, clothes potentiate degree of injury by prolonging contact of hot liquid with the skin, particularly in the case of substances, such as grease or oil, with higher specific heats.[10] The splash or splatter associated with scald injury leads to a significantly heterogeneous burn pattern. Immersion scalds prompt special consideration because of potential for circumferential injury to an involved limb or digit.

Contact burns, caused by heated metal, coals, pavement, and so forth, are generally focal injuries but deep because of the locally concentrated thermal exposure. Chemical burns are mainly alkali or acidic in nature and incite insidious damage until complete dilution and clearance are achieved. Sulfur- and phosphorus-based burns are less commonly encountered chemical injuries. Alkaline products lead to a devastating liquefactive necrosis of the skin causing destruction of integumentary architecture, whereas acids result in coagulative necrosis from which skin can likely recover.[11] Finally, in the setting of electrical burns, the human body acts as a resistor for high-voltage electrical current. On initial evaluation, the site of electrical burn may appear innocuous; however, as electrical energy travels the path of least resistance, the underlying myonecrosis and neuronal damage may be catastrophic.[12] Aside from the cutaneous manifestations, electrical burns have resounding multiorgan system effects that warrant awareness by the treatment team.[13]

CLINICAL EVALUATION OF BURN WOUND DEPTH

Burn depth carries significant implications for wound classification and healing prognosis. The degree of burn is correlated with the corresponding structures involved and is predominantly determined with comprehensive physical examination (**Fig. 1**).[14] However, burn wounds are dynamic and true burn depth may not be evident until hours after the injury or with definition by operative excision.[15] Nonetheless, early clinical evaluation is pivotal not only for successful goal-directed resuscitation but also for expeditious determination of appropriate initial wound management.

First-degree burns affect only the epidermis and are clinically benign, because no blister or scar is formed and management rarely involves surgery. Second-degree injury, also described as partial thickness, extends into the dermis and is characterized by

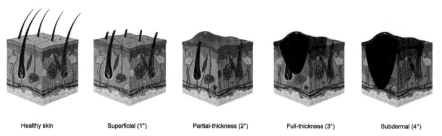

Fig. 1. Burn injury classification and depth.

painful blistering. Second-degree burns range from superficial partial thickness, hyperemic and blanching in nature associated with "weeping," to deep partial thickness, which appear drier and demonstrate a nonblanching pattern.[16] Superficial second-degree wounds can largely be treated with local wound care and topical therapies, whereas deep second-degree burns benefit from surgical excision to facilitate healing. Third-degree, or full-thickness burns, ravage the entirety of the dermis and reach the subcutaneous tissues, whereas fourth-degree injury involves underlying muscle, bone, and other internal structures. Both of these severe burn wounds optimally involve surgical intervention with the latter often prompting loss of affected limb or bodily structure. Given the anatomic components affected by burn injury at each layer, it is widely accepted that depth of injury is largely proportional to the level of sensation present, the extent of excision indicated, risk of wound infection, and severity of scar formation.[14,17]

ZONES OF INJURY AND WOUND CONVERSION

After initial injury, the resulting burn wound may be classified into three zones: (1) the zone of coagulation, (2) zone of stasis or ischemia, and (3) zone of hyperemia.[14,18] The most severe damage occurs in the zone of coagulation, which consists of irreversible necrosis at the center of the wound. Conversely, the zone of hyperemia makes up the outer wound edges and is often the most salvageable region because of compensatory vasodilation.[15,17,19] The intermediate zone, the zone of stasis, is characterized by moderate vascular damage and capillary leakage with reduced levels of perfusion (**Fig. 2**A). It is of extreme importance to burn providers because its degree of injury

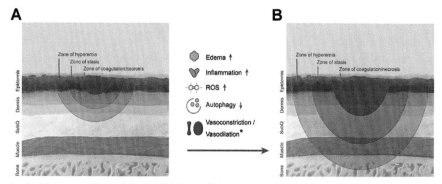

Fig. 2. (*A*) Zones of burn injury. (*B*) Microcellular factors contributing to burn wound conversion. ROS, reactive oxygen species; * initial vasoconstriction followed by vasodilation 6 hours later.

is potentially reversible if early identification, resuscitation, and intervention is achieved.[13,20]

This variable wound reversibility, known as "burn wound conversion," was first identified in the mid-twentieth century.[21] Although the exact pathophysiology has remained elusive, it is thought to be largely multifactorial. As its name suggests, the zone of stasis or ischemia is a region of poor perfusion caused by injury-induced vasoconstriction and cytokine-mediated hypercoagulability.[15,22] This hypoperfusion is further exacerbated by the global increased permeability of capillary beds leading to interstitial fluid shifting and loss of intravascular volume (**Fig. 2B**).[16,17] Thus, prompt resuscitation during the acute burn phase is therapeutically critical for restoring cardiac preload and effective circulating pressures. Important to note, this wound conversion process may continue as long as 2 weeks after initial thermal injury.[17,23] Early excision and debridement of nonviable tissue within the zone of coagulation remains a mainstay of surgical intervention to alleviate the inflammatory burden of the wound while promoting efficient autophagy.[24–26]

BIOLOGY OF WOUND HEALING

Burn wounds have a higher degree of regional inflammation and a complex microenvironment when compared with nonburn wounds; however, the central mechanisms of wound healing still apply.[16,17] Wound healing occurs in three main phases: (1) the inflammatory phase, (2) proliferative phase, and (3) remodeling phase.[27,28] A detailed compilation of various cytokines, growth factors, and cellular components involved in the complex healing process is seen in **Fig. 3**; however, the most predominant ones are highlighted next.

The initial inflammatory response is aimed at stabilizing wound hemostasis and facilitating rapid tissue turnover. Release of proinflammatory cytokines and intracellular substrates, including histamine, bradykinin, and serotonin, causes a profound increase in local vascular permeability, thus permitting extravasation of proteins, fluid, and immune cells into the interstitium.[29,30] Moreover, vasodilation of dermal postcapillary venules in damaged tissue promotes accumulation of transforming growth

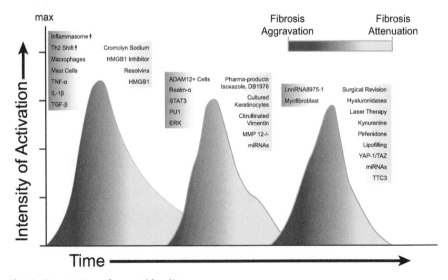

Fig. 3. Progression of wound healing.

factor-β propagating increased delivery of multiple cell types including platelets, neutrophils, macrophages, and lymphocytes to the damaged tissue. Aside from upregulating more chemoattraction, these cells initiate a multitude of phagocytic processes to clear cellular debris and opportunistic pathogens and ensure a wound microenvironment conducive to future re-epithelialization.[19,30,31] Relating to first-degree and superficial second-degree injury, this process is manifested as erythema and local tissue edema of the wound bed. As discussed later, this expected chemotaxis is severely blunted after burns compared with other mechanisms of injury, primarily caused by global immunologic deficiency and dysfunction. The normal acute inflammatory phase generally continues for approximately 1 to 4 days; however, in larger burns these changes continue in a more chronic manner for several weeks.[27,32]

The proliferative phase is marked by construction of the extracellular matrix, which relies heavily on platelet degranulation induced by platelet-derived growth factor.[28,30,33] Platelet-derived growth factor is exceptionally versatile because it promotes assembly of collagenous components and proteoglycan units, while not only attracting fibroblasts but also inducing transformation into myofibroblasts. Accumulation of fibroblasts potentiates secretion of keratinocyte-derived growth factor to activate epithelialization by keratinocytes.[28,34] Perhaps the hallmark of the proliferative phase is angiogenesis. This ongoing neovascularization is facilitated by vascular endothelial growth factor and fibroblast growth factor, and acts to restore cellular integrity and hemostasis.[35-37] Collagen content steadily begins rising, proportionally leading to greater tensile strength.[29] Without early debridement, deep partial-thickness or full-thickness burns wounds have a prolonged progression through the proliferation phase.[38,39] Delay in advancement to the final stage of wound healing has detrimental implications for scar formation.

Wound remodeling marks the final stage of the healing process in which the wound bed is reorganized first by function of collagenases and metalloproteinases. Type III collagen is then replaced by structurally coordinated type I collagen while wound edges undergo contraction by myofibroblasts. This phase is considered a homeostatic maintenance phase because it may last several months to years, although maximum tensile strength is achieved between days 40 and 60 after injury.[28,34]

BURN WOUND CARE AND COVERAGE

Within the acute phase after burn, presence of devitalized tissue, insoluble or foreign material, and persistent ischemia inhibit wound turnover.[29] For this reason, early excision and grafting has become the mainstay of severe burn injury as a means of stimulating the three previously mentioned phases of healing and facilitating wound coverage.[38,40] Optimal timing for early excision is considered by most to be within 1 week of injury, particularly to allow for cellular components within the zones of stasis to reach a new equilibrium. However, for the clearly distinct zone of coagulation, this time frame is increasingly being expedited to occur within 48 hours, immediately following completion of acute resuscitation.[25,26,38,39,41-44] Furthermore, in the case of environmentally contaminated wounds (eg, burns occurring in soil, dirty water), pathologic examination of excised tissue can assist with targeted antimicrobial therapy.[45] If delayed, the wound beds instead become a robust, opportunistic environment for microbial colonization, which further retards healing time, increases risk of systemic infection, lengthens overall hospital stay, and worsens hypertrophic scarring.[42,46-48] Nonetheless, consensus behind systemic antibiotic prophylaxis remains highly variable.[49-53]

Wound dressings are an important component of comprehensive burn care and serve a multitude of functions aside from preventing further wound damage and desiccation. Antimicrobial dressings, often impregnated with silver, mafenide acetate, acetic acid or polymyxin, are commonly used in the acute postoperative period to mitigate or prevent infection.[54,55] Nonetheless, early coverage of deep burn wounds with autologous split-thickness skin grafts has long been, and will likely continue to be, the mainstay of burn surgery.[56] Split-thickness skin grafts are meshed in a range of ratios from 1:1 to 9:1 to maximize graft surface area.[57]

However, in some extensive cases of burn injury healthy skin from which to provide adequate donor tissue is limited. Advancements in biologic dressings and skin substitutes provide viable alternatives to overcome these limitations.[58] Allograft remains the most predominant skin substitute used today, acting to enhance fibroblast proliferation and collagen synthesis once applied to the wound bed. It reduces insensible fluid losses, maintains a moist environment for efficient healing, and even reduces local wound pain.[56,59,60] Alternatively, various dermal substitutes are gaining traction in therapy consideration for deep burns. Integra (Integra LifeSciences Corporation, Plainsboro, NJ), Alloderm (LifeCell Corporation, Branchburg, NJ), and Biodegradable Temporizing Matrix (PolyNovo, Melbourne, Australia) are acellular matrices that mimic some functions of the skin and alleviate risk of cross-species residual antigenicity. All three continue to show promising results for fibrovascular growth within full-thickness burns and maintenance of optimal environments for epithelialization.[40,56,61,62]

It is important to mention a historically popular material, xenograft, typically consisting of porcine skin.[63] Once heavily used, xenograft was removed from the market, leading to the conception of Suprathel (PolyMedics Innovations GmbH, Denkendorf, Germany), another temporary yet durable coverage option. This skin substitute is gaining traction as an innovative dressing that can remain in place until full reepithelization is complete. Its greatest advantage, perhaps, is the progressive transparency of its outer layer to allow for underlying wound inspection and monitoring.[64–66]

Additionally, Mepitel and Mepilex (Mölnlycke, Göteborg, Sweden) are two widely used manufactured dressings. Mepitel is a nonadhesive net that is placed in combination with an additional absorptive dressing. Wound exudate is drained through pores in the Mepitel and absorbed by the overlying dressing to minimize growth interference. By contrast, Mepilex is a bilaminar, adhesive antimicrobial dressing composed of polyurethane foam and a silicone-based adhesive surface.[67] Its benefits extend beyond its composition and cost-effectiveness, because it also may remain in place for several days thus obviating frequent dressing changes.[68]

With the marked demand for accessible yet reliable wound therapy options, innovations within the field are continually developing. Preliminary results with inventive materials, such as acellular fish skin grafts, are encouraging, predicated on their high omega-3 content and long shelf-life span of nearly 3 years.[69–71] Lyophilized tilapia skin is another intriguing therapy, particularly for partial-thickness burns, although investigations are still ongoing.[72,73]

SUMMARY

There continues to be an evolving understanding of the pathophysiology, clinical approach, and coverage options for the burn wound. It is crucial that burn-care providers remain knowledgeable not only about the essential components of burn injury, but also about ongoing advancements in the field, to effectively facilitate healing and recovery.

CLINICS CARE POINTS

- Burn depth depends on temperature of the agent, the specific heat, and contact time.
- Wound healing occurs in three phases: inflammatory (initial), proliferative (process of closure), and remodeling (scarring).
- Wound closure can occur by proliferation of keratinocytes already present in the wound (partial thickness), contracture if the wound is small, or by grafting/flaps when no skin elements are present to secure closure.

DISCLOSURES

No incentives or financial disclosures to report.

REFERENCES

1. Baroni A, Buommino E, De Gregorio V, et al. Structure and function of the epidermis related to barrier properties. Clin Dermatol 2012;30(3):257–62.
2. Sorg H, Tilkorn DJ, Hager S, et al. Skin wound healing: an update on the current knowledge and concepts. Eur Surg Res 2017;58(1–2):81–94.
3. Yousef H, Alhajj M and Sharma S. Anatomy, skin (integument), epidermis, In: Stat-Pearls, 2022, StatPearls Publishing, Available at: https://www.statpearls.com/point-of-care/21212.
4. Rippa AL, Kalabusheva EP, Vorotelyak EA. Regeneration of dermis: scarring and cells involved. Cells 2019;8(6):607.
5. Woodley DT. Distinct fibroblasts in the papillary and reticular dermis. Dermatol Clin 2017;35(1):95–100.
6. Roos A, Weisiger JR, Moritz AR. Studies of thermal injury. VII. Physiological mechanisms responsible for death during cutaneous exposure to excessive heat. J Clin Invest 1947;26(3):505–19.
7. Moritz AR, Henriques FC. Studies of thermal injury. Am J Pathol 1947;23(5):695–720.
8. Loller C, Buxton GA, Kerzmann TL. Hot soup! Correlating the severity of liquid scald burns to fluid and biomedical properties. Burns 2016;42(3):589–97.
9. Chiu TW, Ng DCK, Burd A. Properties of matter Bard in assessment of scald injuries. Burns 2007;33(2):185–8.
10. Log T. Modeling skin injury from hot spills on clothing. Int J Environ Res Publ Health 2017;14(11):1374.
11. Palao R, Monge I, Ruiz M, et al. Chemical burns: pathophysiology and treatment. Burns 2010;36(3):295–304.
12. Lee RC, Astumian RD. The physicochemical basis for thermal and non-thermal 'burn' injuries. Burns 1996;22(7):509–19.
13. Hettiaratchy S, Dziewulski P. Pathophysiology and types of burns. BMJ 2004;328(7453):1427–9.
14. Monstrey S, Hoeksema H, Verbelen J, et al. Assessment of burn depth and burn wound healing potential. Burns 2008;34(6):761–9.
15. Shupp JW, Nasabzadeh TJ, Rosenthal DS, et al. A review of the local pathophysiologic bases of burn wound progression. J Burn Care Res 2010;31(6):849–73.
16. Jeschke MG, van Baar ME, Choudhry MA, et al. Burn injury. Nat Rev Dis Primers 2020;6(1):11.

17. Rowan MP, Cancio LC, Elster EA, et al. Burn wound healing and treatment: review and advancements. Crit Care 2015;19(1):243.
18. Walker NJ and King KC. Acute and chronic thermal burn evaluation and management, In: StatPearls, 2022, StatPearls Publishing. Available at: https://www.statpearls.com/point-of-care/30048.
19. Yeganeh PM, Tahmasebi S, Esmaeilzadeh A. Cellular and biological factors involved in healing wounds and burns and treatment options in tissue engineering. Regen Med 2022;17(6):401–18.
20. Nielson CB, Duethman NC, Howard JM, et al. Pathophysiology of systemic complications and current management. J Burn Care Res 2017;38(1):e469–81.
21. Jackson DM. Second thoughts on the burn wound. J Trauma 1969;9(10):839–62.
22. Singh V, Devgan L, Bhat S, et al. The pathogenesis of burn wound conversion. Ann Plast Surg 2007;59(1):109–15.
23. Gravante G, Palmieri MB, Esposito G, et al. Apoptotic death in deep partial thickness burns vs. normal skin of burned patients. J Surg Res 2007;141(2):141–5.
24. Salibian AA, Rosario ATD, Severo LDAM, et al. Current concepts on burn wound conversion: a review of recent advances in understanding the secondary progressions of burns. Burns 2016;42(5):1025–35.
25. Herndon DN, Barrow RE, Rutan RL, et al. A comparison of conservative versus early excision. Therapies in severely burned patients. Ann Surg 1989;209(5):547–53.
26. Puri V, Khare NA, Chandramouli M, et al. Comparative analysis of early excision and grafting vs delayed grafting in burn patients in a developing country. J Burn Care Res 2016;37(5):278–82.
27. Broughton GI, Janis JE, Attinger CE. Wound healing: an overview. Plast Reconstr Surg 2006;117(7S):1e.
28. Childs DR, Murthy AS. Overview of wound healing and management. Surg Clin 2017;97(1):189–207.
29. Rose LF, Chan RK. The burn wound microenvironment. Adv Wound Care 2016;5(3):106–18.
30. Li J, Chen J, Kirsner R. Pathophysiology of acute wound healing. Clin Dermatol 2007;25(1):9–18.
31. Delavary BM, van der Veer WM, van Egmond M, et al. Macrophages in skin injury and repair. Immunobiology 2011;216(7):753–62.
32. Jeschke MG, Chinkes DL, Finnerty CC, et al. Pathophysiologic response to severe burn injury. Ann Surg 2008;248(3):387–401.
33. Diegelmann RF, Cohen IK, Kaplan AM. The role of macrophages in wound repair: a review. Plast Reconstr Surg 1981;68(1):107–13.
34. Reinke JM, Sorg H. Wound repair and regeneration. ESR (Eur Surg Res) 2012;49(1):35–43.
35. Veith AP, Henderson K, Spencer A, et al. Therapeutic strategies for enhancing angiogenesis in wound healing. Adv Drug Deliv Rev 2019;146:97–125.
36. Demidova-Rice TN, Durham JT, Herman IM. Wound healing angiogenesis: innovations and challenges in acute and chronic wound healing. Adv Wound Care 2012;1(1):17–22.
37. Markiewicz-Gospodarek A, Kozioł M, Tobiasz M, et al. Burn wound healing: clinical complications, medical care, treatment, and dressing types: the current state of knowledge for clinical practice. Int J Environ Res Public Health 2022;19(3):1338.
38. Xiao-Wu W. Effects of delayed wound excision and grafting in severely burned children. Arch Surg 2002;137(9):1049.

39. Ong YS, Samuel M, Song C. Meta-analysis of early excision of burns. Burns 2006; 32(2):145–50.

40. Wang Y, Beekman J, Hew J, et al. Burn injury: challenges and advances in burn wound healing, infection, pain and scarring. Adv Drug Deliv Rev 2018;123:3–17.

41. Sinha S, Schreiner AJ, Biernaskie J, et al. Treating pain on skin graft donor sites: review and clinical recommendations. J Trauma Acute Care Surg 2017;83(5): 954–64.

42. Gallaher JR, Mjuweni S, Shah M, et al. Timing of early excision and grafting following burn in sub-Saharan Africa. Burns 2015;41(6):1353–9.

43. Pietsch JB, Netscher DT, Nagaraj HS, et al. Early excision of major burns in children: effect on morbidity and mortality. J Pediatr Surg 1985;20(6):754–7.

44. Hart DW, Wolf SE, Chinkes DL, et al. Effects of early excision and aggressive enteral feeding on hypermetabolism, catabolism, and sepsis after severe burn. J Trauma Acute Care Surg 2003;54(4):755–64.

45. Norbury W, Herndon DN, Tanksley J, et al. Infection in burns. Surg Infect 2016; 17(2):250–5.

46. Browning JA and Cindass R. Burn debridement, grafting, and reconstruction, In: StatPearls, 2022, StatPearls Publishing. Available at:https://www.statpearls.com/point-of-care/18722.

47. Barret JP, Herndon DN. Effects of burn wound excision on bacterial colonization and invasion. Plast Reconstr Surg 2003;111(2):744–50.

48. Baker RHJ, Townley WA, Mckeon S, et al. Retrospective study of the association between hypertrophic burn scarring and bacterial colonization. J Burn Care Res 2007;28(1):152–6.

49. Branski LK, Al-Mousawi A, Rivero H, et al. Emerging infections in burns. Surg Infect 2009;10(5):389–97.

50. Muthukumar V, Arumugam PK, Bamal R. Role of systemic antibiotic prophylaxis in acute burns: a retrospective analysis from a tertiary care center. Burns 2020; 46(5):1060–5.

51. Csenkey A, Jozsa G, Gede N, et al. Systemic antibiotic prophylaxis does not affect infectious complications in pediatric burn injury: a meta-analysis. PLoS One 2019;14(9):e0223063.

52. Ramos G, Cornistein W, Cerino GT, et al. Systemic antimicrobial prophylaxis in burn patients: systematic review. J Hosp Infect 2017;97(2):105–14.

53. Nunez Lopez O, Cambiaso-Daniel J, Branski LK, et al. Predicting and managing sepsis in burn patients: current perspectives. Ther Clin Risk Manag 2017;13: 1107–17.

54. Jeschke MG, Shahrokhi S, Finnerty CC, et al. Wound coverage technologies in burn care: established techniques. J Burn Care Res 2018;39(3):313–8.

55. Vloemans AFPM, Hermans MHE, van der Wal MBA, et al. Optimal treatment of partial thickness burns in children: a systematic review. Burns 2014;40(2): 177–90.

56. Haddad AG, Giatsidis G, Orgill DP, et al. Skin substitutes and bioscaffolds. Clin Plast Surg 2017;44(3):627–34.

57. Pripotnev S, Papp A. Split thickness skin graft meshing ratio indications and common practices. Burns 2017;43(8):1775–81.

58. Halim A, Khoo T, Shah JumaatMohdY. Biologic and synthetic skin substitutes: an overview. Indian J Plast Surg 2010;43(3):23.

59. Wang C, Zhang F, Lineaweaver WC. Clinical applications of allograft skin in burn care. Ann Plast Surg 2020;84(3S):S158–60.

60. Saffle JR. Closure of the excised burn wound: temporary skin substitutes. Clin Plast Surg 2009;36(4):627–41.
61. Heimbach DM, Warden GD, Luterman A, et al. Multicenter postapproval clinical trial of Integra® dermal regeneration template for burn treatment. J Burn Care Rehabil 2003;24(1):42–8.
62. Palackic A, Duggan RP, Campbell MS, et al. The role of skin substitutes in acute burn and reconstructive burn surgery: an updated comprehensive review. Semin Plast Surg 2022;36(01):033–42.
63. Haller HL, Blome-Eberwein SE, Branski LK, et al. Porcine xenograft and epidermal fully synthetic skin substitutes in the treatment of partial-thickness burns: a literature review. Medicina 2021;57(5):432.
64. Kaartinen IS, Kuokkanen HO. Suprathel causes less bleeding and scarring than Mepilex Transfer in the treatment of donor sites of split-thickness skin grafts. Journal of Plastic Surgery and Hand Surgery 2011;45(4–5):200–3.
65. Schwarze H, Küntscher M, Uhlig C, et al. Suprathel, a new skin substitute, in the management of partial-thickness burn wounds: results of a clinical study. Ann Plast Surg 2008;60(2):181–5.
66. Hundeshagen G, Collins VN, Wurzer P, et al. A prospective, randomized, controlled trial comparing the outpatient treatment of pediatric and adult partial-thickness burns with Suprathel or Mepilex Ag. J Burn Care Res 2018; 39(2):261–7.
67. Tang H, Lv G, Fu J, et al. An open, parallel, randomized, comparative, multicenter investigation evaluating the efficacy and tolerability of Mepilex Ag versus silver sulfadiazine in the treatment of deep partial-thickness burn injuries. J Trauma Acute Care Surg 2015;78(5):1000–7.
68. Gee Kee EL, Kimble RM, Cuttle L, et al. Randomized controlled trial of three burns dressings for partial thickness burns in children. Burns 2015;41(5):946–55.
69. Yoon J, Yoon D, Lee H, et al. Wound healing ability of acellular fish skin and bovine collagen grafts for split-thickness donor sites in burn patients: characterization of acellular grafts and clinical application. Int J Biol Macromol 2022;205: 452–61.
70. Luze H, Nischwitz SP, Smolle C, et al. The use of acellular fish skin grafts in burn wound management: a systematic review. Medicina 2022;58(7):912.
71. Alam K, Jeffery SLA. Acellular fish skin grafts for management of split thickness donor sites and partial thickness burns: a case series. Mil Med 2019; 184(Supplement_1):16–20.
72. Lima Júnior EM, Moraes Filho MO de, Forte AJ, et al. Pediatric burn treatment using tilapia skin as a xenograft for superficial partial-thickness wounds: a pilot study. J Burn Care Res 2019;41(2):241–7.
73. Lima Júnior EM, de Moraes Filho MO, Costa BA, et al. Nile tilapia fish skin–based wound dressing improves pain and treatment-related costs of superficial partial-thickness burns: a phase III randomized controlled trial. Plast Reconstr Surg 2021;147(5):1189–98.

Acute Surgical Management of the Burn Patient

Anju B. Saraswat, MD[a],*, James H. Holmes IV, MD[b]

KEYWORDS

- Burn management • Acute burn care • Surgical burn management • Burn surgery

KEY POINTS

- The goal for burn care is wound closure by 2 to 3 weeks via optimal nonsurgical wound care or excision and grafting.
- Early excision and grafting for large burns leads to improved functional and aesthetic outcomes.
- Deep partial-thickness and full-thickness burns usually require excision and grafting for optimal outcomes.
- Novel techniques have been developed to help achieve wound coverage, especially in patients with larger burns.
- Extensive preoperative preparation, to include open and continuous communication with the operating room and anesthesia teams, leads to a more successful operation.

INTRODUCTION

Burn management has progressed over time to encompass care that includes not just survival but also quality of life and successful reintegration into society. Optimal care includes identifying wounds that will reepithelize within 2 to 3 weeks without an operation, and timely operative intervention for wounds that do require surgery to achieve wound coverage.

Outcome measurements for burn care are no longer isolated to mortalities.[1] Janzekovic[2] in the 1970s demonstrated that surgical excision and grafting can successfully decrease a burn survivor's hospital length of stay, increase functional outcomes, and mitigate overall suffering—thereby establishing a new standard of care for acute burn management. As goals of burn care have shifted to outcome measures that target patient-centered quality metrics, surgical techniques and considerations have

[a] Department of Surgery, AHWFB Burn Center, Wake Forest University School of Medicine, 1 Medical Center Boulevard, 5th Floor Watlington Hall, Winston-Salem, NC 27157, USA; [b] Section of Burns, Department of Surgery, AHWFB Burn Center, Wake Forest University School of Medicine, 1 Medical Center Boulevard, 5th Floor Watlington Hall, Winston-Salem, NC 27157, USA
* Corresponding author. Department of Surgery, Medical Center Boulevard, 5th Floor Watlington Hall, Winston- Salem, NC 27157.
E-mail address: asaraswa@wakehealth.edu

Surg Clin N Am 103 (2023) 463–472
https://doi.org/10.1016/j.suc.2023.01.008
0039-6109/23/© 2023 Elsevier Inc. All rights reserved.

adapted as well.[1] This new perspective includes aspects of wound-bed preparation and aesthetics when surgically managing the acute burn.[3]

NATURE OF THE PROBLEM

The depth of a burn wound predicates whether viable dermal elements exist to achieve wound reepithelization within 2 to 3weeks. Initial evaluation of a burn wound may not accurately reveal the true depth of injured tissue. Over the course of several days, the appearance of the wound will evolve and more closely reflect the severity of the injury. There are many factors that can affect the evolution of a burn wound. The initial injury itself is a primary determinant and includes the duration of exposure and the temperature of the heat source. Initial wound care, location of the burn on the body, age, medical comorbidities, and the systemic response to injury (shock, edema, inflammation) can all affect the evolution of burn-wound depth.[4]

If a wound is assessed as not likely to heal within 3 weeks, surgical management is usually the next step to prevent hypertrophic scarring and to hasten recovery. The exceptions are small burns in which a graft will not achieve a better outcome with surgery when compared with spontaneous healing. Examples of this include a small full-thickness burn on the midthigh. A skin graft would not affect functional or aesthetic outcomes. This burn could be managed with local wound care, and the subsequent scar could be treated with steroid injections and/or laser therapy. Another common scenario is a child with an anterior torso scald burn of variable depth. In this case, most of the burn would heal within 2 to 3 weeks, whereas a small portion thereof (eg, in the middle of the chest) may exceed this timeline. A family discussion should include the possibility that a graft in the middle of the chest would not lead to a better cosmetic outcome and would not change any quality-of-life or functional measures. Again, this scar could be managed afterward with local therapies.

PREOPERATIVE PLANNING

Timing of surgery is important. In general, early excision and grafting will help minimize subsequent hypertrophic scarring. Full-thickness wounds are easily identified, and the decision to proceed with surgery is straightforward. The more elusive problem is differentiating between superficial partial-thickness (those that will heal in 2–3 weeks) and deep partial-thickness burns (those that will not). Early signs of healing, to include epidermal "islands" arising from hair follicles, can help determine the direction of subsequent wound management.

After determining that a patient requires surgery, preoperative preparation should be expeditious and should include the following considerations: comorbidity management, anticipation of blood product needs, obtaining access for fluid resuscitation and hemodynamic monitoring, temperature monitoring, enteral nutrition continuation or discontinuation, patient positioning, anesthetic considerations, and finally, plans for excision and grafting. **Box 1** provides a preoperative checklist.

Comorbidity Optimization

Comorbidity optimization before burn surgery is important, even ifprolonged postponement of surgery is inadvisable.[5] In patients with risk factors, cardiopulmonary evaluation with an electrocardiogram, an echocardiogram, and a chest radiograph should be completed.[6] Special population considerations include patients with foot burns that have diabetic peripheral neuropathy or peripheral vascular disease.

Box 1
Procedural checklist for burn-wound excision

1. Ensure warm room, anticipated transfusion requirements, availability of burn-specific supplies and equipment.

2. Prepare and drape the operative field, to include all areas to be excised and harvested.

3. Perform tangential excision (using instruments of choice) or excision to fascia.

4. Achieve hemostasis with electrocautery, topical epinephrine solution, and/or thrombin.

5. Cover the wound. Harvest autograft with a dermatome; mesh if desired. Alternatives: allograft, RECELL, dermal template.

6. Secure grafts with staples, fibrin glue, or sutures.

7. Apply dressings over grafts, creating a moist environment and limiting sheer forces.

8. Splint or otherwise immobilize grafts for about 5 days, especially over joints.

Evaluation of toe perfusion and vascular flow studies may identify an inflow obstruction that should be corrected before excision and grafting.

Blood Requirements

During a major burn excision (>20% total body surface area [TBSA], >15% TBSA in children), blood loss is predicted, and crossmatched blood products are prepared. Operative blood loss is not easy to estimate because of many factors, but is primarily dependent on the location of the burn and TBSA to be excised. One study reported blood loss of 0.8 mL/cm^2 in adults.[7] A study in children calculated that 3.5% to 5% of the total blood volume is lost per TBSA excised.[8] These estimates can be affected by other factors, such as time elapsed postburn (increased delay means more blood loss), use of a tourniquet or hemostatic agents, use of epinephrine tumescence, and technique of excision.[9,10]

Communication with the anesthesia team before and during the case is essential to a successful operation. There may be times when the surgeon needs to slow the pace of excision to allow the anesthetist to address blood loss. Likewise, it may be necessary to terminate surgery earlier than planned because of patient instability. Intraoperative coagulopathy can be managed with more clarity if thromboelastogram values are followed.[11] Many burn centers transfuse blood in 1:1:1 component ratios, similar to massive transfusion protocols for trauma patients. Whole-blood transfusion is another option.

Vascular Access

In preparation for burn excision, large-bore intravenous lines must be established. This can be accomplished peripherally or centrally. Hemodynamic monitoring may be challenging if all limbs are involved in a burn. An arterial line can assist with both hemodynamic monitoring and assessment of serial arterial blood gases.

Temperature Management

Intraoperative temperature monitoring with an esophageal probe or temperature-sensing urinary catheter should be performed. Prevention of hypothermia is key. Patient temperatures less than 36°C are associated with platelet dysfunction, coagulopathy, increased blood loss, increased infection risk, and dysrhythmias.[12] These physiologic derangements severely limit the patient's ability to withstand prolonged operative times. For major burns, it is important to preheat the operative room before patient arrival and to maintain this throughout the case. Devices to mitigate hypothermia include forced air devices, underbody warming devices, warming lights, and intravenous warming catheters.[13] One can also wrap areas of the body with watertight/plastic material.

Enteral Feeds

Enteral feeds should be continued perioperatively whenever possible. Major burns are associated with a hypermetabolic state that requires increased levels of protein and caloric intake.[14] In burn patients requiring multiple procedures, feeds can be interrupted frequently enough to significantly reduce enteral intake. Studies have demonstrated the safety of continuing tube feeds intraoperatively for postpyloric feeding tubes,[15] as well as for the safety of continuing gastric feeds in patients that are endotracheally intubated or have a tracheostomy—regardless of patient positioning intraoperatively.[16] If feeds are not continued intraoperatively, proactive protocols should be established to catch up on paused feeds and/or to allow for minimal interruption of continuous feeding (eg, pausing feeds en route to the operating room rather than the midnight before).

Positioning

Preoperative planning should include discussion of patient positioning. This is dependent on the location of both the burns and the skin-donor sites. Preoperative discussion allows the team to prepare for various positions; if intraoperative repositioning is planned, a second operating room bed can be prepared.

Anesthetic Considerations

Anesthetic considerations in the burn population should include use of regional anesthesia. This is shown to decrease pain in donor sites, decrease opiate requirements, and facilitate early ambulation.[17] Regional anesthesia can also be used for patients in whom general anesthesia poses high risk. In addition, during prolonged hospital stays, this population can develop tolerance to opiates and sedatives, often requiring higher doses. Ketamine can be used as an analgesic adjunct, as this NMDA-receptor antagonist works synergistically with opiates.[18]

BURN-WOUND EXCISION

Tangential excision is appropriate for partial-thickness burns, and for full-thickness burns of limited extent or on special areas (eg, hands). It can be performed with various instruments. Goulian (Pilling Weck Surgical, Durham, NC, USA) and larger knives (eg, Watson, Humby, Blair, Braithwaite) are used to excise skin at a uniform tangential plane. The VERSAJET hydrosurgery system (Smith & Nephew) can be used as an adjunct to surgical excision in irregularly contoured areas.[19] A powered dermatome, normally used to harvest skin grafts, can also be used to excise burn eschar. As with other instruments, multiple passes should be made until a uniform and diffusely bleeding wound bed is encountered. Bovie electrocautery is used when fascial excision is carried out.

Tangential excision removes devitalized tissue in layers. The resulting wound bed should have uniform and diffuse bleeding and a healthy appearance. Excision and grafting should be performed in a one-step fashion, assuming the patient remains stable from a hemodynamic and temperature standpoint. One study stated that major excisions should be limited to 4 hours or less.[20] To limit blood loss, excision of largeextremity burns should be carried out under tourniquet if possible.[7] When using a tourniquet (after exsanguination with an Esmarch bandage), fine-capillary bleeding will no longer be available as an excision endpoint, mandating attention to the appearance of the wound bed. Other methods to minimizing blood loss include use of hemostatic agents (recombinant human thrombin spray), temporary application of epinephrine-soaked dressings immediately after excision, and electrocautery. For topical application, a 1:200,000 solution of epinephrine in a warmed crystalloid fluid is used.

Excision to fascia is reserved for extensive full-thickness burns. It results in a cosmetically and functionally inferior result. However, skin engrafts much better on fascia than on fat, such that excision to fascia is often required as a lifesaving procedure in patients with deep burns. It can be performed using electrocautery or, in experienced hands, with a scalpel or Mayo scissors.

BURN WOUND CLOSURE

Options for wound coverage include autografts, allografts, xenografts, and dermal substitutes. Autografts can be further categorized into full-thickness skin grafts (FTSGs), split-thickness skin grafts (STSGs), cultured epidermal autografts (CEAs), and autologous-skin-cell suspension.

Full-Thickness Skin Grafts

FTSGs are grafts that include both the epidermis and the dermis from the donor site. They are generally used for smaller full-thickness burns in areas that are highly functional, such as the hands and face. Common donor sites include the inguinal crease and the lower abdomen. Usually this is carried out with an elliptical excision that extends to the subcutaneous fat. The FTSG is then prepared by removing any subcutaneous fat and some dermis if thicker than desired.[21] These grafts have decreased primary contraction compared with STSG and can result in excellent functional outcomes.[22] Preoperative planning should include measurements to determine if an FTSG will cover the desired wound and whether the patient has enough skin laxity at desired harvest sites to successfully close the donor sites primarily. Postoperatively, the graft should be monitored for seroma/hematoma accumulation underneath the graft during the first 24 hours of surgery.

Split-Thickness Skin Grafts

STSGs are most frequently used for acute closure of the excised burn wound. The grafts are usually harvested with a powered dermatome. They include the epidermis and a part of the dermis that can be adjusted by setting the dermatome to a specific depth. Generally, this is set between 8 and 12/1000th of an inch. Grafts are taken from available donor site—preferentially from the thighs and back before other sites. The donor site area can be prepared with subcutaneous injection of a crystalloid solution to achieve tumescence. This creates an even area for harvesting, increasing the firmness of the tissue and decreasing the contours of the body. Epinephrine (at a dose of 1:1 million) can be mixed with the tumescent fluid to decrease blood loss at the donor site.[21] Thicker grafts are taken for areas that are more functional, such as the hands. STSGs can be either used as a sheet without any perforations or meshed in a range of ratios. The skin is meshed with a device that provides meshing ratios from 1:1 to 6:1. More widely meshed STSGs have the advantage of covering larger areas. It also allows for fluid and blood on the wound bed to drain instead of accumulating underneath the graft. A disadvantage is that a meshed STSG will likely heal with a permanent meshed pattern. There also is an increase in wound contraction during healing, as there is less dermis per surface area grafted.[22] Preoperative planning should include whether a dermatome and a mesher are needed for the case.

Cultured Epidermal Autografts

CEAs (Epicel; Vericel Corp, Cambridge, MA, USA) are composed of a sheet of keratinocytes cultured from a small (4 cm²) skin biopsy. This biopsy can be expanded to cover the body surface area of an adult.[23] This is a consideration with massive burns in which TBSA is greater than 70%. These patients are especially challenging, as they will have a finite amount of donor skin and large surface areas that require coverage. A tentative decision to use CEAs should be made as early as possible after injury, because the culture process takes 2 to 3 weeks after receipt of a biopsy.[21] [23] Although CEAs can provide wound coverage, they are susceptible to infection, provide variable graft take, and are subject to early and late graft loss. Nevertheless, they can be useful in selected patients with massive burns.[23,24]

Autologous Skin-Cell Suspension

Autologous skin-cell suspension (RECELL System, Valencia, CA, USA) uses 1 cm² of split-thickness skin from the patient to provide a suspension, which is then sprayed onto up to 80 cm² of excised wound.[25] This typically is sprayed on top of a widely meshed STSG. It has been shown to yield similar acute and long-term outcomes to conventional autografting, while reducing donor site size.[25] This relatively new technology has been studied and evaluated for many different burns. Use on deep dermal burns with contiguous or near-contiguous dermal elements on the wound bed has yielded excellent results. One study demonstrated equivalent or better cosmetic outcomes when this technique was applied to facial burns instead of STSG.[26] This technology is currently being studied for use in combination with dermal skin substitutes as a one-step procedure for full-thickness burn injuries.[27] It can also be applied to burn injuries that heal with hypopigmentation.[28,29] STSG donor sites can be sprayed with RECELL to accelerate reepithelialization.[30]

Allograft

Allograft is an excellent product for temporary wound coverage. This split-thickness cadaveric skin is available meshed or unmeshed and is usually cryopreserved. Allograft provides a barrier to insensible water loss, protects the underlying tissue, and decreases pain by providing wound coverage.[31] Allograft can be used if the patient lacks enough donor sites to permit coverage of all the excised wounds with autograft. It also can be used in situations in which the viability of the wound bed is questionable; in these cases, allograft is used to prepare the wound bed while preserving the patient's donor sites for future use. Following excision, allograft can serve as temporary coverage of an infected wound in which immediate autografting would be contraindicated. Allografts are generally removed before autograft placement. However, if the allograft has become incorporated into the wound bed, it can be partially excised; this should leave behind a layer of allograft dermis, onto which an epidermal autograft is then applied. Finally, use of allograft over widely meshed (3:1 to 6:1) autograft serves to protect the wound while the autograft heals underneath. This "sandwich technique" is highly effective for massive burns.

Xenografts

Xenografts are another option for temporary wound coverage. The leading source of xenograft is porcine skin. Unfortunately, porcine xenograft is not currently available in the United States.[31]

Dermal Substitutes

A variety of these products have become available.[32] They are composed of either a synthetic or an animal-derived dermal template, which is designed to be incorporated into the healing wound. Some, such as the original Integra dermal regeneration template (Integra LifeSciences, Princeton, NJ, USA), also include a temporary epidermal analogue to protect the wound and reduce water loss. Indications for use of a dermal substitute include large areas of full-thickness burns where donor sites are limited, areas of high function where a dermal substitute can help mitigate contraction after autografting, small deep full-thickness burns, and areas of exposed tendons or bone where one-stage excision and autografting will not succeed.

Dermal substitutes are typically used in a two-stage process, in which the burn wound is excised and the dermal substitute is applied to the wound bed. It is then given 2 to 4 weeks to neovascularize and create a "neodermis." Then, a thin epidermal autograft is applied to this bed for wound closure. Alternatively, a one-step procedure can be performed, in which an autograft is immediately applied over the dermal substitute. There has been demonstration of good permanent wound coverage and good scar outcomes.[31,33]

Bioengineered Full-Thickness Skin

Bioengineered full-thickness skin (StrataGraft; Mallinckrodt Pharmaceuticals, Staines-upon-Thames, UK) is a newer option. The advantage to this product is the possibility of wound closure without autografting. This is a bioengineered allogeneic cellularized construct that has proven to be successful in deep partial-thickness burns.[34] Ongoing studies are evaluating its use in full-thickness burns.

RECOVERY

Postoperative dressings for burns include negative-pressure wound therapy (VAC; KCI, San Antonio, TX, USA), mafenide-acetate–soaked dressings, 0.5% silver-nitrate–soaked dressings, silver-impregnated dressings (eg, Silverlon; Argentum Medical, Geneva, IL, USA), and Xeroform gauze (3% bismuth-tribromophenate in petrolatum). Preferences for dressings should be communicated with the operating room team for preparation.

Patients should recover in a warmed environment with attention directed toward identifying any bleeding under bulky dressings and to hemodynamic monitoring. These patients may require larger doses of narcotics and sedatives postoperatively, to limit discomfort and to protect delicate grafts against shearing from excessive activity. These medications can be augmented with ketamine and/or dexmedetomidine infusions in the postoperative period. However, prolonged bedrest following excision and grafting is no longer recommended or necessary, as discussed elsewhere in this issue.

COMPLICATIONS

Graft loss can occur in the early or late stages of wound healing. In the immediate postgrafting period, infection, hematoma/seroma formation, sheer forces, and under-excision of the burn can lead to graft failure. Later during the acute hospitalization, infection and malnutrition can contribute to graft breakdown. Late complications include the development of scar contractures and need for reconstructive tissue surgery as well as laser therapy for hypertrophic scars. These topics are covered elsewhere in this issue.

SUMMARY

Acute surgical management of the burn wound primarily focuses on deep partial-thickness and full-thickness burns. The complexity of burn treatment increases with both the burn size and location. Burn surgery has continued to evolve over the past few decades with emerging technologies to help support the goals of excellent functional and aesthetic outcomes and improved mortality.

CLINICS CARE POINTS

- Optimal burn care includes both identifying wounds that will re-epithelize within 2-3 weeks without an operation with minimal risk for hypertrophic scarring and timely operative intervention for wounds requiring surgery to achieve wound coverage.
- A deeper partial thickness burn may involve most of the dermis without many viable dermal appendages and stem cells for regeneration. A third-degree or full thickness burn affects all layers of the skin. Both of these generally require surgical intervention.
- Pain management involves multimodal therapy. This often includes a combination of NSAIDs, acetaminophen, gabapentin, tricyclic antidepressants, and opioids.
- Preoperative preparation leads to a more successful operation and outcomes that are no longer isolated to just survival but includes patient quality of life and successful reintegration into society.

DISCLOSURE

J.H. Holmes is a consultant for AVITA medical. A.B. Saraswat has nothing to disclose.

REFERENCES

1. Pereira C, Murphy K, Herndon D. Outcome measures in burn care: Is mortality dead? Burns 2004;30(8):761–71.
2. Janzekovic Z. A new concept in the early excision and immediate grafting of burns. J Trauma 1970;10(12):1103–8.
3. Tenenhaus M, Rennekampff HO. Burn surgery. Clin Plast Surg 2007;34(4): 697–715.
4. Harbour P, Song DH. The skin and subcutaneous tissue. In: Schwartz's principles of surgery, 11e. USA: McGraw Hill; 2019.
5. Stoecklin P, Delodder F, Pantet O, et al. Moderate glycemic control safe in critically ill adult burn patients: a 15 year cohort study. Burns 2016;42(1):63–70.
6. King M. Preoperative evaluation. Am Fam Physician 2000;62(2):387–96.
7. Farny B, Fontaine M, Latarjet J, et al. Estimation of blood loss during adult burn surgery. Burns 2018;44(6):1496–501.
8. Housinger TA, Lang D, Warden GD. A prospective study of blood loss with excisional therapy in pediatric burn patients. J Trauma 1993;34(2):262–3.
9. Brown RA, Grobbelaar AO, Barker S, et al. A formula to calculate blood cross-match requirements for early burn surgery in children. Burns 1995;21(5):371–3.
10. Sterling JP, Heimbach DM. Hemostasis in burn surgery—A review. Burns 2011; 37(4):559–65.
11. Welling H, Ostrowski SR, Stensballe J, et al. Management of bleeding in major burn surgery. Burns 2019;45(4):755–62.
12. Rajagopalan S, Mascha E, Na J, et al. The effects of mild perioperative hypothermia on blood loss and transfusion requirement. Anesthesiology 2008;108:71–7.

13. Prunet B, Asencio Y, Lacroix G, et al. Maintenance of normothermia during burn surgery with an intravascular temperature control system: a non-randomised controlled trial. Injury 2012;43(5):648–52.

14. Binnekade JM, Tepaske R, Bruynzeel P, et al. Daily enteral feeding practice on the ICU: attainment of goals and interfering factors. Crit Care 2005;9(3):R218–25.

15. Varon DE, Freitas G, Goel N, et al. Intraoperative feeding improves calorie and protein delivery in acute burn patients. J Burn Care Res 2017;38(5):299–303.

16. Carmichael H, Joyce S, Smith T, et al. Safety and efficacy of intraoperative gastric feeding during burn surgery. Burns 2019;45(5):1089–93.

17. Grunzweig KA, Son J, Kumar AR. Regional anesthetic blocks for donor site pain in burn patients: a meta-analysis on efficacy, outcomes, and cost. Plast Surg (Oakv). 2020;28(4):222–31.

18. Anderson TA, Fuzaylov G. Perioperative anesthesia management of the burn patient. Surg Clin North Am 2014;94(4):851–61.

19. Legemate CM, Goei H, Gostelie OFE, et al. Application of hydrosurgery for burn wound debridement: an 8-year cohort analysis. Burns 2019;45(1):88–96.

20. Ziolkowski N, Rogers AD, Xiong W, et al. The impact of operative time and hypothermia in acute burn surgery. Burns 2017;43(8):1673–81.

21. Greenhalgh DG. Operative management of burns. In: Greenhalgh D.G., *Burn care for general surgeons and general practitioners*. 1st edition. Switzerland: Springer International Publishing; 2016. p. 117–35.

22. Wanner M, Adams C, Ratner D. Skin grafts. In: Rohrer TE, Cook JL, Nguyen TH, editors. *Flaps and grafts in dermatologic surgery.* Amsterdam, Netherlands: Elsevier Inc; 2007. p. 107–16.

23. Atiyeh BS, Costagliola M. Cultured epithelial autograft (CEA) in burn treatment: three decades later. Burns 2007;33(4):405–13.

24. Williamson JS, Snelling CF, Clugston P, et al. Cultured epithelial autograft: five years of clinical experience with twenty-eight patients. J Trauma 1995;39(2):309–19.

25. Holmes JH 4th, Molnar JA, Shupp JW, et al. Demonstration of the safety and effectiveness of the RECELL System combined with split-thickness meshed autografts for the reduction of donor skin to treat mixed-depth burn injuries. Burns 2019;45(4):772–82.

26. Molnar JA, Walker N, Steele TN, et al. Initial experience with autologous skin cell suspension for treatment of deep partial-thickness facial burns. J Burn Care Res 2020;41(5):1045–51.

27. Damaraju SM, Mintz BR, Park JG, et al. Skin substitutes with noncultured autologous skin cell suspension heal porcine full-thickness wounds in a one-stage procedure. Int Wound J 2022;19(1):188–201.

28. Yu N, Liu R, Yu P, et al. Repigmentation of nipple-areola complex after ReCell® treatment on breast vitiligo. J Cosmet Dermatol 2022;21(6):2530–4.

29. Busch KH, Bender R, Walezko N, et al. Combination of medical needling and non-cultured autologous skin cell transplantation (ReNovaCell) for repigmentation of hypopigmented burn scars. Burns 2016;42(7):1556–66.

30. Hu Z, Guo D, Liu P, et al. Randomized clinical trial of autologous skin cell suspension for accelerating re-epithelialization of split-thickness donor sites. Br J Surg 2017;104(7):836–42.

31. Palackic A, Duggan RP, Campbell MS, et al. The role of skin substitutes in acute burn and reconstructive burn surgery: an updated comprehensive review. Semin Plast Surg 2022;36(1):33–42.

32. Hicks KE, Huynh MN, Jeschke M, et al. Dermal regenerative matrix use in burn patients: a systematic review. J Plast Reconstr Aesthet Surg 2019;72(11):1741–51.

33. Demircan M, Cicek T, Yetis MI. Preliminary results in single-step wound closure procedure of full-thickness facial burns in children by using the collagen-elastin matrix and review of pediatric facial burns. Burns 2015;41(6):1268–74.

34. Gibson AL, Holmes JH 4th, Shupp JW, et al. A phase 3, open-label, controlled, randomized, multicenter trial evaluating the efficacy and safety of StrataGraft® construct in patients with deep partial-thickness thermal burns. Burns 2021;47(5):1024–37.

Metabolic and Nutritional Support

Shahriar Shahrokhi, MD, FRCSC[a,b], Marc G. Jeschke, MD, PhD, FCCM, FRCS(C)[a,b,c,d],*

KEYWORDS

• Nutrition • Metabolism • Glucose • Lipid • Proteins

KEY POINTS

• Early and adequate nutrition is key to modulate metabolic responses after burn.
• Hypermetabolism is a central mediator of adverse outcomes after burn.
• Metabolic agents, such as anabolic and anticatabolic agents, may attenuate hypermetabolism and improve outcomes in severely burned patients.

HYPERMETABOLIC RESPONSE

Hypermetabolism is a hallmark of larger burn injuries, that is, burns greater than 40% total body surface area (TBSA); but it can occur even in burns greater than 20% TBSA. The hypermetabolic response is characterized by marked and sustained increases in catecholamines, glucocorticoids, and glucagon.[1] The hypermetabolic response postburn is mediated through a complex interaction of interleukins, tumor necrosis factor, platelet activation factor, reactive oxygen species, and nitric oxide along with other mediators.[2]

Initially after injury (during the first 48 hours), the patients experience an "ebb" phase that is characterized by:

• Decreased cardiac output
• Decreased oxygen consumption
• Decreased metabolic rate
• Impaired glucose tolerance

This is followed by a "flow" phase that is associated with a hyperdynamic circulation and hypermetabolism.[3]

The initial postburn period is marked by low cardiac output; however, in the ensuing 3 to 4 days, cardiac output increases to more than 1.5 times that of healthy volunteers.

[a] Burn Program at Hamilton Health Sciences, Hamilton, Ontario, Canada; [b] Department of Surgery, McMaster University, Hamilton, Ontario, Canada; [c] TaAri Institute, Hamilton Health Sciences Research Institute, Hamilton, Ontario, Canada; [d] David Braley Research Institute, C5-104, 237 Barton Street East, Hamilton, Ontario L8L 2X2, Canada
* Corresponding author. David Braley Research Institute, C5-104, 237 Barton Street East, Hamilton, Ontario L8L 2X2.
E-mail address: marc.jeschke@hhsc.ca

Surg Clin N Am 103 (2023) 473–482
https://doi.org/10.1016/j.suc.2023.01.009
0039-6109/23/© 2023 Elsevier Inc. All rights reserved.

The heart rates of pediatric burn patients can increase further, approaching 1.6 times that of healthy volunteers.[1] Postburn, patients have increased cardiac work, and myocardial oxygen consumption can surpass that of long-distance runners.

Hypermetabolism has been shown to profoundly alter and affect glucose, protein, and fat metabolism. Insulin release during this time period is doubled and plasma glucose levels are markedly elevated, indicating the development of hyperglycemic, hyperinsulinemic insulin resistance.[4] These metabolic alterations are believed to resolve soon after complete wound closure. However, the hypermetabolic response to burn injury may last for more than 24 months after the initial event,[5] and sustained hypermetabolic alterations postburn can persist for up to 3 to 5 years after the initial burn injury.[5] For severely burned patients, the increases in catabolism result in loss of total body protein, which can in turn diminish immune defenses and decrease wound healing capacity.[6]

Postburn, the size of the liver can increase by 225% of normal by 2 weeks and remains enlarged by 200% of normal at the time of discharge.[6]

The elevation in catecholamines, cortisol, and glucagon postburn leads to increased production of free fatty acids, glucose, and amino acids. More significantly, the changes in the glycolysis and gluconeogenesis pathways result in hyperglycemia, and impaired insulin sensitivity. Even though the glucose delivery to peripheral tissue is increased, the inefficiency of anaerobic metabolism drives an increase in lactate production and further increase in glucose production in the liver via breakdown of lactate.[1,5,6]

Recently, adipose tissue was identified as a major contributor to hypermetabolism and catabolism. The adipose tissue undergoes a "browning response," which is characterized by release of energy, lipolysis, and massively increased beta oxidation, all of which worsen the catabolic response.[7]

NUTRITIONAL SUPPORT

Postburn hypermetabolism, resulting in increased oxygen consumption, metabolic rate, urinary nitrogen excretion, lipolysis, and weight loss, directly correlates with increasing burn size. The increase can be 200% of normal. The energy requirements are met by mobilization of carbohydrate, fat, and protein stores leading to muscle mass loss and malnutrition. This malnutrition in burns is undone to some extent by provision of nutritional support, to maintain and improve organ function. To determine the caloric requirements several formulas have been proposed:[8]

- The Harris-Benedict formula:
  - Men: 66.5 + 13.8(weight in kg) + 5(height in cm) − 6.76(age in years)
  - Women: 655 + 9.6(weight in kg) + 1.85(height in cm) − 4.68(age in years)
  - Can be adjusted for activity and stress factor.
  - To meet needs of a pediatric burn patient, will need 1.33 times the predicted basal energy expenditure for burns greater than 40% TBSA.
  - To meet the needs of all the patients will need 1.4 times the measured resting energy expenditure.
- The Curreri formula:
  - Age 16 to 59: 25(weight in kg) + 40(TBSA)
  - Age greater than 60: 20(weight in kg) + 65(TBSA)
  - Often overestimates caloric needs. This formula provides for maintenance in addition to the caloric needs related to the burn wounds.
  - In pediatrics, formulas based on body surface area are more appropriate because of the greater body surface area per kilogram of weight.

- The Toronto formula:
  - $-4343 + 10.5(TBSA) + 0.23$(calorie intake in last 24 h) $+ 0.84$(Harris Benedict estimation without adjustment) $+ 114$(temperature) $- 4.5$(number of postburn days)
  - Must be adjusted with changes in monitoring but useful in the acute phase.

The composition of the nutritional supplementation is of utmost importance. The optimal dietary composition contains 1 to 2 g/kg/d of protein, which can to some extent spare the proteolysis occurring in muscle tissue. Nonprotein calories are given either as carbohydrate or as fat. Carbohydrates have the advantage of stimulating endogenous insulin production and decrease protein oxidation. However, as shown by Hart and colleagues,[9] nutrition in terms of too many carbohydrates can cause hyperglycemia and fatty infiltration of the liver; hence a balanced diet with high carbohydrates, low fat, and significant amount of proteins and amino acids seems to be the ideal nutrition.

Insulin itself has endocrine, paracrine, and anabolic effects after burn. Others and we have shown that insulin increased muscle anabolism, and improves organ function and anti-inflammatory properties.[10]

After severe burn injury, most of the fat transported in very low-density lipoprotein derived from peripheral lipolysis and not from de novo synthesis of fatty acids in the liver. Given the decrease in fat transporters, low-fat diets would be beneficial because additional fat to deliver noncarbohydrate calories has little support. Therefore, the recommended diet would provide less than 15% of total calories from fat content.[11]

Ideally nutritional support should commence within 24 hours postburn and be provided via the enteric route to minimize intestinal mucosal injury and to preserve intestinal barrier function.[6,12] Caloric requirements are based on the formulas mentioned previously and are adjusted based on indirect calorimetry.[13–15] To measure resting energy expenditure is nowadays an important component of clinical burn care. Resting energy expenditure measurement should be conducted once or twice a week to adjust nutrition to the caloric demands and at the same time to avoid overfeeding.

The intricate interplay of feeding composition and monitoring of nutritional demands is important to ensure provision of adequate caloric intake to counter catabolism while preventing overfeeding, which has numerous complications such as:[15]

- Difficulty weaning from ventilatory support
- Fatty liver
- Azotemia
- Hyperglycemia

A more specific insight about body composition and how nutrition and clinical care affects body composition is measured by dual x-ray absorptiometry. However, dual x-ray absorptiometry scan is not readily available for all burn units nor is it always conveniently or safely located to run this test.

OTHER NUTRIENTS

Glutamine is a nonessential amino acid that has been shown by some experimental data to improve outcome in burn-injured patients. Several glutamine clinical trials demonstrated a reduction in gram-negative bacteremia postburn injury. The RE-ENERGIZE trial, however, clearly showed that glutamine supplementation had no effect on outcomes of burn patients.[16]

Vitamins and trace elements are essential for recovery postburn because they are important in immunity and wound healing. Severe burn leads to oxidative stress including significantly increased reactive oxygen species, which combined with the inflammatory response, adds to cellular and organ dysfunction and the depletion of the endogenous defenses.[17,18]

Decreased levels of vitamins A, C, and D and Fe, Cu, Se, and Zn can negatively impact wound healing and skeletal and immune function.[19–22] Studies have demonstrated that severely burned patients receiving antioxidant and trace element supplementation had reduced markers of burn stress–induced inflammation; decreased hypermetabolic response, shorter length of stay, and improved bacterial clearance and hence less morbidity.[23–26]

PHARMACOLOGIC MODALITIES TO ATTENUATE HYPERMETABOLISM

Adequate nutrition and other means, such as environmental temperature, early mobilization, and early excision can only attenuate hypermetabolism and catabolism but are by no means able to prevent or reverse lean body mass loss or the profound protein loss. Therefore, in the search for improving outcomes in burn patients, various pharmacologic agents have been used to reduce the hypermetabolic response postburn.

Growth Hormone

Administration of recombinant human growth hormone (rhGH) (0.1–0.2 mg/kg/d intramuscularly) has been shown to have a host of beneficial effects:

- Increases donor site healing and quality of wound healing[20]
- Diminishes stress responses and inflammation[27,28]
- Elevates levels of insulinlike growth factor 1 (IGF-1)[29]
- Decreases basal energy expenditure and cardiac output[30]
- Augments muscle protein and preserves muscle growth[31,32]

However, a multicenter trial (in nonburn patients) revealed that morbidity and mortality of critically ill patients receiving rhGH were higher than in patients receiving placebo.[33] This was especially true for patients suffering from infections and sepsis, because in this patient group GH profoundly increased multi organ dysfunction syndrome (MODS) and mortality. Exogenous administration of growth hormone has also been linked to hyperglycemia and insulin resistance.[34,35] In addition, rhGH was not found to benefit survival in pediatric patients with severe burns.[36,37] The use of GH in burn patients is at this time not recommended.

Insulinlike Growth Factor

Given that IGF-1 is an effector of growth factor, administering IGF-1/binding protein-3 complex has been shown to ameliorate protein metabolism in burned children and adults with fewer episodes of hypoglycemia than rhGH.[38] Some of the effects of IGF-1/binding protein-3 are[38–41]:

- Reduction in muscle protein breakdown
- Amelioration of gut mucosal integrity
- Improving immune function
- Attenuation of the acute-phase response
- Elevation of constitutive proteins in the serum and decrease in inflammatory response

However, other studies indicate that IGF-1 alone is ineffective in nonburned critically ill patients. IGF-1 did show promise in terms of anabolism and reduction of the hypermetabolic response, but because of its side effects of hypoglycemia, electrolyte abnormalities, and neuro side effects the use of IGF-1 is currently not recommended.[42,43]

Oxandrolone

Oxandrolone is similar to testosterone, but lacks its virilizing effects. Oxandrolone has been shown to stimulate muscle protein synthesis,[44] reduce weight loss, and promote wound healing.[45] Oxandrolone at a dose of 10 mg twice daily has also been shown to decrease hospital stay, morbidity, and mortality.[46] When given at a dose of 0.1 mg/kg twice daily, oxandrolone decreases hospitalization, preserves lean body mass, and enhances protein synthesis in the liver.[47] The dosing for older adults is 0.05 mg/kg twice a day. The long-term effects of oxandrolone are decreased hypermetabolism, and increase in lean body mass and bone mineral content (increasing from 6 to 12 months postburn).[48,49] Therefore, oxandrolone is recommended in burns to be given as an anabolic agent.

Testosterone

Testosterone has been shown to be anabolic in adult burn patients and older adults. The administration of testosterone should be considered when endogenous levels are profoundly depleted. The use in women should be restrictive and considered as a third-line/fourth-line treatment.

Propranolol

Propranolol, a β-adrenergic blocker, is an effective anticatabolic therapy postburn. Acutely, propranolol has anti-inflammatory effect, and can counter loss of skeletal muscle, augment lean body mass, and decrease insulin resistance.[50,51] If given at a dose to decrease heart rate by 15% to 20%, long-term propranolol treatment significantly reduces predicted resting energy expenditure, decreases accumulation of central mass and central fat, prevents bone loss, and improves lean body mass accretion.[50–52] Propranolol seems to be an effective agent to treat catecholamine-induced hypermetabolic stress response postburn. In pediatrics dosing is 1 to 4 mg/kg four times a day, and adults 10 mg four times a day. Adverse events of propranolol are bradycardia, hypotension, and possibly hallucinations. Propranolol mainly acts as an anticatabolic agent and is considered in burn patients that suffer from a substantial inflammatory and hypermetabolic response.

Insulin

Thermally injured patients with hyperglycemia have a greater incidence of bacteremia/fungemia, diminished wound healing capacity, more pronounced protein catabolism, and lower likelihood of survival than burn patients with adequate glucose control.[53,54] Insulin administration seems to promote muscle protein production, helps prevent lean body mass loss, diminishes the acute phase response, and enhances wound healing.[55–61] Care must be taken to avoid hypoglycemia,[62,63] because glucose variability and increased episodes of hypoglycemia tend to lead to greater morbidity and mortality. Hyperglycemia associated with insulin resistance is a clinically significant problem in burn patients and insulin administration while avoiding hypoglycemia improves morbidity and mortality.[62–69]

Metformin

Metformin, an oral hypoglycemic agent, has been suggested as a means to correct hyperglycemia in severely injured patients.[70] Metformin inhibits gluconeogenesis and amplifies peripheral insulin sensitivity, thus countering the main metabolic processes, which lead to postburn hyperglycemia.[70,71] Administration of metformin seems to increase muscle protein synthesis and improve net muscle protein balance.[71] Additionally, metformin seems to have less associated hypoglycemic events, as compared with exogenous insulin administration.[72–75] Metformin reduces plasma glucose concentration, decreases endogenous glucose production, and accelerates glucose clearance in the severely burned.[72–75] Dosing should be 500 mg twice a day to 1000 mg three times a day. Metformin should only be given if glomerular filtration rate is greater than 30 mL/kg.

SUMMARY

Nutrition and metabolic treatment and supplementation are essential for burn patients and have a direct effect on burn outcomes. Early and adequate nutrition is key. Other major interventions that affect metabolism include warm patient rooms and operating rooms, early mobilization and exercise, and early excision and grafting. In terms of adjunctive therapies, we recommend the use of oxandrolone, insulin, metformin, and propranolol, the latter under intensive care unit monitoring. If no adverse effects occur, anabolic agents should be administered, at minimum, for the duration of hospitalization. There is also good evidence for long-term treatment, up to 2 to 3 years postburn, for propranolol and oxandrolone.[76]

FUNDING

The authors received no specific funding for this work.

CLINICS CARE POINTS

- Hypermetabolism is a central component
- Adjuncts have limitations
- To date no single approach has reversed hypermetabolism

ACKNOWLEDGMENTS

Dr M.G. Jeschke received a grant (#R01GM133961) from the National Institutes of Health, United States.

DISCLOSURE

The authors have no disclosures to report.

REFERENCES

1. Williams FN, Jeschke MG, Chinkes DL, et al. Modulation of the hypermetabolic response to trauma: temperature, nutrition, and drugs. J Am Coll Surg 2009; 208:489–502.
2. Gauglitz GG, Herndon DN, Jeschke MG. Insulin resistance postburn: underlying mechanisms and current therapeutic strategies. J Burn Care Res 2008;29: 683–94.
3. Jeschke MG, van Baar ME, Choudhry MA, et al. Burn injury. Nat Rev Dis Primers 2020;6(1):11.

4. Cree MG, Aarsland A, Herndon DN, et al. Role of fat metabolism in burn trauma-induced skeletal muscle insulin resistance. Crit Care Med 2007;35:S476-83.

5. Gauglitz GG, Herndon DN, Kulp GA, et al. Abnormal insulin sensitivity persists up to three years in pediatric patients post burn. J Clin Endocrinol Metab 2009;94: 1656-64.

6. Jeschke MG, Chinkes DL, Finnerty CC, et al. Patholphysiologic response to severe burn injury. Ann Surg 2008;248:387-401.

7. Abdullahi A, Jeschke MG. Taming the flames: targeting white adipose tissue browning in hypermetabolic conditions. Endocr Rev 2017;38(6):538-49.

8. Hall KL, Shahrokhi S, Jeschke MG. Enteral nutrition support in burn care: a review of current recommendations as instituted in the Ross Tilley Burn Centre. Nutrients 2012;4(11):1554-65.

9. Hart DW, Wolf SE, Herndon DN, et al. Energy expenditure and caloric balance after burn: increased feeding leads to fat rather than lean mass accretion. Ann Surg 2002;235(1):152-61.

10. Bogdanovic E, Jeschke MG. Insulin therapy improves protein metabolism in the critically ill. Crit Care 2012;16(3):125.

11. Pereira CT, Jeschke MG, Herndon DN. Beta-blockade in burns. Novartis Found Symp 2007;280:238-48 ; discussion 248-51.

12. Rousseau A-F, Losser M-R, Ichai C, et al. ESPEN endorsed recommendations: nutritional therapy in major burns. Clin Nutr 2013;32(4):497-502.

13. Hart DW, Wolf SE, Chinkes DL, et al. Effects of early excision and aggressive enteral feeding on hypermetabolism, catabolism, and sepsis after severe burn. J Trauma 2003;54(4):755-61, discussion 761-754.

14. Ireton-Jones CS, Turner WW Jr, Liepa GU, et al. Equations for the estimation of energy expenditures in patients with burns with special reference to ventilatory status. J Burn Care Rehabil 1992;13(3):330-3.

15. Hart DW, Wolf SE, Zhang XJ, et al. Efficacy of a high-carbohydrate diet in catabolic illness. Crit Care Med 2001;29(7):1318-24.

16. McClave SA, Snider HL. Use of indirect calorimetry in clinical nutrition. Nutr Clin Pract 1992;7(5):207-21.

17. Saffle JR, Medina E, Raymond J, et al. Use of indirect calorimetry in the nutritional management of burned patients. J Trauma 1985;25(1):32-9.

18. Wischmeyer PE. Glutamine in burn injury. Nutr Clin Pract 2019;34(5):681-7.

19. Gamliel Z, DeBiasse MA, Demling RH. Essential microminerals and their response to burn injury. J Burn Care Rehabil 1996;17(3):264-72.

20. Berger MM. Antioxidant micronutrients in major trauma and burns: evidence and practice. Nutr Clin Pract 2006;21(5):438-49.

21. Gottschlich MM, Mayes T, Khoury J, et al. Hypovitaminosis D in acutely injured pediatric burn patients. J Am Diet Assoc 2004;104(6):931-41, quiz 1031.

22. Gottschlich MM, Mayes T, Khoury J, et al. Clinical trial of vitamin D_2 vs D_3 supplementation in critically ill pediatric burn patients. JPEN - J Parenter Enter Nutr 2017;41(3):412-21.

23. Berger MM, Shenkin A. Trace element requirements in critically ill burned patients. J Trace Elem Med Biol 2007;21(Suppl 1):44-8.

24. Berger MM, Binnert C, Chiolero RL, et al. Trace element supplementation after major burns increases burned skin trace element concentrations and modulates local protein metabolism but not whole-body substrate metabolism. Am J Clin Nutr 2007;85(5):1301-6.

25. Meyer NA, Muller MJ, Herndon DN. Nutrient support of the healing wound. New Horiz 1994;2(2):202-14.

26. Berger MM, Baines M, Raffoul W, et al. Trace element supplementation after major burns modulates antioxidant status and clinical course by way of increased tissue trace element concentrations. Am J C Am J Clin Nutr 2007;85(5): 1293–300.

27. Rehou S, Shahrokhi S, Natanson R, et al. Antioxidant and trace element supplementation reduce the inflammatory response in critically ill burn patients. J Burn Care Res 2018;39(1):1–9.

28. Herndon DN, Hawkins HK, Nguyen TT, et al. Characterization of growth hormone enhanced donor site healing in patients with large cutaneous burns. Ann Surg 1995;221:649–56.

29. Jeschke MG, Herndon DN, Wolf SE, et al. Recombinant human growth hormone alters acute phase reactant proteins, cytokine expression, and liver morphology in burned rats. J Surg Res 1999;83:122–9.

30. Wu X, Thomas SJ, Herndon DN, et al. Insulin decreases hepatic acute phase protein levels in severely burned children. Surgery 2004;135:196–202.

31. Jeschke MG, Chrysopoulo MT, Herndon DN, et al. Increased expression of insulin-like growth factor-I in serum and liver after recombinant human growth hormone administration in thermally injured rats. J Surg Res 1999;85:171–7.

32. Branski LK, Herndon DN, Barrow RE, et al. Randomized controlled trial to determine the efficacy of long-term growth hormone treatment in severely burned children. Ann Surg 2009;250(4):514–23.

33. Aili Low JF, Barrow RE, Mittendorfer B, et al. The effect of short-term growth hormone treatment on growth and energy expenditure in burned children. Burns 2001;27:447–52.

34. Hart DW, Wolf SE, Beauford RB, et al. Determinants of blood loss during primary burn excision. Surgery 2001;130:396–402.

35. Takala J, Ruokonen E, Webster NR, et al. Increased mortality associated with growth hormone treatment in critically ill adults. N Engl J Med 1999;341:785–92.

36. Gore DC, Honeycutt D, Jahoor F, et al. Effect of exogenous growth hormone on whole-body and isolated-limb protein kinetics in burned patients. Arch Surg 1991;126:38–43.

37. Demling R. Growth hormone therapy in critically ill patients. N Engl J Med 1999; 341:837–9.

38. Przkora R, Herndon DN, Suman OE, et al. Beneficial effects of extended growth hormone treatment after hospital discharge in pediatric burn patients. Ann Surg 2006;243:796–801 ; discussion 3.

39. Ramirez RJ, Wolf SE, Barrow RE, et al. Growth hormone treatment in pediatric burns: a safe therapeutic approach. Ann Surg 1998;228:439–48.

40. Herndon DN, Ramzy PI, Debroy MA, et al. Muscle protein catabolism after severe burn, effects of IGF-1/IGFBP3 treatment. Ann Surg 1999;229:713–20.

41. Spies M, Wolf SE, Barrow RE, et al. Modulation of types I and II acute phase reactants with insulin-like growth factor-1/binding protein-3 complex in severely burned children. Crit Care Med 2002;30:83–8.

42. Jeschke MG, Barrow RE, Herndon DN. Insulin-like growth factor I plus insulin-like growth factor binding protein 3 attenuates the proinflammatory acute phase response in severely burned children. Ann Surg 2000;231:246–52.

43. Cioffi WG, Gore DC, Rue LW III, et al. Insulin-like growth factor-1 lowers protein oxidation in patients with thermal injury. Ann Surg 1994;220(3):310–9.

44. Hart DW, Wolf SE, Ramzy PI, et al. Anabolic effects of oxandrolone after severe burn. Ann Surg 2001;233:556–64.

45. Demling RH, Seigne P. Metabolic management of patients with severe burns. World J Surg 2000;24:673–80.
46. Wolf SE, Edelman LS, Kemalyan N, et al. Effects of oxandrolone on outcome measures in the severely burned: a multicenter prospective randomized double-blind trial. J Burn Care Res 2006;27:131–41.
47. Jeschke MG, Finnerty CC, Suman OE, et al. The effect of oxandrolone on the endocrinologic, inflammatory, and hypermetabolic responses during the acute phase postburn. Ann Surg 2007;246:351–62.
48. Pham TN, Klein MB, Gibran NS, et al. Impact of oxandrolone treatment on acute outcomes after severe burn injury. J Burn Care Res 2008;29:902–6.
49. Przkora R, Herndon DN, Suman OE. The effects of oxandrolone and exercise on muscle mass and function in children with severe burns. Pediatrics 2007;119: e109–16.
50. Gore DC, Honeycutt D, Jahoor F, et al. Propranolol diminishes extremity blood flow in burned patients. Ann Surg 1991;213:568–73 ; discussion 73–74.
51. Herndon DN, Hart DW, Wolf SE, et al. Reversal of catabolism by beta-blockade after severe burns. N Engl J Med 2001;345:1223–9.
52. Baron PW, Barrow RE, Pierre EJ, et al. Prolonged use of propranolol safely decreases cardiac work in burned children. J Burn Care Rehabil 1997;18:223–7.
53. Gore DC, Chinkes D, Heggers J, et al. Association of hyperglycemia with increased mortality after severe burn injury. J Trauma 2001;51:540–4.
54. Gore DC, Chinkes DL, Hart DW, et al. Hyperglycemia exacerbates muscle protein catabolism in burn-injured patients. Crit Care Med 2002;30:2438–42.
55. Ferrando AA, Chinkes DL, Wolf SE, et al. A submaximal dose of insulin promotes net skeletal muscle protein synthesis in patients with severe burns. Ann Surg 1999;229:11–8.
56. Pierre EJ, Barrow RE, Hawkins HK, et al. Effects of insulin on wound healing. J Trauma 1998;44:342–5.
57. Thomas SJ, Morimoto K, Herndon DN, et al. The effect of prolonged euglycemic hyperinsulinemia on lean body mass after severe burn. Surgery 2002;132:341–7.
58. Zhang XJ, Chinkes DL, Wolf SE, et al. Insulin but not growth hormone stimulates protein anabolism in skin would and muscle. Am J Physiol 1999;276:E712–20.
59. Jeschke MG, Klein D, Bolder U, et al. Insulin attenuates the systemic inflammatory response in endotoxemic rats. Endocrinology 2004;145:4084–93.
60. Jeschke MG, Rensing H, Klein D, et al. Insulin prevents liver damage and preserves liver function in lipopolysaccharide-induced endotoxemic rats. J Hepatol 2005;42:870–9.
61. Klein D, Schubert T, Horch RE, et al. Insulin treatment improves hepatic morphology and function through modulation of hepatic signals after severe trauma. Ann Surg 2004;240:340–9.
62. Langouche L, Vanhorebeek I, Van den Berghe G. Therapy insight: the effect of tight glycemic control in acute illness. Nat Clin Pract Endocrinol Metab 2007;3: 270–8.
63. Brunkhorst FM, Engel C, Bloos F, et al. Intensive insulin therapy and pentastarch resuscitation in severe sepsis. N Engl J Med 2008;358:125–39.
64. Jeschke MG, Kraft R, Emdad F, et al. Glucose control in severely thermally injured pediatric patients: what glucose range should be the target? Ann Surg 2010;252: 521–8.
65. Van den Berghe G, Wouters PJ, Bouillon R, et al. Outcome benefit of intensive insulin therapy in the critically ill: insulin dose versus glycemic control. Crit Care Med 2003;31:359–66.

66. Vlasselaers D, Milants I, Desmet L, et al. Intensive insulin therapy for patients in pediatric intensive care: a prospective, randomized controlled study. Lancet 2009;373:547–56.

67. Pidcoke HF, Wanek SM, Rohleder LS, et al. Glucose variability is associated with high mortality after severe burn. J Trauma 2009;67:990–5.

68. Pisarchik AN, Pochepen ON, Pisarchyk LA. Increasing blood glucose variability is a precursor of sepsis and mortality in burned patients. PLoS One 2012;7. e46582.

69. Jeschke MG. Clinical review: glucose control in severely burned patients. Current best practice. Crit Care 2013;17(4):232.

70. Gore DC, Wolf SE, Herndon DN, et al. Metformin blunts stress-induced hyperglycemia after thermal injury. J Trauma 2003;54:555–61.

71. Gore DC, Wolf SE, Sanford A, et al. Influence of metformin on glucose intolerance and muscle catabolism following severe burn injury. Ann Surg 2005;241:334–42.

72. Moon RJ, Bascombe LA, Holt RI. The addition of metformin in type 1 diabetes improves insulin sensitivity, diabetic control, body composition and patient well-being. Diabetes Obes Metab 2007;9:143–5.

73. Staels B. Metformin and pioglitazone: effectively treating insulin resistance. Curr Med Res Opin 2006;22(Suppl 2):S27–37.

74. Musi N, Goodyear LJ. Insulin resistance and improvements in signal transduction. Endocrine 2006;29:73–80.

75. Hundal RS, Inzucchi SE. Metformin: new understandings, new uses. Drugs 2003; 63:1879–94.

76. Stanojcic M, Finnerty CC, Jeschke MG. Anabolic and anticatabolic agents in critical care. Curr Opin Crit Care 2016;22(4):325–31.

Critical Care Rehabilitation of the Burn Patient

Jill M. Cancio, OTD, OTR/L, CHT*, William S. Dewey, BS, PT, CHT

KEYWORDS

- Critical care • Rehabilitation • Burns

KEY POINTS

- Burn rehabilitation is an essential component of burn critical care and begins on admission to the burn intensive care unit (ICU).
- Out-of-bed mobilities are a crucial component of burn rehabilitation in the ICU.
- Simultaneously, concerted attention to monitoring, maintaining, and restoring hand function in the burn ICU is critical to postburn recovery.
- Further work on the physiologic, functional, and long-term impact of this care is needed.

INTRODUCTION

Burns are among the most devastating forms of trauma, with both immediate and long-lasting physiologic and functional effects.[1] Despite the fact that modern burn care has significantly reduced the mortality associated with severe burn injuries,[2,3] the rehabilitation and community reintegration of survivors continues to be a challenge.[3] Given the complex nature of burn injury, an interprofessional team approach is essential for optimal outcomes.[4] This team approach includes early occupational and physical rehabilitation in the burn intensive care unit (BICU).

CONSEQUENCES OF PROLONGED BED REST

Long-term bed rest is a major issue during the acute phase following severe traumatic injury to include severe burn injury. These patients are often heavily sedated with a major focus on maintaining maximum physiologic stability that often requires bed rest.[5] In the nineteenth century, bed rest was first introduced as a medical treatment with a goal to decrease metabolic demand on the body and emphasize healing and rest to promote recovery.[6] However, prolonged bed rest has substantial consequences on musculoskeletal, cardiovascular, respiratory, integumentary, and cognitive systems and may be associated with damage and/or harm to the body.[7]

US Army Institute of Surgical Research, 3698 Chambers Pass Suite B, JBSA Fort Sam Houston, TX 78234-7767, USA
* Corresponding author.
E-mail address: jill.m.cancio.civ@health.mil

Surg Clin N Am 103 (2023) 483–494
https://doi.org/10.1016/j.suc.2023.01.010
0039-6109/23/Published by Elsevier Inc.

surgical.theclinics.com

A long-recognized characteristic of the physiologic adaptation to long-term bed rest in patients is cardiovascular deconditioning[8] as well as ICU-acquired weakness (ICUAW). The combined effect of prolonged bed rest and the body's stress response to burn injury is reduced lean-body mass,[9] decreased bone mineral density,[10] diminished muscle strength and cardiopulmonary endurance,[11,12] increased prevalence of burn scar contracture,[13] and reduced functional outcomes and health-related quality of life (HRQOL).[14]

REHABILITATION IN THE BURN INTENSIVE CARE UNIT

Recent studies in non-burn ICUs[15–18] suggest that beginning rehabilitation and mobilization early in the course of critical illness may reduce the odds of complications such as ICUAW,[15,18] ventilator-associated pneumonia,[18] and deep vein thrombosis[18] and may decrease ICU length of stay.[17,18] Early mobilization in the critical care environment is generally considered safe,[19] has been shown to result in improved physical function,[20,21] reduces the need for mechanical ventilation,[22] and improves self-perceived HRQOL.[21] Many professional societies and organizations have published clinical practice guidelines that recommend early mobilization of ICU patients.[19,23–26] Although critically ill burn patients share many of the characteristics of other critically ill populations, it is unclear if these guidelines can be specifically applied to the burn population with their unique medical, surgical, and rehabilitative needs.

Rehabilitation in the BICU is risky and labor-intensive. There are many factors that may interfere with burn rehabilitation to include pain, stiffness, bulky dressings, postoperative restrictions after skin grafting, and the effects of analgesics and anxiolytics.[27] No standard of care currently exists regarding the frequency, duration, intensity, progression, and types of exercise for severely burned patients in the ICU.[28] The following sections describe burn rehabilitation in the critical care setting to include edema management, positioning, mobilization, perioperative care, and management of hand burns.

Phases of Rehabilitation

Therapy planning for patients in the BICU should be specific to the recovery phase. Richard and colleagues[29] describe three such phases—acute, intermediate, and long-term. These phases should be an integral component of care planning and help guide rehabilitation priorities. The acute phase occurs at the time of admission through the start of skin grafting.[29] The intermediate period extends to wound closure and commonly involves postoperative immobilization.[29] The long-term phase consists of an extensive duration from wound closure to a plateau in therapy. This article focuses on the interventions in the acute and intermediate phases of recovery as patients are commonly within these stages when in the BICU.

Positioning

The initial priorities in the acute phase are edema control and pressure relief. The swelling peak usually occurs 12 to 48 hours after a burn.[30,31] Thus, it is imperative to rapidly position patients for optimal edema control with adequate elevation.[32] Open wounds, friction, and relative immobility all contribute to the high propensity for compromised skin integrity.[32,33] Interventions should be used to off-load high-risk areas and skin should be frequently inspected to ensure devices are not causing excessive pressure. Although patients will not develop a contracture in the initial days following a burn, it is important that positioning in the acute phase also consider anti-contracture placement as the wounds will contract over time and could result in a loss of motion. Hedman and colleagues[32] provide a comprehensive list of positioning devices and techniques to manage edema and excessive pressure to sensitive body parts in patients who have been severely burned.

Edema control and measurement

Patients who sustain large surface area burns and/or deep circumferential burns are at a high risk of developing substantial edema. The presence of edema increases susceptibility to comorbidities such as neuropathies, tissue compromise, and stiffness.[34] Burn resuscitation in the initial hours of care, and issues with volume management during subsequent critical care, may compound and prolong edema. Burn therapists assist the interdisciplinary team in assessment and management of edema through edema reduction techniques (ie, positioning, motion, compression) and examining for signs of vascular compromise.[32] Edema can initially be managed by elevation of the affected areas. The hands and feet should be placed above the knees and elbows, that is, at or above the level of the heart. Range-of-motion exercises can also assist the reduction of edema.[35] Prompt and consistent utilization of an efficient method to measure edema is crucial. The figure-of-eight measurement technique is a practical, valid, and rapid method that can assist the care team with edema assessment, particularly in burned hands and upper limbs.[36] Objective edema measurements help support decisions for optimal positioning and device selection.

Mobility

Out-of-bed (OOB) activities are crucial for reducing mortality and morbidity for patients in the BICU. A retrospective study determined that individuals who accomplished certain mobility targets during the first week of the BICU stay (eg, out of bed to a cardiac chair the first full day of the hospital stay, sitting edge of bed by admission day 5, and ambulating by day 8) demonstrated decreased mortality.[37] Ambulation is traditionally one of the earliest functional tasks in burn rehabilitation. Although the benefits of early ambulation are well-established, it is challenging to ascertain when it is safe for these patients, and evidence-based guidelines are lacking. Daily rounds provide an optimal forum to discuss OOB plans so all perspectives can be considered.

Mobility should be initiated as soon as the patient is deemed medically stable by the physician. The type of mobility used will vary based on the patient's medical and cognitive status. The patients' surgical status must also be taken into consideration when making mobility decisions. Recent graft sites in areas prone to high amounts of friction during mobility need to be considered. For instance, if a graft was placed on the plantar surface of a foot, it may be necessary for the patient to mobilize in a non-weight-bearing status for this extremity. A survey study aimed at tracking current trends in early mobility in the burn population determined that time to OOB mobility after surgery was significantly different for different body locations, with grafts placed above the waist resuming OOB mobility earliest.[38]

Sedated patients require the use of passive interventions that provide improved upright positioning needed for multisystem stimulation and respiratory function. These interventions can include a tilt table and/or sitting OOB in a device such as a TotalLift II Chair (**Figs. 1** and **2**). Physiologic monitoring is necessary when assessing a patient's response to upright positioning, so that tolerance to orthostatic response, pain, and weight bearing can be assessed. We recommend that although the patient is on a tilt table, vital signs be recorded when in the supine position and at 15° increments (0°–60°). Heart rate, respiratory rate, mean arterial pressure, and oxygen saturation values are assessed 5 minutes after reaching each angle. Knowledge of patients'

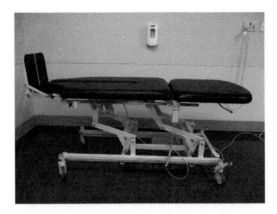

Fig. 1. Tilt table.

current medications, particularly vasoactive drugs, should also be considered when determining or anticipating a patient's response to mobilization. The tilt table session should be a multidisciplinary effort to include rehabilitation, nursing, and respiratory therapy.

A study was conducted on early passive tilting and its efficacy in treating ICUAW.[39] There was no improvement noted in muscle strength at ICU discharge for this particular study.[39] However, the study population was adults admitted to a surgical ICU and was largely not comparable to BICU patients. Furthermore, the focus was largely on improved muscle strength and tolerance of tilt treatments. Data to define whether a tilt treatment was successful were not reported. Another study reported that standing with the assistance of a tilt table improves minute ventilation in chronically ill patients during and immediately after the intervention.[40] Further study is needed to better understand the physiologic impact of tilt treatments and their potential ability to inform critical care decision-making (eg, by interrogating the patient's intravascular volume status).

If the patient is more alert but still requires a considerable amount of physical assistance to achieve a standing position, a modified tilt table or Moveo can be an effective mobilization device (**Fig. 3**). The Moveo is a tilt table that allows patients to perform

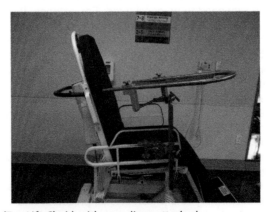

Fig. 2. Care chair (TotaLift Chair) with arm slings attached.

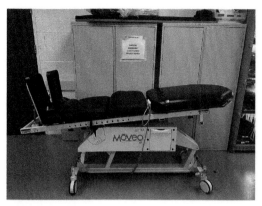

Fig. 3. Moveo or modified tilt table.

squat exercises at various levels of head and trunk elevation. The use of this modality as opposed to the use of maximal physical assistance by two or more rehabilitation staff offers a safe and controlled method to transition from bed rest to ambulation. It requires fewer staff and less risk of injury to both the patient and staff. A case series on the use of a modified tilt table for preambulation strength training is reported in the burn literature.[41] It allowed patients to perform weight-bearing squat exercises in a gravity-reduced environment. Therapists tracked objective progress through the measures of incline and number of repetitions. The authors observed additional psychological benefits as the patients were empowered to take more of an active role during the early stage of recovery.[41]

A standing frame is another option for an alert patient that is unable to safely stand and needs to engage in active trunk control. The standing frame can take a patient from a seated to a standing position using a hydraulic lift via a sling under the buttocks. These devices are commonly used as a progression to more conventional standing transfers and ambulation as the patient's status permits.

Compression
Compression of extremities when they are in a dependent position helps counteract the increased hydrostatic pressures in the distal limbs. The vascular support provided by elastic compression is valuable not only for controlling a diminished orthostatic response, but also for supporting healing tissues that are susceptible to microvascular hemorrhage when limbs are dependent. Such fluid shifts can also cause increased pressure on exposed nerve endings and cause significant pain during mobility. Applying elastic bandages in a figure-of-eight pattern can help prevent the elastic compression from unrolling during mobility attempts (**Fig. 4**).[32] Compression should be applied in a distal to proximal direction and can be placed over wound dressings. Compression can also be used for edema control when the patient is no longer in the acute resuscitation phase; however, caution should be used as burn patients have many risk factors for skin breakdown. Close visual inspection is needed to assess tissue integrity, and the response to the compression should be regularly assessed using the figure-of-eight edema measurement technique.[36]

Contracture
A burn scar contracture features a lack of motion resulting from a lack of extensible tissue.[29] Burn scar contractures are common[42] and significantly impact function

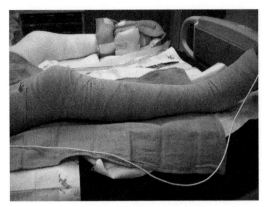

Fig. 4. Figure-of-eight compression wrap of a lower extremity.

and quality of life.[43,44] Early identification, communication, and documentation of contracture risk areas are crucial for treatment planning. To help with contracture risk assessment, Richard and colleagues[45] identified the cutaneous functional unit (CFU) concept.[45] CFUs are areas of skin that permit range of motion (ROM), proximal to the moving joint. The skin moves serially in the direction of joint motion.[46,47] The position of adjacent joints also impacts the skin recruitment necessary to perform joint motion.[48,49]

These cutaneokinematic concepts were considered when Parry and colleagues[50] developed a goniometric method for measuring joint motion in burn patients. This technique should be used to help identify burn scar contractures. It is imperative to incorporate knowledge of skin movement and the impact of adjacent joint position when developing orthotics, positioning devices and exercises to prevent and treat burn scar contracture.

Hands

Hands have the highest incidence of contracture[51] and have a significant impact on function and quality of life.[52] Hand contractures are difficult to manage due to the multiplicity of CFUs (over 30 CFUs in each hand) and complex anatomy.[53] A lack of active movement associated with sedation increases contracture risk. This necessitates the use of a comprehensive splinting program that places the tissue in an elongated state.[54] Bulky dressings can make it difficult to place the hands in an anti-contracture position[55]; thus, it is imperative to limit dressing girth to enable optimal splint fit.

The superficial nature of tendons and their relative avascularity leads to challenges with deep hand burns, especially on the dorsal surface. Exposed tendons are at great risk for drying and subsequent rupture; thus, finger joints are commonly immobilized.[54] Prompt tissue coverage over exposed tendons can accelerate ROM activity, particularly at the proximal interphalangeal (PIP) joint.

Tendon adherence is another complication associated with deep burns of the hand and forearm. Tendon excursion is required to produce active movement. The combination of the dermal wound-healing process and concomitant immobility associated with sedated patients can result in significant tendon adherence. Adherence should be suspected when active ROM is less than passive ROM. The active movement of the involved flexor or extensor extrinsic muscles should be emphasized when adherence is suspected.

Another complication that can limit active motion is motor loss resulting from peripheral neuropathy.[56] Motor loss can be difficult to assess when a patient cannot follow commands. Neuropathies cause muscle imbalance, and the lack of active movement of the affected area compounds contracture risk. Goals for managing neuropathies should be (1) prevent soft-tissue tightness that results from muscle imbalance and (2) substitute for motor loss with functional splinting. Early recognition is a key for successful management.

Finally, the immobility of sedated patients that suffer hand burns also places their joint capsules and muscle-tendon units at contracture risk. Joint contracture can occur due to capsular and collateral ligament shortening, particularly at the metacarpophalangeal (MCP) joint. The ideal position of the digits is in a "safe" position when splinting to protect these anatomical structures.[54] The safe position consists of positioning the wrist in approximately 20° of extension, MCP joints of the index to small fingers in 70° to 90° of flexion, PIP and distal interphalangeal (DIP) joints in full extension, and the thumb in palmar abduction. This position ensures pretension on the collateral ligaments of the wrist and the MCP, PIP, and DIP joints of the hand, thus prolonging the development of stiffness and contracture.

Activities of daily living
Patient participation in activity of daily living (ADL) promotes active movement to help restore quality of life.[57] This can be challenging in an ICU where the patient may not have sufficient alertness to participate in these activities. Treatment plans should incorporate patient participation in ADL as their cognitive status allows. Success helps restore motion and reestablish a sense of normalcy.[58]

Delirium
Delirium in critically ill patients has the potential to develop from multiple predisposing and precipitating factors[59]; it prolongs hospitalization and increases mortality.[60] Evidence supports the reduction of incident delirium using non-pharmacological multicomponent interventions.[61,62] Concurrent implementation of more than one intervention is demonstrated to be more effective than the use of any single intervention.[63,64] Rehabilitation therapists, functioning as part of a multidisciplinary burn team, can play a significant role in addressing this problem. Therapists can deliver a "disorder of consciousness message" to sedated patients as a standard intervention to support improved consciousness.[65,66] Scripted elements should include information related to orientation, safety, and security, encouraging a sense of control, and reduction of confusion.[67] Soothing elements can be loosely scripted to allow for therapist preference but will focus on a sense of comfort. Sleep deprivation or loss of circadian rhythm (exacerbated by excessive noise and lighting) is another potentially modifiable risk factor.[68] Patient care activities, metabolic consequences of critical illness, mechanical ventilation, and sedative and analgesic medications complicate these issues.[60] Interventions can focus on cognition or orientation, early mobility, hearing, sleep-wake cycle preservation, vision, and hydration.[62]

FUTURE DIRECTIONS

Relatively little is known about the effects of instituting active exercise, whereas the patient is in the BICU. The ACT (Acuity, Contracture, and Time) study was a prospective, observational multicenter study in burn patients. These data showed that increased burn rehabilitation treatment time results in improved functional outcomes, that is, decreased burn scar contracture and loss of motion, but the study was not specific to the BICU.[69] Richard and colleagues[29] reported that research is needed to define the efficacy of early mobility of the critically ill burn patient; there are no pro-spective studies that directly address the use of the tilt table and/or early ambula-tion.[70,71] Thus, it is unknown whether a successful tilt influences morbidity and mortality (ie, BICU length of stay, amount of mechanical support, functional status on discharge).

SUMMARY

Given the complex nature of thermal injury, an interprofessional team approach is essential for optimal outcomes. This includes early occupational and physical rehabil-itation, beginning in the ICU. Burn-specific techniques (focused on edema manage-ment, wound healing, and contracture prevention) are successfully integrated into BICU care. Research demonstrates that early intensive rehabilitation of critically ill burn patients is safe and effective. Further work on the physiologic, functional, and long-term impact of this care is needed.

CLINICS CARE POINTS

- No standard of care currently exists regarding the frequency, duration, intensity, progression, and types of exercise for severely burned patients in the ICU.
- Hands have the highest incidence of contracture and have a significant impact on function and quality of life. Careful attention to and management of hand burns should be a priority beginning in the BICU upon admission.
- Criticailly ill patients have a high potental to develop delirium. Evidence supports the reduction of incident delirium using non-pharmacological multicomponent interventions. This warrents further exploration in the burn popluation.

DISCLOSURE

The opinions or assertions contained herein are the private views of the author and are not to be construed as official or as reflecting the views of the Department of the Army or the Department of Defense.

REFERENCES

1. Church D, Elsayed S, Reid O, et al. Burn wound infections. Clin Microbiol Rev 2006;19(2):403–34.
2. Capek KD, Sousse LE, Hundeshagen G, et al. Contemporary burn survival. J Am Coll Surg 2018;226(4):453–63.
3. Jeschke MG, Pinto R, Kraft R, et al. Morbidity and survival probability in burn pa-tients in modern burn Care. Crit Care Med 2015;43(4):808–15.
4. Cambioso-Daniel J, Suman OE, Jaco M, et al. Treatment for total burn care: burn centers and multidisciplinary burn teams. In: Herdon DN, editor. Total burn care. 5th edition. Edinburgh: Elsevier; 2018. p. 8–13.
5. Brower RG. Consequences of bed rest. Crit Care Med 2009;37(10):S422–8.
6. Pavy-Le Traon A, Heer M, Narici MV, et al. From space to earth: advances in hu-man physiology from 20 years of bed rest studies (1986–2006). Eur J Appl Phys-iol 2007;101(2):143–94.
7. Allen C, Glasziou P, Del Mar C. Bed rest: a potentially harmful treatment needing more careful evaluation. Lancet 1999;354(9186):1229–33.

8. Wieser M, Gisler S, Sarabadani A, et al. Cardiovascular control and stabilization via inclination and mobilization during bed rest. Med Biol Eng Comput 2014; 52(1):53–64.

9. Przkora R, Barrow RE, Jeschke MG, et al. Body composition changes with time in pediatric burn patients. J Traum 2006;60(5):968–71.

10. Klein GL, Herndon DN, Langman CB, et al. Long-term reduction in bone mass after severe burn injury in children. J Pediatr 1995;126(2):252–6.

11. Cambiaso-Daniel J, Rivas E, Carson JS, et al. Cardiorespiratory capacity and strength remain attenuated in children with severe burn injuries at over 3 years postburn. J Pediatr 2018;192:152–8.

12. Ganio MS, Pearson J, Schlader ZJ, et al. Aerobic fitness is disproportionately low in adult burn survivors years after injury. J Burn Care Res 2015;36(4):513–9.

13. Oosterwijk AM, Mouton LJ, Schouten H, et al. Prevalence of scar contractures after burn: A systematic review. Burns 2017;43(1):41–9.

14. Klein MB, Lezotte DC, Heltshe S, et al. Functional and psychosocial outcomes of older adults after burn injury: Results from a multicenter database of severe burn injury. J Burn Care Res 2011;32(1):66–78.

15. Anekwe DE, Biswas S, Bussières A, et al. Early rehabilitation reduces the likelihood of developing intensive care unit-acquired weakness: A systematic review and meta-analysis. Physiotherapy 2020;107:1–10.

16. Doiron KA, Hoffmann TC, Beller EM. Early intervention (mobilization or active exercise) for critically ill adults in the intensive care unit. Cochrane Database Sys Rev 2018;3(3):CD010754.

17. Schujmann DS, Teixeira Gomes T, Lunardi AC, et al. Impact of a progressive mobility program on the functional status, respiratory, and muscular systems of ICU patients: A randomized and controlled trial. Crit Care Med 2020;48(4):491–7.

18. Wang J, Ren D, Liu Y, et al. Effects of early mobilization on the prognosis of critically ill patients: a systematic review and meta-analysis. Int J Nurs Stud 2020; 110:103708.

19. Hodgson CL, Stiller K, Needham DM, et al. Expert consensus and recommendations on safety criteria for active mobilization of mechanically ventilated critically ill adults. Crit Care 2014;18(6):1–9.

20. Tipping CJ, Harrold M, Holland A, et al. The effects of active mobilisation and rehabilitation in ICU on mortality and function: A systematic review. Intensive Care Med 2017;43(2):171–83.

21. Kayambu G, Boots R, Paratz J. Early physical rehabilitation in intensive care patients with sepsis syndromes: a pilot randomised controlled trial. Intensive Care Med 2015;41(5):865–74.

22. Schweickert WD, Pohlman MC, Pohlman AS, et al. Early physical and occupational therapy in mechanically ventilated, critically ill patients: A randomised controlled trial. Lancet 2009;373(9678):1874–82.

23. Bein T, Bischoff M, Brückner U, et al. S2e guideline: positioning and early mobilisation in prophylaxis or therapy of pulmonary disorders: Revision 2015: S2e guideline of the German Society of Anaesthesiology and Intensive Care Medicine (DGAI). Anaesthesist 2015;64(Suppl 1):1–26.

24. Agency for Healthcare Research and Quality. Early mobility guide for reducing ventilator-associated events in mechanically ventilated patients. Johns Hopkins Medicine/Armstrong Institute for Patient Safety and Quality. 2022. Available at: https://www.ahrq.gov/sites/default/files/wysiwyg/professionals/quality-patient-safety/hais/tools/mvp/modules/technical/early-mobility-mvpguide.pdf. Accessed September 02, 2022.

25. Devlin JW, Skrobik Y, Gélinas C, et al. Clinical practice guidelines for the prevention and management of pain, agitation/sedation, delirium, immobility, and sleep disruption in adult patients in the ICU. Crit Care Med 2018;46(9):e825–73.
26. National Institute for Health and Care Excellence (NICE). Rehabilitation after critical illness. Available at: https://www.nice.org.uk/guidance/cg83. Accessed September 02, 2022.
27. Cartotto R, Johnson L, Rood JM, et al. Clinical practice guideline: early mobilization and rehabilitation of critically Ill burn patients. J Burn Care Res 2023;44(1):1–15.
28. Cambiaso-Daniel J, Parry I, Rivas E, et al. Strength and cardiorespiratory exercise rehabilitation for severely burned patients during intensive care units: a survey of practice. J Burn Care Res 2018;39(6):897–901.
29. Richard RL, Hedman TL, Quick CD, et al. A clarion to recommit and reaffirm burn rehabilitation. J Burn Care Res 2008;29(3):425–32.
30. Kramer G, LUND T, Herndon DN. Pathophhysiology of burn shock and burn edema. In: Herdon DN, editor. *Total burn care*. 2nd edition. Philadelphia: WB Saunders; 2002. p. 78–87.
31. Demling RH. The burn edema process: current concepts. J Burn Care Rehabil 2005;26(3):207–27.
32. Hedman TL, Quick CD, Richard R, et al. Rehabilitation of burn casulaties. In: Pasquina PF, Cooper RA, editors. Textbooks in military medicine: Care of the combat amputee. Office of the Surgeon General, United States Army. Washington, D.C.: Falls Churuch & Borden Institute; 2009. p. 277–380.
33. Gordon MD, Gottschlich MM, Helvig EI, et al. Review of evidenced-based practice for the prevention of pressure sores in burn patients. J Burn Care Rehabil 2004;25(5):388–410.
34. Edgar DW, Fear M, Wood FM. A Descriptive study of the temporal patterns of volume and contents change in human acute burn edema: Application in evidence-based intervention and research design. J Burn Care Res 2016;37(5):293–304.
35. Richard R, Miller S, Finley R Jr, et al. Comparison of the effect of passive exercise v static wrapping on finger range of motion in the burned hand. J Burn Care Rehabil 1987;8(6):576–8.
36. Dewey WS, Hedman TL, Chapman TT, et al. The reliability and concurrent validity of the figure-of-eight method of measuring hand edema in patients with burns. J Burn Care Res 2007;28(1):157–62.
37. Shields BA, Carpenter JN, Bustillos BD, et al. The interplay of nutrition, physical activity, severity of illness, and mortality in critically ill burn patients: Is there a connection? J Burn Care Res 2019;40(6):936–42.
38. Parry I, Sen S, Palmieri T, et al. Current Trends in practice for early mobility with the burn population. J Burn Care Res 2018;40(1):29–33.
39. Sarfati C, Moore A, Pilorge C, et al. Efficacy of early passive tilting in minimizing ICU-acquired weakness: a randomized controlled trial. J Crit Care 2018;46:37–43.
40. Chang AT, Boots RJ, Hodges PW, et al. Standing with the assistance of a tilt table improves minute ventilation in chronic critically ill patients. Arch Phys Med Rehabil 2004;85(12):1972–6.
41. Trees DW, Ketelsen CA, Hobbs JA. Use of a modified tilt table for preambulation strength training as an adjunct to burn rehabilitation: a case series. J Burn Care Rehabil 2003;24(2):97–103.
42. Schneider JC, Holavanahalli R, Helm P, et al. Contractures in burn injury: Defining the problem. J Burn Care Res 2006;27(4):508–14.

43. Sheffield CG 3rd, Irons GB, Mucha P Jr, et al. Physical and psychological outcome after burns. J Burn Care Rehabil 1988;9(2):172–7.
44. Leblebici B, Adam M, Bağiş S, et al. Quality of life after burn injury: the impact of joint contracture. J Burn Care Res 2006;27(6):864–8.
45. Richard RL, Lester ME, Miller SF, et al. Identification of cutaneous functional units related to burn scar contracture development. J Burn Care Res 2009;30(4):625–31.
46. Richard R, Lester M, Dewey S. Natural skin and burn scar biomechanic investigation. J Burn Care Res 2012;33(Suppl_1):S126.
47. Richard R, Lester M, Dewey W, et al. Reliability of a video analysis software system to assess dowal hand skin movement. J Burn Care Res 2013;34(suppl_1):S185.
48. Richard R, Ford J, Miller SF, et al. Photographic measurement of volar forearm skin movement with wrist extension: The influence of elbow position. J Burn Care Rehabil 1994;15(1):58–61.
49. Richard R, Parry IS, Santos A, et al. Burn hand or finger goniometric measurements: sum of the isolated parts and the composite whole. J Burn Care Res 2017;38(6):e960–5.
50. Parry I, Richard R, Aden JK, et al. Goniometric measurement of burn scar contracture: a paradigm shift challenging the standard. J Burn Care Res 2019;40(4):377–85.
51. Schneider JC, Holavanahalli R, Helm P, et al. Contractures in burn injury part II: investigating joints of the hand. J Burn Care Res 2008;29(4):606–13.
52. van Zuijlen PP, Kreis RW, Vloemans AF, et al. The prognostic factors regarding long-term functional outcome of full-thickness hand burns. Burns 1999;25(8):709–14.
53. Richard R, Jones JA, Parshley P. Hierarchical decomposition of burn body diagram based on cutaneous functional units and its utility. J Burn Care Res 2015;36(1):33–43.
54. Barillo DJ, Paulsen SM. Management of burns to the hand. Wounds 2003;15(1):4–9.
55. Richard R, Schall S, Staley M, et al. Hand burn splint fabrication: correction for bandage thickness. J Burn Care Rehabil 1994;15(4):369–71.
56. Tu Y, Lineaweaver WC, Zheng X, et al. Burn-related peripheral neuropathy: a systematic review. Burns 2017;43(4):693–9.
57. Colaianni DJ, Provident I, DiBartola LM, et al. A phenomenology of occupation-based hand therapy. Austral Occup Ther J 2015;62(3):177–86.
58. Mata H, Humphry R, Sehorn S, et al. Meaningful occupations impacted by burn injuries. Am J Occup Ther 2017;71(4 Supplement 1). 7111520302p1.
59. Zaal I. Epidemiology of delirium in the intensive care unit, Doctoral dissertation, 2014, Utrecht University.
60. Pun BT, Ely EW. The importance of diagnosing and managing ICU delirium. Chest 2007;132(2):624–36.
61. Bannon L, McGaughey J, Verghis R, et al. The effectiveness of non-pharmacological interventions in reducing the incidence and duration of delirium in critically ill patients: a systematic review and meta-analysis. Intensive Care Med 2019;45(1):1–12.
62. Hshieh TT, Yue J, Oh E, et al. Effectiveness of multicomponent nonpharmacological delirium interventions: a meta-analysis. JAMA Inter Med 2015;175(4):512–20.
63. Mulkey MA, Olson DM, Hardin SR. Top four evidence-based nursing interventions for delirium. Medsurg Nurs 2019;28(6):357–62.

64. Happ MB, Tuite P, Dobbin K, et al. Communication ability, method, and content among nonspeaking nonsurviving patients treated with mechanical ventilation in the intensive care unit. Am J Crit Care 2004;13(3):210–8.

65. Henricson M, Segesten K, Berglund A-L, et al. Enjoying tactile touch and gaining hope when being cared for in intensive care—A phenomenological hermeneutical study. Intensive Crit Care Nurs 2009;25(6):323–31.

66. Puggina ACG, da Silva MJP, Santos JLF. Use of music and voice stimulus on patients with disorders of consciousness. J Neurosci Nurs 2011;43(1):E8–16.

67. Meghani S, Punjani NS. Does communication really a matter of concern in unconscious patients? J Nurs 2014;4(3):16–9.

68. Pulak LM, Jensen L. Sleep in the intensive care unit: a review. J Intensive Care Med 2016;31(1):14–23.

69. Richard R, Dewey W, Anyan W, et al. Increased burn rehabilitation treatment time improves patient outcome. J Burn Care Res 2014;35(3):S100.

70. de Figueiredo TB, Utsunomiya KF, de Oliveira A, et al. Mobilization practices for patients with burn injury in critical care. Burns 2020;46(2):314–21.

71. O'Neil AM, Rush C, Griffard L, et al. 5 -year retrospective analysis of a vented mobility algorithm in the burn ICU. J Burn Care Res 2022;43(5):1129–34.

Pharmacologic Management of Pain, Agitation, and Delirium in Burn Patients

Kaitlin A. Pruskowski, PharmD, BCPS, BCCCP, FCCM[a,b,*],
Maximilian Feth, MD[a,c], Linda Hong, MD[a],
Amanda R. Wiggins, MD[a]

KEYWORDS

- Burn • Pain • Agitation • Delirium • Critical care

KEY POINTS

- A multimodal analgesic regimen should include long-acting opioids, a gabapentinoid, acetaminophen, and as-needed opioids and other adjuncts.
- In most patients, the use of benzodiazepines should be avoided or minimized.
- Non-pharmacologic strategies should be implemented for the prevention of delirium, as pharmacologic strategies have not been shown to prevent or shorten its duration. Pharmacologic agents may need to be considered if extreme symptoms of hyperactive delirium are present to ensure the safety of the patient, staff members, and fresh autografts.

INTRODUCTION

Pain, agitation, and delirium are common during postburn hospitalization. Often, one of these complications can exacerbate the others, causing greater distress for the patient. Furthermore, critically ill patients present with additional layers of complexity. A multidisciplinary team with a multimodal approach can help mitigate symptoms and prevent further harm. This review aims to guide in managing these complicated patients in a critical-care setting.

PAIN

Burns are among the most painful types of injuries one can experience. Pain that is not appropriately or adequately managed can lead to anxiety and delirium in the acute

[a] US Army Institute of Surgical Research, 3698 Chambers Pass, ATTN: FCMR-SRT, JBSA Fort Sam, Houston, TX 78234, USA; [b] Uniformed Services University, 4301 Jones Bridge Road, Bethesda, MD 20814, USA; [c] Department of Anaesthesiology, Intensive Care Medicine, Emergency Medicine and Pain Therapy, Federal Armed Forces Hospital Ulm, Oberer Eselsberg 40, 89081, Ulm, Germany
* Corresponding author. US Army Institute of Surgical Research, 3698 Chambers Pass, ATTN: FCMR-SRT, JBSA Fort Sam, Houston, TX 78234.
E-mail address: Kaitlin.a.pruskowski.civ@health.mil

Surg Clin N Am 103 (2023) 495–504
https://doi.org/10.1016/j.suc.2023.02.003
0039-6109/23/© 2023 Elsevier Inc. All rights reserved.
surgical.theclinics.com

setting. Burn pain can be categorized as background pain, neuropathic pain, procedural pain, and breakthrough pain. As such, a multimodal approach to pain management must be taken.

Patient Evaluation

If able, self-report is the preferred method of evaluating pain.[1] For patients who are unable to self-report pain, a validated non-verbal pain scale, such as the Critical Care Pain Observation Tool, should be used to ensure that pain is being appropriately managed.[1] Pain assessments should be performed several times per day. After every change in a patient's analgesic regimen, the patient must be re-evaluated not only for improvement in pain control, but also for any untoward effects of the change. In addition, the American Burn Association recommends that the Burn-Specific Pain Anxiety Scale be used as one of the assessment tools.[1] This scale employs nine different components to evaluate: feelings of worry about wound healing, tension and fear of losing control during dressing changes, anxious anticipation of pain during or after medical procedures, and feeling 'on edge' because of enduring pain.[2]

Goal Setting

Goal setting and expectation management are paramount in pain management. Burn patients should understand that medical management will not alleviate all pain. Instead, the goal should be to make pain manageable so that they can participate in their own care, including rehabilitation and dressing changes.

Non-pharmacologic options

Non-pharmacologic strategies for pain management, including music, massage, aromatherapy, and virtual reality have been studied in the burn population with some positive results.[3] As this review focuses on pharmacologic management, these strategies will not be discussed in detail.

Pharmacologic Options

Background pain is the pain that is constantly felt after a burn injury. Agents that are typically used to address background pain include long-acting opioids, methadone, and acetaminophen. If long-acting opioids are not feasible, a scheduled short-acting opioid may be considered. Methadone is an attractive option for background pain, as it has multiple mechanisms of action, including agonism at the mu-opioid receptors and antagonism at the N-methyl-D-aspartate (NMDA) receptors. Additionally, methadone has a long half-life, ranging from 8 to 59 hours.[4] When methadone is initiated early postburn, it may reduce the duration of mechanical ventilation.[5] This agent can prolong the corrected QT interval (QTc) and is metabolized by multiple cytochrome P 450 (CYP) enzymes, which can lead to drug interactions.[4]

Acetaminophen is a non-opioid adjunct that has not been well-studied in burns. Meyer and colleagues[6] showed that the background pain could be controlled with acetaminophen alone in pediatric burn patients. In non-burn adult surgical populations, acetaminophen dosed at 1 g every 6 hours decreased the amount of opioids required.[7–9] Although these studies utilized intravenous acetaminophen, a study by Jibril and colleagues[10] showed that intravenous acetaminophen was not more effective than enterally administered acetaminophen. Despite the lack of literature, acetaminophen should be considered as an adjunct for background postburn pain management.

Neuropathic pain can be characterized as burning dysesthesia, hyperalgesia, and neuralgic episodes.[11] This can be due to direct nerve damage or inflammation of the nerves after injury. The gabapentinoids, gabapentin and pregabalin, are the mainstays of neuropathic pain management in non-burn patients. However, these agents have shown mixed results in burn patients. Gray and colleagues reported that the addition of gabapentin improved neuropathic pain, but Wibbenmeyer and colleagues reported that it did not affect neuropathic pain or opioid consumption.[11,12] Pregabalin has been studied less. Gray and colleagues[13] saw a decrease in neuropathic pain after burn injury, but no difference in opioid consumption. Despite the conflicting literature, gabapentinoids should be considered for the management of postburn neuropathic pain.

Procedural pain is associated with procedures including dressing changes, rehabilitation sessions, and line changes. With long hospital stays and repeated procedures, patients can have anxiety about upcoming procedures, which in turn can intensify their pain. In this event, anxiolytics and other strategies to address anxiety should be administered. These agents will be discussed below. For the pain component of procedural pain, as-needed opioids should be administered. Patients can be premedicated with an enteral opioid approximately 45 to 60 minutes before the start of the procedure; opioids can be re-dosed as needed throughout the procedure. Additionally, ketamine, dexmedetomidine, or intravenous lidocaine can be used during the procedure.[14–16]

Breakthrough pain is the intensification of pain not associated with a procedure or rehabilitation. This type of pain should be managed with an as-needed intravenous or enteral opioid.

Regional anesthesia, to include peripheral-nerve blocks, can be utilized in multimodal pain-management strategies in the perioperative period. Peripheral-nerve blocks can be performed as a single-shot injection that results in approximately 12 to 18 hours of analgesia, or through the insertion of a continuous peripheral-nerve catheter which provides analgesia for up to 7 days.[17] Such blocks reduce general anesthesia requirements, improve postoperative pain, facilitate rehabilitation,[18] reduce systemic analgesic consumption, and decrease opioid side effects.[19] It is important to weigh the need for analgesia against the need to minimize motor weakness to allow for rehabilitation.

Summary

There are several components of burn pain, and each one is treated with different agents. A multimodal pain regimen should be employed to address all aspects of burn pain. A typical regimen may include a long-acting opioid or methadone, acetaminophen, a gabapentinoid, and as-needed opioids.

AGITATION

Agitation is defined as an elevation of psychomotor activity leading to a loss of control or a cognitive disturbance. It is seen in up to 70% of intensive care unit (ICU) patients.[20,21] Agitation is associated with an increase in sedation, ICU and ventilator days, ICU-related infections, and ICU-acquired weakness. Inadequate agitation management predisposes ICU patients to an increased risk of falls and of accidental or self-removal of devices, tubes, and lines. Agitation also poses a risk for the critical-care team and increases their workload significantly. The assessment and treatment of agitation and delirium should always be based on decisions by a multidisciplinary team (nurses, doctors, pharmacists).[22]

Risk factors for agitation include patient factors as well as setting-specific aspects (**Table 1**). Almeida and colleagues[23] identified pain and delirium during critical care as

Table 1
Common causes of agitation in ICU settings

Medical causes	• Metabolic disorders (hypo/hypernatremia, hypo/hyperglycemia) • Sepsis • Ventilator dyssynchrony • Respiratory distress (hypoxia, hypercapnia) • Neurological events (stroke, seizures) • Urinary or fecal retention
Medication or substance withdrawal	• Alcohol • Opioids • Hypnotics
Drug-induced causes	• Ketamine • Opioids • Anti-infectives (eg, fluroquinolones) • Anti-convulsives (eg, valproic acid) • Corticosteroids
Burn-specific causes	• Anxiety induced by the burn itself • Anxiety induced by painful burn-care procedures
ICU-specific causes	• Painful ICU procedures • Anxiety induced by the ICU setting • Sleep deprivation • Miscommunication between provider team and patient

well as mechanical ventilation and smoking habits as risk factors for agitation. Anxiety is frequently seen in burn patients and can be another cause of agitation. In the acute phase after burn injury, common causes of anxiety are fear of death, the loss of control, or an upcoming burn-care procedure. Additionally, pre-injury anxiety disorders can also increase anxiety levels during critical care.[24]

According to the 2018 Pain, Agitation and Delirium guidelines by the Society of Critical Care Medicine, the treatment of agitation, anxiety, and sedation in critically ill patients should follow a standardized multi-step approach.[25] Anxiety and pain share a bidirectional relationship: pain might lead to anxiety and anxiety might lead to a sensation of pain.[26] However, both anxiety and pain might result in higher agitation levels. Hence, approaches in the management of critically ill patients should not focus on agitation exclusively, but evaluate the complex of agitation, pain, and anxiety.

Patient Evaluation

Routine assessment of agitation and sedation levels should be performed several times per day. For agitation and sedation, the Richmond Agitation and Sedation Scale (RASS) can be utilized as a monitoring tool in ICU settings with RASS +2 as a cut-off for intervention.[27]

Non-Pharmacologic Options

Non-pharmacological approaches, such as the evaluation and resolution of treatable causes, should always be the first step in the management of agitation. This should be tailored to a patient's needs instead of providing a standard pharmacological treatment without focusing on the underlying condition. Even in intubated patients, good communication between the medical team and the patient increases patient comfort. Non-pharmacological treatment of agitation might also focus on sleep (quality, rhythmicity), early mobilization, noise management, family comfort, and patient positioning.

For intubated patients, ventilator settings should be checked in case of sudden agitation to detect ventilator dyssynchrony. Restraint of patients should only be used when non-pharmacological and pharmacological interventions are not successful.[28]

Pharmacologic Options

Pharmacologic agents used for the management of agitation can cause excessive or prolonged sedation in the ICU and lead to adverse events, including short-term and long-term cognitive impairment or mortality.[29,30] Before initiating such agents, organic causes should be evaluated and corrected. Sedative agents have been administered intensively to reduce anxiety and distress in the critically ill for decades. However, certain sedatives and the depth of sedation increase morbidity and mortality and impair cognitive outcomes after ICU discharge. Therefore, current guidelines recommend lighter sedation targets (RASS -1 to +1), or avoidance of sedative agents.[31] A daily sedation interruption according to a local protocol should be performed.[32]

Short-acting drugs should be utilized as first-line agents. Light sedation levels can be achieved by multimodal approaches, reducing doses of single sedative agents, and avoiding accumulation and tolerance.[33] Sedation regimens should be based on a patient's circadian rhythm. They might consist of a baseline sedative plus a titratable sedative as needed to adjust sedation levels, for example, to enable procedures. Although they have been used extensively in the ICU, benzodiazepines lead to prolonged mechanical ventilation; increase the risk for and duration of delirium; and should, therefore, be avoided for most ICU patients.[34] However, in special populations, such as patients with alcohol withdrawal syndrome, benzodiazepines might be used as an adjunct in a multimodal treatment approach.[35] Despite the evidence, midazolam was shown in 2018 to be the leading sedative agent used in burn units.[36,37] Instead of benzodiazepines, propofol, ketamine, or dexmedetomidine should be considered,[38-40] but dexmedetomidine and propofol may cause hypotension in the burn shock period.

Due to its neutral effects on hemodynamics and its analgesic potential, ketamine is an attractive option for sedation in critically ill burn patients. In recent years, some retrospective studies have found that ketamine reduced opioid and other analgesic requirements.[41-43] Crowley and colleagues[44] found valproic acid to reduce the incidence of agitation and delirium in ICU patients without increased rates of adverse events. Gagnon and colleagues[45] demonstrated a reduction in the incidence of agitation with a course of valproic acid in critically ill patients.

Summary

Recent research has focused on alternatives to sedative agents such as benzodiazepines in the management of agitation, especially in non-intubated patients. Larger trials on agitation management are needed.

DELIRIUM

Delirium is a temporary disturbance in cognition, attention, and awareness.[46] Delirium is a common hospital-acquired condition; up to 80% of burn ICU patients will develop delirium.[47] There are numerous risk factors for the development of delirium in burn patients, including older age, receipt of higher doses of benzodiazepines, alcohol use before injury, burn size larger than 10% Total Body Surface Area (TBSA), need for surgical intervention, and American Society of Anaesthesiologists Physical Status Classification System (ASA) score of 3 or greater.[47,48] Additional risk factors for delirium seen in critically ill patients include receipt of multiple blood transfusions, prior coma, dementia, and use of psychoactive medications.[25] Agarwal and colleagues[47] showed that higher doses of opiates and the addition of methadone showed a decreased risk of delirium.

Patient Evaluation

Patients should be routinely (at least once per shift) assessed for delirium using a tool such as the Confusion Assessment Method for the ICU or the Intensive Care Delirium Screening Checklist.[25] They should be used in conjunction with a sedation scale to determine whether a patient is experiencing hypoactive, hyperactive, or mixed delirium. Despite these recommendations, a recent survey among burn providers showed that 57.5% of respondents did not use a specific or validated tool when assessing patients for delirium.[36]

Prevention

The Society of Critical Care Medicine does not recommend the use of pharmacologic agents, including haloperidol, dexmedetomidine, or risperidone, for the prevention of delirium. These agents do not reduce the incidence of delirium or improve other outcomes. Instead, non-pharmacologic strategies should be implemented. For example, the ABCDEF Bundle includes assessing, managing, and treating pain; performing spontaneous awakening and breathing trials daily; choosing analgesics and sedatives that do not increase the risk of delirium; assessing, preventing, and managing delirium if/when it occurs; early mobility and exercise; and family engagement.[49]

Pharmacologic Options

If a patient develops delirium, the routine use of pharmacologic agents is not recommended.[25] Pharmacologic agents including atypical antipsychotics have not been shown to decrease the duration of delirium or improve outcomes.[50–52] However, if the patient is exhibiting extreme symptoms of hyperactive delirium, a pharmacologic agent, including dexmedetomidine or atypical antipsychotics, may be considered to ensure the safety of the patient, staff members, and any fresh autografts. Agents such as dexmedetomidine may also be considered if hyperactive delirium is precluding extubation.[25]

Outcomes

In burn patients, the development of delirium has been associated with longer ICU and hospital lengths of stay, longer duration of mechanical ventilation, increased cost of hospitalization, and increased risk of mortality.[47,48,53] Additionally, delirium has been associated with cognitive impairment up to 12 months after ICU discharge.[54]

Summary

The majority of patients admitted to a burn ICU will develop delirium. The routine use of pharmacologic agents to prevent or treat delirium is not recommended. Instead, non-pharmacologic strategies, including the ABCDEF Bundle should be implemented.

CLINICS CARE POINTS

Pain
- A multimodal analgesic regimen should include long-acting opioids, a gabapentinoid, acetaminophen, and as-needed opioids and other adjuncts.
- The patient's self-report of pain is the key. Pain should be assessed several times per day using a validated pain tool.

- The team should set goals for pain control and manage expectations; it is unlikely that medical management will completely alleviate pain, but the goal should be to make the pain tolerable so that the patient can participate in their care.

Anxiety
- In most patients, the use of benzodiazepines should be avoided or minimized.
- The use of ketamine infusions can be considered to provide sedation and analgesia, but there is limited literature to support this.
- The use of dexmedetomidine and propofol should be avoided during the burn shock phase due to the adverse effects of hypotension and bradycardia. Later, in a burn patient's hospital stay, these agents may be safe.

Delirium
- Non-pharmacologic strategies should be implemented for prevention, as pharmacologic strategies have not been shown to prevent or shorten the duration of delirium.
- Pharmacologic agents may need to be considered if extreme symptoms of hyperactive delirium are present to ensure the safety of the patient, staff members, and fresh autografts.

SUMMARY

Both clinical and functional outcomes in burn patients are affected by symptoms of pain, agitation, and delirium. Due to the complexity of burn injuries, a multimodal pain approach is often most effective. This entails both pharmacologic and non-pharmacologic treatments. When addressing anxiety and delirium, first trialing non-pharmacologic management is recommended. Pharmacologic treatment of delirium and anxiety in these patients is dependent on the risk to the patient and the underlying cause. Treating these problems will help decrease ICU length of stay, duration of mechanical ventilation, and hospital costs; and improve quality of life.

DISCLOSURE

The opinions or assertions contained herein are the private views of the author and are not to be construed as official or as reflecting the views of the Department of the Army or the Department of Defense. The authors have nothing to disclose.

REFERENCES

1. Romanowski KS, Carson J, Pape K, et al. American Burn Association guidelines on the management of acute pain in the adult burn patient: a review of the literature, a compilation of expert opinion, and next steps. J Burn Care Res 2020; 41(6):1129–51.
2. Taal LA, Faber AW. The burn specific pain anxiety scale: introduction of a reliable and valid measure. Burns 1997;23(2):147–50.
3. Kim DE, Pruskowski KA, Ainsworth CR, et al. A review of adjunctive therapies for burn injury pain during the opioid crisis. J Burn Care Res 2019;40(6):983–95.
4. Dolophine [package insert]. NJ: West-Ward Pharmaceuticals Corp. Eatontown; 2018.
5. Jones GM, Porter K, Coffey R, et al. Impact of early methadone initiation in critically injured burn patients: a pilot study. J Burn Care Res 2013;34(3):342–8.
6. Meyer WJ 3rd, Nichols RJ, Cortiella J, et al. Acetaminophen in the management of background pain in children post-burn. J Pain Symptom Manage 1997;13(1):50–5.
7. Memis D, Inal MT, Kavalci G, et al. Intravenous paracetamol reduced the use of opioids, extubation time, and opioid-related adverse effects after major surgery in intensive care unit. J Crit Care 2010;25(3):458–62.

8. Pettersson PH, Jakobsson J, Owall A. Intravenous acetaminophen reduced the use of opioids compared with oral administration after coronary artery bypass grafting. J Cardiothorac Vasc Anesth 2005;19(3):306–9.

9. Jelacic S, Bollag L, Bowdle A, et al. Intravenous acetaminophen as an adjunct analgesic in cardiac surgery reduces opioid consumption but not opioid-related adverse effects: a randomized controlled trial. J Cardiothorac Vasc Anesth 2016;30(4):997–1004.

10. Jibril F, Sharaby S, Mohamed A, et al. Intravenous versus oral acetaminophen for pain: systematic review of current evidence to support clinical decision-making. Can J Hosp Pharm 2015;68(3):238–47.

11. Gray P, Williams B, Cramond T. Successful use of gabapentin in acute pain management following burn injury: a case series. Pain Med 2008;9(3):371–6.

12. Wibbenmeyer L, Eid A, Liao J, et al. Gabapentin is ineffective as an analgesic adjunct in the immediate postburn period. J Burn Care Res 2014;35(2):136–42.

13. Gray P, Kirby J, Smith MT, et al. Pregabalin in severe burn injury pain: a double-blind, randomised placebo-controlled trial. Pain 2011;152(6):1279–88.

14. Asmussen S, Maybauer DM, Fraser JF, et al. A meta-analysis of analgesic and sedative effects of dexmedetomidine in burn patients. Burns 2013;39(4):625–31.

15. Kundra P, Velayudhan S, Krishnamachari S, et al. Oral ketamine and dexmedetomidine in adults' burns wound dressing–A randomized double blind cross over study. Burns 2013;39(6):1150–6.

16. Wasiak J, Mahar P, McGuinness SK, et al. Intravenous lidocaine for the treatment of background or procedural burn pain. Cochrane Database Syst Rev 2012;(6): Cd005622.

17. Sheckter CC, Stewart BT, Barnes C, et al. Techniques and strategies for regional anesthesia in acute burn care-a narrative review. Burns Trauma 2021;9:tkab015.

18. Bittner EA, Shank E, Woodson L, et al. Acute and perioperative care of the burn-injured patient. Anesthesiology 2015;122(2):448–64.

19. Grunzweig KA, Son J, Kumar AR. Regional anesthetic blocks for donor site pain in burn patients: a meta-analysis on efficacy, outcomes, and cost. Plast Surg (Oakv). 2020;28(4):222–31.

20. Jaber S, Chanques G, Altairac C, et al. A prospective study of agitation in a medical-surgical ICU: incidence, risk factors, and outcomes. Chest 2005; 128(4):2749–57.

21. Fraser GL, Prato BS, Riker RR, et al. Frequency, severity, and treatment of agitation in young versus elderly patients in the ICU. Pharmacotherapy 2000;20(1): 75–82.

22. Heim M, Draheim R, Krupp A, et al. Evaluation of a multidisciplinary pain, agitation, and delirium guideline in mechanically ventilated critically ill adults. Hosp Pharm 2019;54(2):119–24.

23. Almeida TM, Azevedo LC, Nosé PM, et al. Risk factors for agitation in critically ill patients. Rev Bras Ter Intensiva 2016;28(4):413–9.

24. Obed D, Schroeter A, Gruber L, et al. Outcomes following burn injury in intensive care patients with major psychiatric disorders. Burns. Epub 20220630.

25. Devlin JW, Skrobik Y, Gélinas C, et al. Clinical practice guidelines for the prevention and management of pain, agitation/sedation, delirium, immobility, and sleep disruption in adult patients in the ICU. Crit Care Med 2018;46(9):e825–73.

26. Taal LA, Faber AW. Post-traumatic stress, pain and anxiety in adult burn victims. Burns 1997;23(7–8):545–9.

27. Sessler CN, Gosnell MS, Grap MJ, et al. the richmond agitation-sedation scale: validity and reliability in adult intensive care unit patients. Am J Respir Crit Care Med 2002;166(10):1338–44.
28. Cui N, Yan X, Zhang Y, et al. Non-Pharmacological interventions for minimizing physical restraints use in intensive care units: An umbrella review. Front Med 2022;9:806945.
29. Kollef MH, Levy NT, Ahrens TS, et al. The use of continuous i.v. sedation is associated with prolongation of mechanical ventilation. Chest 1998;114(2):541–8.
30. Shehabi Y, Bellomo R, Reade MC, Bailey M, Bass F, Howe B, et al. Early intensive care sedation predicts long-term mortality in ventilated critically ill patients. Am J Respir Crit Care Med 2012;186(8):724–31.
31. Shehabi Y, Bellomo R, Reade MC, Bailey M, Bass F, Howe B, et al. Early goal-directed sedation versus standard sedation in mechanically ventilated critically ill patients: a pilot study. Crit Care Med 2013;41(8):1983–91.
32. Mehta S, Burry L, Cook D, Fergusson D, Steinberg M, Granton J, et al. Daily sedation interruption in mechanically ventilated critically ill patients cared for with a sedation protocol: a randomized controlled trial. JAMA 2012;308(19):1985–92.
33. Zhou Y, Jin X, Kang Y, et al, Liang G, Liu T, Deng N. Midazolam and propofol used alone or sequentially for long-term sedation in critically ill, mechanically ventilated patients: a prospective, randomized study. Crit Care 2014;18(3):R122.
34. Riker RR, Shehabi Y, Bokesch PM, Ceraso D, Wisemandle W, Koura F, et al. Dexmedetomidine vs midazolam for sedation of critically ill patients: a randomized trial. JAMA 2009;301(5):489–99.
35. Weinberg JA, Magnotti LJ, Fischer PE, Edwards NM, Schroeppel T, Fabian TC, et al. Comparison of intravenous ethanol versus diazepam for alcohol withdrawal prophylaxis in the trauma ICU: results of a randomized trial. J Trauma 2008;64(1):99–104.
36. Depetris N, Raineri S, Pantet O, et al, Lavrentieva A. Management of pain, anxiety, agitation and delirium in burn patients: a survey of clinical practice and a review of the current literature. Ann Burns Fire Disasters 2018;31(2):97–108.
37. Lavrentieva A, Depetris N, Rodini I. Analgesia, sedation and arousal status in burn patients: the gap between recommendations and current practices. Ann Burns Fire Disasters 2017;30(2):135–42.
38. Srivastava VK, Agrawal S, Kumar S, et al, Mishra A, Sharma S, Kumar R. Comparison of dexmedetomidine, propofol and midazolam for short-term sedation in postoperatively mechanically ventilated neurosurgical patients. J Clin Diagn Res 2014;8(9):Gc04–7.
39. Hall RI, Sandham D, Cardinal P, Tweeddale M, Moher D, Wang X, et al. Propofol vs midazolam for ICU sedation : a Canadian multicenter randomized trial. Chest 2001;119(4):1151–9.
40. Enomoto Y, Iwagami M, Tsuchiya A, Morita K, Abe T, Kido T, et al. Dexmedetomidine use and mortality in mechanically ventilated patients with severe burns: A cohort study using a national inpatient database in Japan. Burns 2021;47(7):1502–10.
41. Pruskowski KA, Harbourt K, Pajoumand M, et al, Chui SJ, Reynolds HN. Impact of ketamine use on adjunctive analgesic and sedative bedications in critically ill trauma patients. Pharmacotherapy 2017;37(12):1537–44.
42. Groetzinger LM, Rivosecchi RM, Bain W, Bahr M, Chin K, McVerry BJ, et al. Ketamine infusion for adjunct sedation in mechanically ventilated adults. Pharmacotherapy 2018;38(2):181–8.

43. Garber PM, Droege CA, Carter KE, et al, Harger NJ, Mueller EW. Continuous Infusion Ketamine for adjunctive analgosedation in mechanically ventilated, critically ill patients. Pharmacotherapy 2019;39(3):288–96.
44. Crowley KE, Urben L, Hacobian G, et al, Geiger KL. Valproic acid for the management of agitation and delirium in the intensive care setting: a retrospective analysis. Clin Ther 2020;42(4):e65–73.
45. Gagnon DJ, Fontaine GV, Smith KE, Riker RR, Miller RR 3rd, Lerwick PA, et al. Valproate for agitation in critically ill patients: a retrospective study. J Crit Care 2017;37:119–25.
46. Association AP. Diagnostic and statistical manual of mental disorders (DSM-5). Arlington, VA: American Psychiatric Pub; 2013.
47. Agarwal V, O'Neill PJ, Cotton BA, Pun BT, Haney S, Thompson J, et al. Prevalence and risk factors for development of delirium in burn intensive care unit patients. J Burn Care Res 2010;31(5):706–15.
48. Stanley GHM, Barber ARJ, O'Brien AM, Hamill C, Boardman G, Frear CC, et al. Delirium in hospitalised adults with acute burns - A systematic review. Burns 2022;48(5):1040–54.
49. Marra A, Ely EW, Pandharipande PP, et al, Patel MB. The ABCDEF bundle in critical care. Crit Care Clin 2017;33(2):225–43.
50. Girard TD, Pandharipande PP, Carson SS, Schmidt GA, Wright PE, Canonico AE, et al. Feasibility, efficacy, and safety of antipsychotics for intensive care unit delirium: The MIND randomized, placebo-controlled trial. Crit Care Med 2010; 38(2):428–37.
51. Page VJ, Ely EW, Gates S, Zhao XB, Alce T, Shintani A, et al. Effect of intravenous haloperidol on the duration of delirium and coma in critically ill patients (Hope-ICU): A randomised, double-blind, placebo-controlled trial. Lancet Respir Med 2013;1(7):515–23.
52. Devlin JW, Roberts RJ, Fong JJ, Skrobik Y, Riker RR, Hill NS, et al. Efficacy and safety of quetiapine in critically ill patients with delirium: a prospective, multi-center, randomized, double-blind, placebo-controlled pilot study. Crit Care Med 2010;38(2):419–27.
53. Holmes EG, Jones SW, Laughon SL. A retrospective analysis of neurocognitive impairment in older patients with burn injuries. Psychosomatics 2017;58(4): 386–94.
54. Wolters AE, van Dijk D, Pasma W, Cremer OL, Looije MF, de Lange DW, et al. Long-term outcome of delirium during intensive care unit stay in survivors of critical illness: a prospective cohort study. Crit Care 2014;18(3):R125.

Long-Term Outcomes in Burn Patients

Julia Bryarly, MD, Karen Kowalske, MD*

KEYWORDS

- Burn • Outcomes • Complication • Function • Rehabilitation

KEY POINTS

- Burn survivors have many complications unrelated to skin closure including contracture, neuropathy, and heterotopic ossification.
- Significant psychological distress, difficulty with return to work, and community reentry are common.
- Major burn injury is a chronic disease and survivors are at risk for systemic complications such as recurrent pneumonia, renal failure, venous stasis, and musculoskeletal impairment.

INTRODUCTION

Since the 1970s, there has been an increased awareness of the importance of nonsurgical interventions for burn care. Physical and occupational therapies have become mainstays in the burn unit. The importance of positioning to prevent contractures and early mobilization has been well described. More recently, attention has turned to looking beyond the acute hospitalization at issues that are ongoing challenges for burn survivors. This was emphasized at the 2012 American Burn Association (ABA) Burn Quality Consensus conference.[1] This forum published a series of recommendations regarding important quality-of-care requirements to improve patient outcomes. This article will review approaches to complications and discuss the emerging information related to long-term outcomes.

CONTRACTURE

Contraction occurs naturally during wound healing following a burn. This can lead to scar contracture, loss of range of motion (ROM), and eventual joint contracture if contraction continues beyond reepithelialization.[2] Following a hospitalization for burn, scar contracture is present in 38% to 54% at discharge. More than a third had major joint contracture, most commonly affecting the shoulder, elbow, or knee.[3,4]

Physical Medicine and Rehabilitation, University of Texas, Southwestern Medical Center, 5323 Harry Hines Boulevard, Dallas, TX 75235-9055, USA
* Corresponding author.
E-mail address: Karen.kowalske@utsouthwestern.edu

Surg Clin N Am 103 (2023) 505–513
https://doi.org/10.1016/j.suc.2023.02.004
0039-6109/23/© 2023 Elsevier Inc. All rights reserved.

Treatment is largely preventative, directed at minimization of the formation of the contracture. However, more research is needed with respect to timing, frequency, or aggressiveness of therapy. There is some evidence that mechanical tension or stretch can induce fibroblast differentiation into myofibroblasts leading to scar hypertrophy.[2] However, most clinicians would agree that scar management, stretching, splinting, serial casting, and surgery are useful to help preserve ROM or correct contracture. Massage therapy and manual elongation techniques have shown some evidence of benefit, decreasing pain and pruritus. There is less objective evidence for use of massage than for some other conservative measures such as pressure and silicon therapy with respect scar quality but guidelines on timing, amount of pressure, or duration are lacking.[5–7] For cases in which contracture has already formed, serial casting may be used to regain ROM. In our experience, use of botulinum toxin (Botox) coupled with casting and physiotherapy may improve ROM and limit progression of contracture in certain cases when spasticity is not present. Progressive treatment techniques alone, such as dynamic or static progressive splinting or serial casting, appear able to rapidly correct contracture compared with a multimodal approach; however, there is little consensus on optimal timing of initiation, duration, or positioning of splints. Varied techniques have been described, suggesting more research is needed before evidence-based protocols are developed.[8–11]

When conservative methods fail to correct contracture, more invasive methods such as intralesional steroid injections, laser treatments and surgical techniques can improve scar quality and improve ROM.

NEUROPATHY

Burn-related peripheral neuropathy can lead to substantial impairment resulting in limb weakness, sensory disturbance, pruritus, and/or neuropathic pain. Symptoms of neuropathy can develop as early as the first-week postburn (as with neuropathic pain) but more frequently emerge through the course of recovery (as with compressive neuropathy).[12] Insult to the nerves directly occurs with flame and electrical injury, whereas indirect means of injury can also occur in the context of compression, metabolic derangements, vascular occlusion, neurotoxic factors, and circulating inflammatory cytokines.[13] The association between burn injury and peripheral neuropathy in the literature varies considerably, with studies reporting rates ranging from 2% to 84% of patients—depending on the methodology and inclusion criteria used. In a large retrospective study of patients with major burn injury, Kowalske and colleagues found the incidence of generalized peripheral neuropathy and/or mononeuropathy to be approximately 10%.[13] More severe burns are associated with a higher incidence of peripheral neuropathy. Electrical injury frequently causes nerve injury, with 90% of such patients presenting with mononeuropathy.[13]

The typical patterns seen following burn are consistent with mononeuropathy, mononeuritis multiplex, or generalized polyneuropathy, with median sensory mononeuropathy being the most common of these.[14] Generalized peripheral neuropathy is the least common pattern among burn patients. It is reported to occur 3% of those severely burned, particularly those with extended intensive care unit stays, and presents similarly to critical-illness neuropathy.[13]

Iatrogenic compression injuries—caused by splinting, positioning, or bulky dressings—can all result in neuropathy. Most neuropathies are actually present within the first-week postburn, and thus are more likely due to injury-related factors such as microvascular ischemia.[15] With time, hypertrophic scarring, contracture, and heterotopic ossification (HO) can also cause compressive neuropathy.[12] Because HO most commonly occurs at the posterior elbow in burn patients, there is potential for compromise of the ulnar nerve at that location. Ulnar nerve palsy can result in intrinsic hand weakness, impaired sensation, and pain, leading to significant functional impairment.

Neuropathic pain can develop in the context of any of the above neuropathies. It may be poorly characterized by patients but is often described as a sharp, pins-and-needles, electric, or burning sensation. In a large retrospective study, Klifto concluded that the prevalence of chronic neuropathic pain (CNP) was 6% in those with upper extremity burns at a single center. CNP was associated with older age, alcohol or substance abuse, current daily smoking, larger total body surface area (TBSA) burned, third-degree burns, inhalation injury, more surgery, and longer hospital stay.[16] CNP combined with postburn pruritus can be devastating for patients, lowering quality of life. The incidence is reported as high as 93% at hospital discharge and as high as 70% at more than a decade postburn.[17–20] Pruritus can be so bothersome for patients that it is associated with increased rates of depression and suicidality.[21,22] Risks include TBSA and number of surgical interventions but it is also related to female gender and symptoms of PTSD.[19]

Treatment modalities of neuropathy and related neuropathic pain include the use of pharmaceuticals, autologous fat grafting, early wound excision, and surgical decompression. Opioids are not indicated for neuropathic pain or itch after burn injury. Gabapentin or pregabalin are the drugs of choice.[23,24] Topical lidocaine has been effective in treating pain in animal models and also can be effective at treating pruritus but seems less effective in most burn survivors. Other topicals including doxepin and ketamine-lidocaine-amitriptyline have also shown promise.[20] Physiotherapy can improve ROM of the joints associated with compression of the nerve and can improve weakness and impaired function through compensatory strategies. Somatosensory rehabilitation has also been proposed as novel nonpharmacologic treatment. In a case series, Nedelec and colleagues found that about 50% of patients from a group of 17 either had resolution of allodynia or had improved sensation for light touch.[25] Massage along the length of the scar is also associated with decreased reports of pain and pruritus.[5] Furthermore addressing underlying exacerbating comorbidities such as smoking, alcohol use, diabetes, and poor nutritional status are important to improving the health of the nerve.

Approximately half of the patients with chronic pain did not respond to treatment.[16] A significant subset of burn patients continue to experience debilitating symptoms long after injury, suggesting that there is a need for better treatment of neuropathy and associated neuropathic pain.[26,27]

HETEROTOPIC OSSIFICATION

Heterotopic ossification (HO) is a process in which osseous lesions develop within soft tissue and develop into mature lamellar bone.[28] The pathophysiology of HO is not known. Cases generally occur following severe trauma or neurologic injury. Those who are severely burned can develop HO in sites distal to their burn injury but it most commonly appears in a joint with overlying burns, and it occurs more frequently in areas of persistently open wounds.[29] The most common areas for HO in burn are the elbow followed by the shoulder, hip, and knee.[30] HO typically occurs before 2 months, with one case reported as early as 12 days postburn.[31] Although HO is uncommon among the general burn population (occurring in only about 1%–4% of patients), it been reported in up to 50% in those with large TBSA.[29,32] Through Burn Model System database analysis, Levi and colleagues found that patients with greater than 30%

TBSA were more than 11 times more likely to develop HO than those with smaller burns. Furthermore, the risk of HO is associated with an increased number of surgeries, time with open wounds, days on mechanical ventilation, arm burns requiring skin grafting, infection, immobility, and male sex.[33,34] Interestingly, the incidence of HO in military burns is 40%, despite care similar to the civilian population. This suggests that trauma at the time of injury may be linked to the formation of HO.

Complications of HO include pain, nerve compression, open wounds, restricted ROM, and eventual contracture, all leading to decreased function and mobility.

Treatment strategies commonly used for nonburn HO, such as prophylactic radiation therapy, nonsteroidal anti-inflammatory drugs, and bisphosphonates, are typically not used in burn patients because of potential adverse effects or poor efficacy in this population.[31,35] These interventions may be more suitable as prophylaxis against recurrence following HO resection, although the recurrence rate of HO after surgery is very low.[36]

Many efforts are directed at the prevention of HO. Early postburn ROM is essential. No scientific evidence supports the concept that overaggressive ROM is a risk factor for HO.[31] Although some patients with HO respond to ROM exercise, ultimately a subset of patients will develop refractory ankylosis requiring surgical excision.[37] In contrast to other populations with HO, burn survivors show good outcomes with early resection followed by physiotherapy.[29] If for some reason HO cannot be corrected, use of orthotics should be considered.[30]

AMPUTATION

Burn-related amputation is rare, accounting for only about 2% of burn cases regardless of mechanism. Much of the literature on burn-related amputations is focused on electrical injury. The risk of amputation following electrical injury is reported as high as 68%. Other studies have reported the cause of amputation is more frequently flame injury.[38] In a 5-year retrospective study, 24% of electrical burn patients underwent amputations, with digits being the most common site.[39] In another study of a burn center in Portugal, 6.8% of elderly burn patients required amputation.[40] Patients with diabetes are at increased risk for osteomyelitis, which in turn increases likelihood of amputation.

Several studies have shown that many burn patients with an amputation can be successfully fitted with prosthetics, and that overall quality-of-life indicators are comparable to those for nonamputee burn patients. General care is similar to that of other burn patients, including wound care, edema control, preservation of ROM, and pain control. However, special consideration must be taken when it comes to placing patients into prosthetics because the injury and repair can alter limb shape and delay prosthetic fitting.[41]

Early amputation has been associated with better outcomes, shorter LOS, and more prosthetic use compared with amputation greater than 48 hours postburn.[42] Patients who were employed before their injuries were more likely to return to work even if amputated.[43]

HEAT SENSITIVITY AND TOLERANCE

Heat sensitivity is very common after burn injury, affecting up to two-thirds of burn survivors. It is more common with larger TBSA and is strongly associated with decreased satisfaction with life and lower physical health scores.[44] Crandall showed that burn survivors with greater than 40% TBSA sustain twice the temperature elevation during heat stress of more than 2 hours duration, compared with those with less than 40%

TBSA and to healthy controls. Interestingly, there was no difference in core temperature elevation within the initial 30 minutes of exercise during heat stress.[45]

OUTCOMES

Mortality was the outcome evaluated in almost all burn studies before 1980. As infection control, skin coverage, nutrition, and fluid management improved, survival became the expectation even after extensive burns. According to the American Burn Association's 2021 Burn Injury Summary Report, overall mortality of admitted burn patients was 3.1%; it was less than 1% for those aged younger than 16 years; and it was 10% for those aged older than 70 years.[46] Hospital LOS is another outcome that most centers evaluate. Although this number is usually around 1 day per percent burn, many factors such as lack of social support or stable housing and distance from the burn center influence it. Another variable that may affect LOS is the ready availability of inpatient rehabilitation (IPR). In the national dataset, 8.5% of patients are discharged to another facility; however, discharge to a psychiatric unit, IPR, or skilled nursing facility (SNF) are lumped together. A study by Pham showed that a center with a physiatrist as part of the burn team discharged 30% of patients aged older than 55 years to IPR and 10% to SNF, whereas a similar center without a physiatrist discharged 11% to IPR and 24% to SNF.[47] This difference is important for a couple of reasons. First, Medicare requires that 60% of patients admitted fall into 1 of 12 categories, one of which is burns. Admitting burn survivors would help IPRs meet this criterion. Second, a study by Palmieri showed that for patients aged older than 60 years at the time of burn, 5-year mortality was more than twice as high for those sent to an SNF compared with those who were sent home (58% vs 24%).[48] Interesting national data show that burn patients have lower cognition scores on IPR admission but these scores improve dramatically during the stay.[49] This is likely related to delirium, which clears in the structured environment of IPR. Mistaking delirium for dementia may be one reason why burn patients are not routinely discharged to IPR.

Once burn survivors are discharged from the hospital, rehabilitation, and follow-up are critical. The 2012 ABA Burn Quality Consensus Conference advocated for standardized quality metrics, including documenting time to return to work/school, physical function, and quality of life.[1] Multiple return-to-work studies have shown a variety of predictors, including preburn employment, TBSA, LOS, hand burn, work conditions, and personality traits. Recently, Carrougher's report on almost 1000 subjects showed a strong correlation with preburn employment but not with hand burns or TBSA. In our experience, issues such as wanting to work, liking the job, or needing money are more significant than injury characteristics. Another interesting factor from Carrougher's article was that 1 of the 3 sites had significantly higher return-to-work rates in all analyses. This site is the only one that has a vocational counselor as part of the burn team.[50]

Return to school is a challenge for children with a burn injury. Studies show increased issues with frustration and irritability and greater risk of being bullied.[51] Both burn severity and demographic factors affect adjustment. School reentry can have a significant mitigating effect on these challenges by helping teachers and students to have a better understanding of the issues related to a burn injury and clearing up any misperceptions.[52]

Patient-reported outcomes have become a common way of evaluating outcome after burn injury, with 13 generic tools validated for burn patients and 4 burn-specific tools.[53] Patients report that hypertrophic scarring interferes with the quality of life. Patients with head and neck burns have decreased satisfaction with appearance.[54,55] Positive body image is associated with improved community integration. Symptoms of distress correlate with decreased body image, community integration, and the sense of social stigma.[56] As important as it is to describe causal factors, it is essential to now migrate toward the study of interventions to improve outcomes.

Paying more attention to long-term burn survivors has led to the realization that burn injury is a chronic condition.[57] Satisfaction with life never recovers to preburn levels. There is a steep decline in mental and physical health in the first 5 years postburn. Pruritus, issues with temperature regulation, joint pain, and fatigue persist.[30] Burn survivors with inhalation injury are predisposed to pneumonia. Those who required dialysis at the time of burn are at greater risk for long-term renal failure.[57] It is essential that burn clinicians educate themselves and their patients on these issues so appropriate preventive steps can be taken. The Phoenix Society for Burn Survivors has been an excellent resource for facilitating a better understanding of the acute challenges of burn survivors, as well as the new understanding of burns as a chronic condition.

SUMMARY

Now that more individuals are surviving larger burns, clinicians should develop a working knowledge of complications, outcomes, and long-term challenges. The modern burn center needs a robust infrastructure to meet these challenges, and the burn community needs diligent investigation into treatment approaches to guide best practices and to support evidence-based protocols.

CLINICS CARE POINTS

- Contractures are common and require prevention and early treatment.
- Neuropathy is most often seen in electrical injury and usually recovers.
- Itch and neuropathic pain are best treated with gabapentin or pregabalin.
- HO occurs in large burns and can be successfully treated.
- Burn surivors continue to have life long issues related to the burn injury. It is essential that a treating physician be aware of involvement of other body systems beyond the skin which may create long term medial challenges.

DECLARATION OF INTERESTS

Neither author has any financial disclosure.

REFERENCES

1. Gibran NS, Wiechman S, Meyer W, et al. Summary of the 2012 ABA Burn Quality Consensus conference. J Burn Care Res 2013;34(4):361–85.
2. Junker JP, Kratz C, Tollback A, et al. Mechanical tension stimulates the transdifferentiation of fibroblasts into myofibroblasts in human burn scars. Burns 2008; 34(7):942–6.
3. Oosterwijk AM, Mouton LJ, Schouten H, et al. Prevalence of scar contractures after burn: A systematic review. Burns 2017;43(1):41–9.
4. Schneider JC, Holavanahalli R, Helm P, et al. Contractures in burn injury: defining the problem. J Burn Care Res 2006;27(4):508–14.

5. Khansa I, Harrison B, Janis JE. Evidence-Based Scar Management: How to Improve Results with Technique and Technology. Plast Reconstr Surg 2016; 138(3 Suppl):165S–78S.

6. Anthonissen M, Daly D, Peeters R, et al. Reliability of Repeated Measurements on Post-Burn Scars with Corneometer CM 825((R)). Skin Res Technol 2015;21(3): 302–12.

7. Tredget EE, Shupp JW, Schneider JC. Scar Management Following Burn Injury. J Burn Care Res 2017;38(3):146–7.

8. Richard R, Miller S, Staley M, et al. Multimodal versus progressive treatment techniques to correct burn scar contractures. J Burn Care Rehabil 2000;21(6): 506–12.

9. Richard R, Ward RS. Splinting strategies and controversies. J Burn Care Rehabil 2005;26(5):392–6.

10. Peng W, Zhang X, Kong X, et al. The efficacy and safety of fractional CO_2 laser therapy in the treatment of burn scars: A meta-analysis. Burns 2021;47(7): 1469–77.

11. Rodriguez-Menocal L, Davis SS, Becerra S, et al. Assessment of Ablative Fractional CO_2 Laser and Er:YAG Laser to Treat Hypertrophic Scars in a Red Duroc Pig Model. J Burn Care Res 2018;39(6):954–62.

12. Ferguson JS, Franco J, Pollack J, et al. Compression neuropathy: a late finding in the postburn population: a four-year institutional review. J Burn Care Res 2010; 31(3):458–61.

13. Kowalske K, Holavanahalli R, Helm P. Neuropathy after burn injury. J Burn Care Rehabil 2001;22(5):353–7.

14. Gabriel V, Kowalske KJ, Holavanahalli RK. Assessment of recovery from burn-related neuropathy by electrodiagnostic testing. J Burn Care Res 2009;30(4): 668–74.

15. Margherita AJ, Robinson LR, Heimbach DM, et al. Burn-associated peripheral polyneuropathy. A search for causative factors. Am J Phys Med Rehabil 1995; 74(1):28–32.

16. Klifto KM, Yesantharao PS, Dellon AL, et al. Chronic Neuropathic Pain Following Hand Burns: Etiology, Treatment, and Long-Term Outcomes. J Hand Surg Am 2021;46(1):67 e1–e67 e9.

17. Carrougher GJ, Martinez EM, McMullen KS, et al. Pruritus in adult burn survivors: postburn prevalence and risk factors associated with increased intensity. J Burn Care Res 2013;34(1):94–101.

18. Holavanahalli RK, Helm PA, Kowalske KJ. Long-term outcomes in patients surviving large burns: the skin. J Burn Care Res 2010;31(4):631–9.

19. Van Loey NE, Bremer M, Faber AW, et al. Itching following burns: epidemiology and predictors. Br J Dermatol 2008;158(1):95–100.

20. Chung BY, Kim HB, Jung MJ, et al. Post-Burn Pruritus. Int J Mol Sci 2020;21(11).

21. Halvorsen JA, Dalgard F, Thoresen M, et al. Itch and mental distress: a cross-sectional study among late adolescents. Acta Derm Venereol 2009;89(1):39–44.

22. Silverberg JI, Hinami K, Trick WE, et al. Itch in the General Internal Medicine Setting: A Cross-Sectional Study of Prevalence and Quality-of-Life Effects. Am J Clin Dermatol 2016;17(6):681–90.

23. Lee J, Jang D, Bae J, et al. Efficacy of pregabalin for the treatment of chronic pruritus of unknown origin, assessed based on electric current perception threshold. Sci Rep 2020;10(1):1022.

24. Gilron I, Bailey JM, Tu D, et al. Morphine, gabapentin, or their combination for neuropathic pain. N Engl J Med 2005;352(13):1324–34.

25. Nedelec B, Calva V, Chouinard A, et al. Somatosensory Rehabilitation for Neuropathic Pain in Burn Survivors: A Case Series. J Burn Care Res 2016;37(1): e37–46.

26. Sheridan RL, Hurley J, Smith MA, et al. The acutely burned hand: management and outcome based on a ten-year experience with 1047 acute hand burns. J Trauma 1995;38(3):406–11.

27. Skoog T. Electrical injuries. J Trauma 1970;10(10):816–30.

28. Vanden Bossche L, Vanderstraeten G. Heterotopic ossification: a review. J Rehabil Med 2005;37(3):129–36.

29. Chen JY, Fu CW, Ho HY, et al. Surgical treatment of postburn heterotopic ossification around the elbow: Three case reports. Medicine (Baltim) 2019;98(6): e14403.

30. Holavanahalli RK, Helm PA, Kowalske KJ. Long-Term Outcomes in Patients Surviving Large Burns: The Musculoskeletal System. J Burn Care Res 2016;37(4): 243–54.

31. Kornhaber R, Foster N, Edgar D, et al. The development and impact of heterotopic ossification in burns: a review of four decades of research. Scars Burn Heal 2017;3. 2059513117695659.

32. Sun Y, Lin Y, Chen Z, et al. Heterotopic Ossification in Burn Patients. Ann Plast Surg 2022;88(2 Suppl 2):S134–7.

33. Levi B, Jayakumar P, Giladi A, et al. Risk factors for the development of heterotopic ossification in seriously burned adults: A National Institute on Disability, Independent Living and Rehabilitation Research burn model system database analysis. J Trauma Acute Care Surg 2015;79(5):870–6.

34. Klein MB, Logsetty S, Costa B, et al. Extended time to wound closure is associated with increased risk of heterotopic ossification of the elbow. J Burn Care Res 2007;28(3):447–50.

35. Shafer DM, Bay C, Caruso DM, et al. The use of eidronate disodium in the prevention of heterotopic ossification in burn patients. Burns 2008;34(3):355–60.

36. Hunt JL, Arnoldo BD, Kowalske K, et al. Heterotopic ossification revisited: a 21-year surgical experience. J Burn Care Res 2006;27(4):535–40.

37. Peterson SL, Mani MM, Crawford CM, et al. Postburn heterotopic ossification: insights for management decision making. J Trauma 1989;29(3):365–9.

38. Bartley CN, Atwell K, Purcell L, et al. Amputation Following Burn Injury. J Burn Care Res 2019;40(4):430–6.

39. Ghavami Y, Mobayen MR, Vaghardoost R. Electrical burn injury: a five-year survey of 682 patients. Trauma Mon 2014;19(4):e18748.

40. Caetano P, Brandao C, Campos I, et al. Aging and burn: a five-year retrospective study in a major burn centre in Portugal. Ann Burns Fire Disasters 2018;31(3): 163–7.

41. Thananopavarn P, Hill JJ 3rd. Rehabilitation of the Complex Burn Patient with Multiple Injuries or Comorbidities. Clin Plast Surg 2017;44(4):695–701.

42. Williams ZF, Bools LM, Adams A, et al. Early versus delayed amputation in the setting of severe lower extremity trauma. Am Surg 2015;81(6):564–8.

43. Carrougher GJ, McMullen K, Mandell SP, et al. Impact of Burn-Related Amputations on Return to Work: Findings From the Burn Injury Model System National Database. J Burn Care Res 2019;40(1):21–8.

44. Oh J, Madison C, Flott G, et al. Temperature Sensitivity After Burn Injury: A Burn Model System National Database Hot Topic. J Burn Care Res 2021;42(6):1110–9.

45. Crandall CG, Cramer MN, Kowalske KJ, et al. Adolph Distinguished Lecture. It's more than skin deep: thermoregulatory and cardiovascular consequences of severe burn injuries in humans. J Appl Physiol (1985) 2021;131(6):1852–66.
46. American Burn Association. 2021 Summary Report. 2022. Available at. https://ameriburn.org/education/publications/. Accessed 10/2/22.
47. Pham TN, Carrougher GJ, Martinez E, et al. Predictors of Discharge Disposition in Older Adults With Burns: A Study of the Burn Model Systems. J Burn Care Res 2015;36(6):607–12.
48. Palmieri TL, Molitor F, Chan G, et al. Long-term functional outcomes in the elderly after burn injury. J Burn Care Res 2012;33(4):497–503.
49. Purohit M, Goldstein R, Nadler D, et al. Cognition in patients with burn injury in the inpatient rehabilitation population. Arch Phys Med Rehabil 2014;95(7):1342–9.
50. Carrougher GJ, Bamer AM, Mandell SP, et al. Factors Affecting Employment After Burn Injury in the United States: A Burn Model System National Database Investigation. Arch Phys Med Rehabil 2020;101(1S):S71–85.
51. McGarry S, Elliott C, McDonald A, et al. Paediatric burns: from the voice of the child. Burns 2014;40(4):606–15.
52. Pan R, Dos Santos BD, Nascimento LC, et al. School reintegration of pediatric burn survivors: An integrative literature review. Burns 2018;44(3):494–511.
53. Griffiths C, Guest E, White P, et al. A Systematic Review of Patient-Reported Outcome Measures Used in Adult Burn Research. J Burn Care Res 2017;38(2):e521–45.
54. Goverman J, He W, Martello G, et al. The Presence of Scarring and Associated Morbidity in the Burn Model System National Database. Ann Plast Surg 2019;82(3 Suppl 2):S162–8.
55. Sinha I, Nabi M, Simko LC, et al. Head and neck burns are associated with long-term patient-reported dissatisfaction with appearance: A Burn Model System National Database study. Burns 2019;45(2):293–302.
56. Mercado AE, Donthula D, Thomas JE, et al. Mediators and moderators of the relationship between body image and community integration among burn survivors. Burns 2022;48(4):932–40.
57. Barrett LW, Fear VS, Waithman JC, et al. Understanding acute burn injury as a chronic disease. Burns Trauma 2019;7:23.

Burn Scar Management and Reconstructive Surgery

Noor Obaidi, MD, PhD[a], Corey Keenan, DO[a], Rodney K. Chan, MD, FRCSC[a,b,*]

KEYWORDS

- Burn scars • Scar management • Surgical scar techniques • Reconstructive surgery
- Functional reconstruction • Keloid • Hypertrophic scars • Scar contracture

KEY POINTS

- Planning for reconstruction begins from the acute burn admission. Adequate debridement and proper coverage of open wounds and deep burns minimizes late reconstructive needs.
- Nonsurgical and surgical scar management modalities should complement one another to manage early and late sequalae after burn.
- A comprehensive and longitudinal plan to address the burn survivor's postburn deformities should include the survivor's expectations, priorities, risk tolerance, and donor availability.

BACKGROUND

Cutaneous scaring is an inevitable consequence following burns deeper than the dermis. Although burn scars from more superficial injuries can resemble normal skin in appearance and function after a period of remodeling, scars from deeper burns can cause debilitating symptoms such as pain, itching, tightness, and restricted range of motion. Many of these complaints are localized to the head and neck and upper extremities, not just because these areas are commonly burned but also because of their functional significance and the demand for precise movements in basic activities. Most burn survivors find the appearance of their scars undesirable, especially when they are raised, red, texturally irregular, and rough.[1] It is important for surgeons treating burn scars to be aware of the techniques to control scar formation and manage their late sequalae.[1,2]

We have often heard burn scars described as either functional or cosmetic, a categorization we do not endorse. Scarring from burns has significant psychosocial consequences. Depression and posttraumatic stress disorder are common psychological sequelae and are present respectively in 13% to 23% and 13% to 45% of burn

[a] The Metis Foundation, 84 NorthEast 410 Loop, STE 325, San Antonio, TX 78216, USA; [b] United States Army Institute of Surgical Research, Fort Sam Houston, TX, USA
* Corresponding author.
E-mail address: chan@metisfoundationusa.org

Surg Clin N Am 103 (2023) 515–527
https://doi.org/10.1016/j.suc.2023.01.012
0039-6109/23/© 2023 Elsevier Inc. All rights reserved.

surgical.theclinics.com

survivors after deep dermal injuries.[3] Simply because a burn scar does not result in restricted range of motion does not mean that it has no functional consequence and should be deemed purely cosmetic. Rather, we advocate for using the term "reconstructive" to describe burn scar treatments that attempt to restore normal appearance and function. The word "cosmetic" should be isolated to treatments that attempt to improve from normal appearance to "better-than-normal" (think face-lift, breast augmentation, and so forth).

Scars change over time. Some scars will improve with maturation, but some will worsen. They never disappear entirely. How a scar changes over time depends on location, size, and type. Proper management of the acute wound in the early stages of healing is the best way to diminish late morbidity from scarring.[3] The body's scar response also relies a great deal on skin tension and scar location. Naturally occurring vectors created on the skin surface from movement of the underlying structures create lines of tension known as Langer lines. Scars are worse when there is high skin tension.[4,5]

Another determining factor of scar healing is blood supply. The area of the skin with a rich supply of vasculature is known to heal with finer scars given the same degree of insult.[6,7] Genetics and ethnicity further influence postoperative scar response. Lighter-skin individuals (Fitzpatrick scale: 1, 2, and 3) are more likely to scar less, whereas people of darker skin color (Fitzpatrick scale: 4, 5, and 6) such as those of African/Asian/Hispanic descent seem more genetically predisposed to hypertrophic scars and keloids.[4,8]

DEVELOPING A COMPREHENSIVE TREATMENT PLAN

We begin our conversation with a new patient aiming to gain an understanding of their background, social situation, and priorities. We explain that reconstruction is a moderately lengthy journey. We photograph the burns and take note of potential donor areas. This is important because donor sites can be scarce and certain ones need to be reserved for specific problems (ie, for color-matched skin or regional flaps). After a period of consideration, which may be beyond the first visit, we propose to the burn survivor (and family if available) short- and long-term goals, taking into consideration their priorities but also their propensity for risks, repeated procedures, and hospitalizations. The timing of procedures also depends on the interval from their acute injury. Residual systemic inflammation can worsen scarring and negatively affect results. Early on, we rely on nonsurgical modalities such as compression, topical moisturizers, and lasers to temporize scarring while emphasizing rehabilitation and reintegration. We use 6 months as a rough time interval for when to begin more invasive procedures to correct these postburn deformities, with the exception of periocular and perioral deformities when we typically intervene earlier.

DESCRIPTION OF BURN SCARS

Often, scars are described based on appearance such as color (red, purple, blanching), texture, thickness, raised/depressed, or elasticity. There are scales, most common of which is the Vancouver Scar Scale (VSS) and the Patient and Observer Scar Assessment Scale (POSAS), that assign a numerical value based on these criteria.[1–3] Although helpful when conducting a study, these numbers are rarely used in clinical practice. Rather, we find it most useful to describe scars based on type, biology, and the severity of associated symptoms.

Description Based on Type

Some may argue that the type of burn scarring is irrelevant, as it does not dictate the treatment plan. We disagree, as the type of scar often instructs the depth of injury and allows for better surgical planning. Knowledge of the types of burn scars also enriches understanding of the factors influencing their formation, which can be used to prevent scar formation.

1. *Scarring from deep partial-thickness burns that heal conservatively*: the underlying question of whether a burn is capable of "healing on its own" really has to do with whether there remains an adequate amount of dermal regenerative elements for a healed scar to retain the skin's native function without a rampant fibrotic response (**Fig. 1**). Because currently there is no better tool than clinical gestalt, one can mistakenly assess that a burn has adequate regenerative elements but subsequently result in poor scar outcomes. For late reconstruction, however, these scars tend to be superficial to the deep fascia, and there is generally a helpful layer of adipose tissue beneath the scar.
2. *Recipient-site scarring*: this refers to scarring at the site of skin-graft placement (**Fig. 2**). There are 2 distinct types of recipient-site scars. Firstly, there are "mesh-pattern" scars; this is a pattern that results from the meshing and expansion of split-thickness skin grafts in order to increase the surface area of coverage.[9]

The second type of recipient-site scarring refers to islands of raised scar that are present within a grafted area. In comparison to "mesh-pattern" scars, these scars are more mosaic and irregular. They correspond to wounds where there was either insufficient amount of skin graft applied or the overlying graft failed to take (**Fig. 3**). This phenomenon is also commonly seen on the edges of a skin graft placed adjacent to normal skin or the seams where 2 pieces of skin graft are pieced together. There are similarities between this type of scarring and deep partial-thickness burns that are left to heal on their own.[10]

3. *Donor-site scarring*: the degree of scarring after a skin-graft harvest depends not only on the genetic predisposition of the patient but also on the degree of local and systemic inflammation at the time of healing (**Fig. 4**). For instance, systemic inflammation is exacerbated by a larger total burn size, and skin grafts harvested from such a patient are more prone to poor scarring. Local inflammation is also a contributor and is exacerbated by repeated or thick skin-graft harvests.[10]

Description Based on Biology

1. *Keloid scars*: keloid scarring is a genetic condition in which the degree of scarring is out of proportion to the degree of injury (**Fig. 5**).[11] In contrast to hypertrophic scars, keloid scars are typically more scattered, larger, extend beyond the borders of original injury, and do not fade over time.[12] Although there are many treatment modalities, including steroid injections, lasers, radiotherapy, and surgery, recurrence is common.[11,13]
2. *Hypertrophic scars.* Hypertrophic scars are the most common type of burn scarring. These are pathologic scars that result from an abnormal response to wound healing in which extra connective tissue is formed. These scars are itchy and painful, causing severe functional and psychosocial disabilities.[3,14,15] Hypertrophic scars are elevated but do not spread into the surrounding tissue. They proliferate from dermal tissue due to excessive fibroblast-derived extracellular matrix and collagen deposition.[8,16] Hypertrophic scars are also sometimes referred to as burn-scar contractures, if anatomic structures are displaced or the range of motion is limited.[17–22]

Description Based on Severity of Symptoms

Two people can have the same injury pattern and present with varying complaints regarding their scar. One determinant of how scars affect an individual is the degree

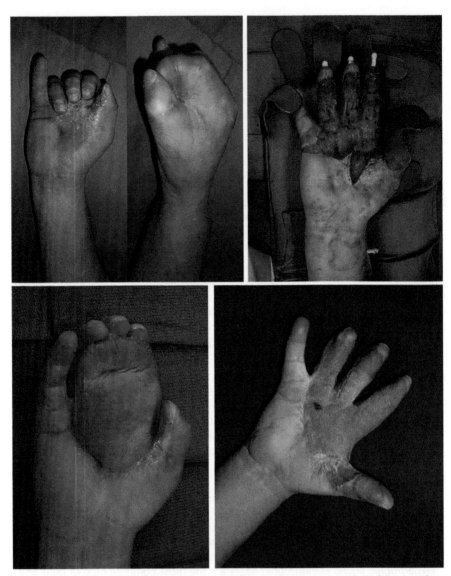

Fig. 1. An example of right-hand palmar burn left to heal on its own and resulting in palmar contracture and nonfunctional hand. Pedicled groin flap was used for initial coverage after a release operation. Multiple debulking and division and inset operations were needed to separate the fingers.

to which they would like their scars to return to normal skin appearance. Although there are exceptions to this rule, we have found that the preinjury level of activity plays an important role. Before embarking on a treatment plan, it is important to make sure the expectations of the burn survivor can be met with the proposed plan. Furthermore, with each treatment, we try to understand the manner and degree to which a particular scar affects their daily routine. Albeit imperfect, the success of a treatment is ultimately determined based on amelioration of these symptoms.

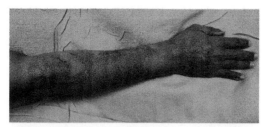

Fig. 2. Example of mesh-pattern scar on recipient site of a meshed and expanded split-thickness skin graft. The skin follows a regular but rough pattern.

TREATMENT MODALITIES
Nonsurgical

Early scar management is commonly achieved with less invasive methods such as stretching, massage, sunscreens, moisturizers, and compression. Although topical agents such as silicone sheeting and intralesional steroid injections are useful for post-traumatic or postsurgical scars, we have not often found them to be useful for burn-scar management. Hydration is best achieved with daily application of moisturizers.[23–25]

Massage: massage can improve the skin's structural properties to regain the strength and elasticity required for normal mobility. Research showed an immediate

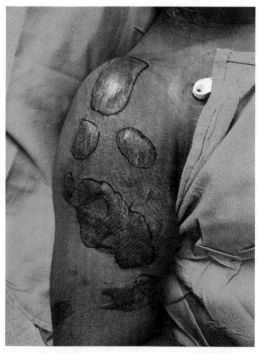

Fig. 3. An example of recipient-site scarring within a meshed skin graft. The skin graft follows a regular but rough pattern that is like the initial meshing pattern of the skin applied. In addition, there are islands of raised scars (marked) that may correspond to areas of poor graft take.

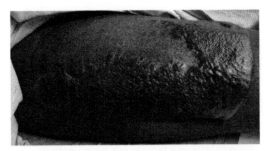

Fig. 4. Example of donor-site hypertrophic scarring. The degree of scarring depends on genetic factors and the degree of local and systemic inflammation at the time of healing.

increase in elasticity in response to massage. Massage can also decrease pain and pruritus.[26–31]

Topical products: products such as ointments, creams, oils, and patches with hydration effects can be an important adjunct. Silicone-based creams and sheets create an adjunct to the skin barrier to prevent further loss of moisture.

Steroids: intralesional steroid injections are commonly used to treat small areas of raised scars. Burn scars are rarely candidates for steroid injection because of the vast area of involvement. It can be helpful when there is a scar that is limited in size. The local application of steroids will decrease the inflammation and proliferation response and helps to slow excessive collagen production. This technique softens and flattens scars, helping them blend in with the surrounding tissue. Delayed adverse effects include hyper- or hypopigmentation, acne, or excessive hair growth at the treated site. Another delayed side effect is lipoatrophy (localized fat tissue loss), which can leave minor depressions in the patient's skin postinjection.[32–34]

Dermabrasion: dermabrasion is a skin-resurfacing technique that uses a rapidly rotating device to remove the outer layer of skin. The newly formed skin layer usually grows smoother and healthier. Dermabrasion in the management of burn scar has largely been used for decreasing textural irregularity, particularly in mesh-pattern scars. Dermabrasion can be done alone or in combination with other procedures.[35–37]

Laser Scar Ablation

Laser has become a mainstay of early intervention for burn scars.[38] Several commercially available lasers are available. In general, early immature burn scars are red and

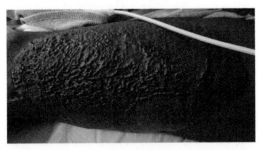

Fig. 5. Example of keloid scarring in recipient site after reconstruction. The mesh pattern scar seen here is far out of proportion to the typical skin graft recipient. These scars extend outside the margins of the affected cutaneous injury and are typically raised.

inflamed and may proceed to become fibrotic. Nonablative laser that can decrease inflammation via obliteration of small blood vessels is helpful in this early period. Pulse-dye lasers use a chromophore that targets 595 nm, corresponding to the heme moiety. Several centers report using intense pulse light lasers with good success as well. The success of these laser treatments is incremental and generally requires 3 to 6 treatments for optimal results.

More mature scars are characterized by their thickness and stiffness. We find that scars that are tight and texturally irregular without limitation of range of motion benefit from ablative lasers such as the carbon dioxide (CO_2) laser or the erbium (Er:YAG) laser. Laser scar revision is based on the principle of controlled thermal injury to induce healing. Fractional lasers produce arrays of nonselective microscopic thermal damage zones throughout the skin layers. This thermal energy penetrates deeply, stimulates collagen production, and promotes tissue remodeling.[1,38–40]

EMERGING SCAR MANAGEMENT STRATEGIES

Recent studies of fat grafting into scars have shown promise to improve function and appearance. Patients reported satisfactory results 6 months after the procedure, and histology demonstrated new collagen deposition, neovascularization, and dermal hyperplasia, which mimicked surrounding undamaged skin. Nevertheless, a randomized, multisite study investigating mature scars noted that when microfat was injected as compared with an equivalent volume of saline and matched for number of cannula passes, there were no notable differences in outcomes (Katz/Chan, Ref); this may indicate that the effect seen with autologous fat injection is merely mechanical.

Another emerging technique is the implantation of full-thickness skin columns into scars. Full-thickness skin columns including sweat glands and hair follicles can facilitate addition of normal skin into scarred areas devoid of normal skin function. This technique provides for additional skin function with little-to-no donor site requirements and without any significant down time.[37,41–49]

SURGICAL BURN-SCAR MANAGEMENT

The main goal of surgical burn-scar treatment is to restore normal anatomy by relieving tension while minimizing morbidity. There are 2 main options to consider— release using local tissue flaps and release using a skin graft.

Release with Local Adjacent Tissue

Z-plasty is a commonly used form of local tissue rearrangement to release linear burn scar contractures. In addition to lengthening scars, it is also useful in redirecting scars, flattening raised or depressed scars, and recreating a webspace. The classic Z-plasty design incorporates angles of 60° with 3 equal limbs to achieve a theoretic 75% lengthening (**Fig. 6**). This configuration achieves the desired increase in length of the contracture by taking advantage of available lateral skin laxity. Positioning of this classic Z-plasty in series and in opposition are both reliable methods to improve burn-scar contractures. The double-opposing or "jumping man" Z-plasty combines 2 Z-plasties oriented along a common central limb axis, with advancement of a triangular flap into a releasing incision made perpendicular to the central axis (**Fig. 7**). This technique is particularly useful for releasing webspace contractures in which there is significant transverse skin laxity. Clever variations including W-plasty and Trapeze-plasty have also been described.

The advantage of a Z-plasty is that a donor site is not needed and recovery is short. However, not all burn scars are ideal candidates. Use in broad contractures often

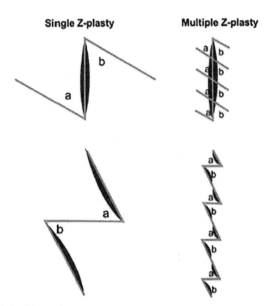

Fig. 6. Single and double Z-plasty.

results in less than a satisfactory release. Surgeons must weigh the benefits against the risks of inadequate correction and need for additional operations. Meticulous handling of the flaps and preservation of the subdermal blood supply are paramount to a successful outcome and minimizing tip necrosis.

Incisional Release with Graft

Broad burn-scar contractures require a generous transverse release to restore structures to their normal anatomic positions. As a rule of thumb, most burn-scar

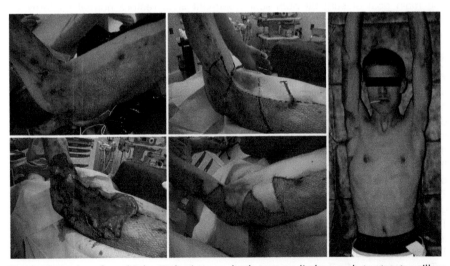

Fig. 7. Example of multiple Z-plasties on both upper limbs used to treat axillary contractures.

contractures involving a mobile structure, such as an eyelid or a joint, will require an incision across the entire axis of rotation. For instance, an eyelid release requires an incision from just medial to the medial canthus to the lateral orbital rim. An antecubital fossa release traverses the medial epicondyle to the lateral epicondyle.

Generally, the contracture should be released on the table with a single attempt. However, when there is a severe long-standing contracture, considerable shortening of musculotendinous units and neurovascular structures occurs. In addition, immediate complete release may not be possible when the joints are subluxated or dislocated.[10,16] The shortening of deeper structures can result in a less-than-optimal release. Patients should be forewarned about the possible need for additional procedures.

A question often arises whether a broad scar contracture should be excised, either in lieu of or concurrent with a release. Scar excision should rarely be contemplated when dealing with contracture. A contracture implies a lack of skin, and scar excision increases the amount of skin replacement needed. Scar excision may be considered for hypertrophic scarring of the face when the subunit concept is indicated. Even then, the use of CO_2 laser scar resurfacing as an alternative to scar excision should be considered.[50]

Many options exist for skin coverage of the resulting defect after a transverse release. Color-matched full-thickness skin in the form of a graft is ideal but not always available. Thick split-thickness skin graft (STSG) is a good second choice. Dermal substitutes have been touted to augment the performance of a thin STSG with reasonable success. The superiority of a thicker graft reflects that fact that the quantity of transferred dermis correlates with skin quality. Thin grafts engraft more easily but at the cost of an increase in secondary graft contraction. Full-thickness skin grafts require ideal conditions to survive but the result is excellent (**Fig. 8**).

Pedicled flaps, tissue expansion, and the use of previously burned or grafted skin as flaps: just as thicker skin grafts provide a greater amount of tissue for higher quality results, proponents of flap coverage of burn releases argue that flaps contain the most tissue and have the added advantage of not having to rely on the blood supply of the recipient bed to survive. Indeed, should a release necessitate the exposure of nongraftable structures, a pedicled flap will provide the most durable option. However, before using a flap for the coverage of a graftable wound bed, one must balance donor-site morbidity against the potential benefits, especially if muscle, nerve, or an axial blood vessel will be sacrificed. Furthermore, flap debulking is almost guaranteed. Therefore, although pedicled flaps have been described for just about any type of burn

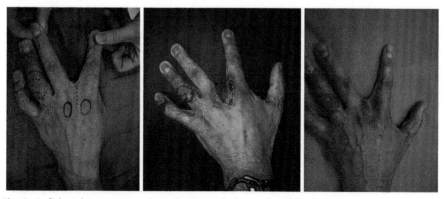

Fig. 8. Left-hand transverse release between index and middle finger joints.

reconstruction, fasciocutaneous flaps predominate, and the use of preoperative tissue expansion as a delay strategy has gained popularity.

Tissue expansion is a valuable tool when a large contiguous piece of skin is needed either as a full-thickness graft or as a flap. The amount of expanded skin has to be enough to cover the width of the tissue expander as well as the width of the eventual defect. The incision used for placement of the tissue expander should be carefully planned so as not to compromise the blood flow to any future flaps. Furthermore, the surgeon should have a plan for how the expanded skin will be advanced before the placement of the expander. Several investigators have described techniques for maximizing advancements from rectangular tissue expanders. Complications of tissue expansion include infection, implant exposure, and flap ischemia.

Use of pedicled flaps to reconstruct defects in areas of functional importance or those with exposed critical structures is often limited by the presence of previously burned skin in the surrounding tissues. Many surgeons are reluctant to include this previously burned or previously grafted skin as part of a local or regional flap due to concerns about vascularity. These concerns are often unfounded, as the underlying fascia and its axial blood supply are often spared. Many cases have been performed incorporating previously burned or grafted skin into fasciocutaneous flaps for trunk, hand, and upper-extremity reconstruction. Previously burned skin flaps were compared with controls in the pediatric population, with no difference in flap necrosis rates.[50–55] Previously burned flaps can be particularly useful in the upper extremity. Therefore, highly mobile areas with vital underlying structures such as the olecranon, antecubital fossa, and digital webspaces can be reconstructed using local fasciocutaneous flaps, such as the distally or proximally based radial forearm flap, posterior interosseous flap, or lateral arm flap. The resultant donor site defects can typically be skin grafted; given that the donor sites often consist of previously grafted tissue, donor-site morbidity is minimal. One must be careful to do a thorough preoperative and intraoperative assessment of the flap to ensure preserved vascularity[50–55]; This assessment includes preoperative Doppler ultrasonography to identify the axial artery as well as intact perforators within the skin territory incorporated into the flap; this should be supplemented by intraoperative assessment of bleeding from the flap edges to ensure preserved vascular supply from the axial source vessels. In addition, careful attention should be paid to minimize factors that may compromise blood supply of the flap. Technical pearls include inclusion of underlying fascia in areas of prior skin graft, atraumatic handling of tissues, minimal use of electrocautery, and tension-free closure. Vigilance for early venous congestion is paramount.

TREATMENT RESISTANCE AND COMPLICATIONS

After surgical scar revisions, common postsurgical risks and side effects apply, including infection and bleeding. One of the common risks that is unique to burn scar management is the possibility of recurrence. This risk is particularly common when the scar release is performed in the early postburn period while there is rampant systemic inflammation and robust fibroblast response, although skin grafts are more profoundly affected.[56] Skin grafts and flaps are also subject to failure due to infection or poor blood supply. Scar releases may also result in partial success, leaving a portion of the problem unresolved, necessitating repeated operations.[51,57–59]

SUMMARY

Burn-scar management is a complex and often time-consuming, longitudinal process for burn survivors. Patient education, compliance, and expectation management are essential for success. Surgeons treating burn scars must take into account not only the deformities present but also the survivor's expectations, priorities, risk tolerance, and donor availability. A sound rehabilitation plan following each reconstructive operation is needed to maximize success.

CLINICS CARE POINTS

- Scar management plan begins with a thorough preoperative discussion.
- Adherence to the management plan is essential to achieve reliable results.
- The patient should be aware of risks for recurrence and partial correction.

REFERENCES

1. Alam Murad, Jeffrey S, Dover JW, et al. Treatment of scars from burns and trauma. New York: McGraw-Hill; 2021.
2. Mustoe TA, Cooter RD, Gold MH, et al. International clinical recommendations on scar management. Plast Reconstr Surg 2002;110(2):560–71.
3. Van Loey NE, Van Son MJ. Psychopathology and psychological problems in patients with burn scars: epidemiology and management. Am J Clin Dermatol 2003; 4(4):245–72.
4. Bae SH, Bae YC, Nam SB, et al. A skin fixation method for decreasing the influence of wound contraction on wound healing in a rat model. Arch Plast Surg 2012;39:457–62.
5. Wilgus TA, Ferreira AM, Oberyszyn TM, et al. Regulation of scar formation by vascular endothelial growth factor. Lab Invest 2008;88(6):579–90.
6. Kim HY, Kim JW, Park JH, et al. Personal factors that affect the satisfaction of female patients undergoing esthetic suture after typical thyroidectomy. Arch Plast Surg 2013;40:414–24.
7. Toll EC, Loizou P, Davis CR, et al. Scars and satisfaction: do smaller scars improve patient-reported outcome? Eur Arch Oto-Rhino-Laryngol 2012;269: 309–13.
8. González N, Goldberg DJ. Update on the Treatment of Scars. J Drugs Dermatol 2019;18(6):550–5.
9. Shevchenko RV, James SL, James SE. A review of tissue-engineered skin bioconstructs available for skin reconstruction. J R Soc Interface 2010;7(43):229–58.
10. Thomas JR, Somenek M. Scar revision review. Arch Facial Plast Surg 2012;14(3): 162–74.
11. Hawash AA, Ingrasci G, Nouri K, et al. Pruritus in Keloid Scars: Mechanisms and Treatments. Acta Derm Venereol 2021;101(10):adv00582.
12. Ogawa R. Keloid and Hypertrophic Scars Are the Result of Chronic Inflammation in the Reticular Dermis. Int J Mol Sci 2017;18(3):606.
13. Lee JY-Y, Yang C-C, Chao S-C, et al. Histopathological Differential Diagnosis of Keloid and Hypertrophic Scar. Am J Dermatopathol 2004;26(5):379–84.
14. Ngaage M, Agius M. The Psychology of Scars: A Mini-Review. Psychiatr Danub 2018;30(Suppl 7):633–8.
15. Mekeres GM, Voita-Mekeres F, Tudoran C, et al. Predictors for Estimating Scars' Internalization in Victims with Post-Traumatic Scars versus Patients with Postsurgical Scars. Healthcare (Basel) 2022;10(3):550.

16. Stekelenburg CM, Marck RE, Tuinebreijer WE, et al. A systematic review on burn scar contracture treatment: searching for evidence. J Burn Care Res 2015;36(3): e153–61.

17. Wainwright DJ. Burn reconstruction: the problems, the techniques, and the applications. Clin Plast Surg 2009;36(4):687–700.

18. MacLennan SE, Corcoran JF, Neale HW. Tissue expansion in head and neck burn reconstruction. Clin Plast Surg 2000;27(1):121–32.

19. https://onlinelibrary.wiley.com/doi/10.1111/ajd.12715.

20. Rendon MI, Berson DS, Cohen JL, et al. Evidence and considerations in the application of chemical peels in skin disorders and aesthetic resurfacing. J Clin Aesthet Dermatol 2010;3(7):32–43.

21. Fabbrocini G, De Padova MP, Tosti A. Chemical peels: what's new and what isn't new but still works well. Facial Plast Surg 2009;25(5):329–36.

22. Hruza GJ. Dermabrasion. Facial Plast Surg Clin North Am 2001;9(2):267–ix.

23. Onselen JV. Scars: impact and management, with a focus on topical silicone-based treatments. Br J Nurs 2018;27(Sup12):S36–40.

24. Widgerow AD, Chait LA, Stals R, et al. New innovations in scar management. Aesthetic Plast Surg 2000;24(3):227–34.

25. Chen MA, Davidson TM. Scar management: prevention and treatment strategies. Curr Opin Otolaryngol Head Neck Surg 2005;13(4):242–7.

26. Cho YS, Jeon JH, Hong A, et al. The effect of burn rehabilitation massage therapy on hypertrophic scar after burn: a randomized controlled trial. Burns 2014;40(8): 1513–20.

27. Klosová H, Němečková Crkvenjaš Z, Štětinský J. Meek Micrografting Technique and its use in the Treatement of Severe Burn Injuries at the University hospital Ostrava Burn Center. Acta Chir Plast 2017;59(1):11–7.

28. Quintero EC, Machado JFE, Robles RAD. Meek micrografting history, indications, technique, physiology and experience: a review article. J Wound Care 2018; 27(Sup2):S12–8.

29. Holmes Iv JH, Molnar JA, Carter JE, et al. A Comparative Study of the ReCell® Device and Autologous Spit-Thickness Meshed Skin Graft in the Treatment of Acute Burn Injuries. J Burn Care Res 2018;39(5):694–702.

30. DeBruler DM, Blackstone BN, McFarland KL, et al. Effect of skin graft thickness on scar development in a porcine burn model. Burns 2018;44(4):917–30.

31. Gronet EM, Chan R, Cooper L, et al. Full-thickness Skin Microcolumns Implanted into a Dermal Regeneration Template: A Novel Method for "Donor-free" Skin Replacement Therapy. Plast Reconstr Surg Glob Open 2020;8(9 Suppl):151.

32. Ekstein SF, Wyles SP, Moran SL, et al. Keloids: a review of therapeutic management. Int J Dermatol 2021;60(6):661–71. https://doi.org/10.1111/ijd.15159.

33. Zoumalan CI. Topical Agents for Scar Management: Are They Effective? J Drugs Dermatol 2018;17(4):421–5.

34. Khatri KA, Mahoney DL, McCartney MJ. Laser scar revision: A review. J Cosmet Laser Ther 2011;13(2):54–62.

35. Bradley DT, Park SS. Scar revision via resurfacing. Facial Plast Surg 2001;17(4): 253–62.

36. Fulton JE Jr. Dermabrasion, chemabrasion, and laserabrasion. Historical perspectives, modern dermabrasion techniques, and future trends. Dermatol Surg 1996;22(7):619–28.

37. Son D, Harijan A. Overview of surgical scar prevention and management. J Korean Med Sci 2014;29(6):751–7.

38. Alster T, Zaulyanov L. Laser scar revision: a review. Dermatol Surg 2007;33(2): 131–40.
39. Zhang DD, Zhao WY, Fang QQ, et al. The efficacy of fractional CO_2 laser in acne scar treatment: A meta-analysis. Dermatol Ther 2021;34(1):e14539.
40. Nedelec B, Couture MA, Calva V, et al. Randomized controlled trial of the immediate and long-term effect of massage on adult postburn scar. Burns 2019;45(1): 128–39.
41. Al-Shaqsi S, Al-Bulushi T. Cutaneous Scar Prevention and Management: Overview of current therapies. Sultan Qaboos Univ Med J 2016;16(1):e3–8.
42. Hayashida K, Akita S. Surgical treatment algorithms for post-burn contractures. Burns Trauma 2017;5:9.
43. Russell J, Pateman K, Batstone M. Donor site morbidity of composite free flaps in head and neck surgery: a systematic review of the prospective literature. Int J Oral Maxillofac Surg 2021;50(9):1147–55.
44. Davis WE, Boyd JH. Z-plasty. Otolaryngol Clin North Am 1990;23(5):875–87.
45. Bernstein L. Z-plasty in head and neck surgery. Arch Otolaryngol 1969;89(4): 574–84.
46. Lenoir P, Lallemant M, Vilchez M, et al. V-Y advancement flap to correct a perineal defect after an episiotomy dehiscence. Int Urogynecol J 2021;32(7):1935–7.
47. Kang AS, Kang KS. Rhomboid flap: Indications, applications, techniques and results. A comprehensive review. Ann Med Surg (Lond) 2021;68:102544.
48. Bach A, Sanchez-Gonzalez M, Warman R. Double Rhomboid Suture Technique for Congenital Ptosis. J Pediatr Ophthalmol Strabismus 2018;55(2):117–21.
49. Hendriks TCC, Botman M, de Haas LEM, et al. Burn scar contracture release surgery effectively improves functional range of motion, disability and quality of life: A pre/post cohort study with long-term follow-up in a Low- and Middle-Income Country. Burns 2021;47(6):1285–94.
50. Cho SB, Lee SJ, Chung WS, et al. Treatment of burn scar using a carbon dioxide fractional laser. J Drugs Dermatol 2010;9:173–5.
51. Cherup L, Zachary L, Gottlieb L, et al. The radial forearm skin graft-fascial flap. Plast Reconstr Surg 1990;85:898–902.
52. Hultman CS, Friedstat JS, Edkins RE, et al. Laser resurfacing and remodeling of hypertrophic burn scars: the results of a large, prospective, before-after cohort study, with long-term follow-up. Ann Surg 2014;260(3):519–29.
53. Pribaz J, Pelham J. Use of previously burned skin in local fasciocutaneous flaps for upper extremity reconstruction. Ann Plast Surg 1994;33:272–80.
54. Tolhurst D, Haeseker B, Zeeman R. The development of the fasciocutaneous flap. Plast Reconstr Surg 1983;71:597–605.
55. Barret J, Herndon D, McCauley R. Use of previously burned skin as random cutaneous local flaps in pediatric burn reconstruction. Burns 2002;28:500–2.
56. Herskovitz I, Hughes OB, Macquhae F, et al. Epidermal skin grafting. Int Wound J 2016;13(Suppl 3):52–6.
57. Lei YM, Sepulveda M, Chen L, et al. Skin-restricted commensal colonization accelerates skin graft rejection. JCI Insight 2019;5(15):e127569.
58. Suman O, McEntire S, Cowan A, et al. Chapter 47 - Comprehensive rehabilitation of the burn patient. In: Herndon DN, editor. *Total burn care*. 4th edition. Amsterdam: Elsevier Health Sciences; 2012. p. 517–49.
59. Brusselaers N, Pirayesh A, Hoeksema H, et al. Burn scar assessment: a systematic review of different scar scales. J Surg Res 2010;164(1):e115–23.

Military Burn Care and Burn Disasters

Booker King, MD[a], Leopoldo C. Cancio, MD[b], James C. Jeng, MD[c],*

KEYWORDS

- Burns • Mass-casualty disaster • Military personnel • Armed conflict
- Aeromedical evacuation

KEY POINTS

- A common feature of both wars and disasters is the need to optimize care despite inadequate local resources.
- Triage aims to provide the best possible care for the greatest number of burn survivors and considers burn size, age, and comorbidities.
- Movement of patients through successively higher echelons of care offloads facilities at the point of injury but also exposes patients to the risks of transport. Thorough reassessment of patients is needed at each echelon.
- Few personnel have current knowledge and experience in mass-casualty or military burn care. Training at both the individual and system levels is critical to preparedness.

INTRODUCTION

In this article, we will examine burn care because it is superimposed on the complex environments of the battlefield and mass-casualty disasters. Care in these environments has similarities to include potential to overwhelm first-responder resources, lack of specialized burn training of personnel, need for effective triage of patients at the point of injury (POI), and exceeding the capacity of local medical facilities. In burn mass-casualty events, state and regional coordination is essential because local manpower and equipment may need to be resupplied after operating several hours at high tempo. The battlefield is an equally unpredictable environment. As past incidents have proven, proper training and preparedness are essential for optimal outcomes in both environments.

^a North Carolina Jaycee Burn Center, University of North Carolina Chapel Hill, Burnett Womack Building, Campus Box 7206, Chapel Hill, NC 27599-7206, USA; ^b U.S. Army Burn Center, U.S. Army Institute of Surgical Research, Fort Sam Houston, San Antonio, TX 78234-6315, USA; ^c University of California Irvine, 3800 West Chapman Avenue, Suite 6200, Orange, CA 92868, USA
* Corresponding author:
E-mail address: jcjeng@hs.uci.edu

Surg Clin N Am 103 (2023) 529–538
https://doi.org/10.1016/j.suc.2023.01.013
0039-6109/23/© 2023 Elsevier Inc. All rights reserved.

MILITARY BURN CARE

Burn injury traditionally comprises 5% to 20% of combat wounded. These proportions can vary depending on the phase of the military operation.[1] The modern battlefield is an asymmetric, fluid, and hostile environment. The complexity of delivery of care in this environment is highlighted by the difficulties of caring for several patients with poly-traumatic injuries and the need to transport them through higher echelons of care.[2] Military facilities in the theater of operations will have limited resources, staffing, and holding capacity. Burn care on the battlefield will pose several additional chal-lenges. First, many of the first responders, physicians, and nurses do not have training in the care of burn patients. Second, the coordination of burn resuscitation, wound care, and aeromedical transport of burn casualties on the battlefield requires a high level of strategic medical planning and a keen understanding of the battlespace. Third, the care of host nation civilians to include children will present a significant challenge to the military medical team. The battlefield can be the most complex environment for a medical team to operate in.[3] This environment often poses threats to the safety and security of the medical team, the burn patient, and other support or security elements within the team.

A common mode of injury during recent conflicts was the improvised explosive de-vice (IED). IEDs can cause combination of multisystem blast, thermal, and chemical injuries. The injury patterns changed from Operation Iraqi Freedom (OIF) in the early 2000s to Operation Enduring Freedom (OEF) several years later. In early OIF, a com-mon scenario was severe burn and blast injury that occurred after a military vehicle struck an IED or an IED detonated near a crowd or gathering. Severe thermal injury, multiple amputations, and a variety of other injuries were sustained. Moreover, the ser-vice member was at risk from severe thermal and inhalation injury caused by being trapped in a burning vehicle. Extrication from the vehicle was often delayed because the uninjured members of the team were engaging other threats.[4] In OEF, IED explo-sions often were triggered by dismounted soldiers who sustained traumatic lower ex-tremity amputations, perineal, pelvic, and occasional thermal injuries. Personal protective equipment such as helmet, body armor, ballistic eye protection, and so forth, will mitigate some of the injuries sustained. However, no amount of equipment will prevent all injuries. Local national casualties will likely not have such equipment and will have a more severe injury pattern.[5]

Rockets, rocket-propelled grenades, and other munitions can cause devastating injury to a large number of casualties. Polytrauma and burns are often a part of the injury pattern. The severity of burn injury can be variable but the combination of large surface area burn and severe traumatic injury portends the highest morbidity and mor-tality.[6] Munitions from previous conflicts to include the Soviet–Afghan War and Iran–Iraq War may contain white phosphorous that can cause severe burns and life-threatening hypocalcemia.[7] The use of chlorine gas was also documented. Chlorine gas can cause severe eye and skin injury and can result in severe inhalation injury in the unprotected patient.[8]

ROLE I (PREHOSPITAL) CARE

The initial task of the first responder (combat medic or Navy corpsman) on the battle-field is to assess the tactical situation, aide in securing perimeter, identify, quickly eval-uate, and stabilize the wounded. This task is difficult under ideal situations but even more so during active combat. The first responder has limited resources but must triage service members, coalition troops, host nation personnel, and local civilians for care. They will often decide who should be evacuated, method of evacuation (ground vs rotary), and the order in which patients will be evacuated. The presence of local national elderly and pediatric patients can complicate triage efforts. Severe burns can be a distraction and delay the identification and treatment of immediately life-threatening injuries.[9]

Rotary evacuation with the HH60 Blackhawk helicopter was the "work horse" of US medical evacuation in recent conflicts. The flight medic is trained to stabilize the patient and provide security as needed during the mission. Obtaining a stable airway is difficult in this circumstance due to the limited space, noise, and poor lighting. A definite airway is often not obtained until arrival at a Role II or III facility (Forward Resuscitative Surgical Team, Combat Support Hospital, Field Hospital). This delay should not be prolonged in patients suspected to have inhalation injury. Intravenous access should be obtained quickly but potential sites for access are limited in patients with large burns. Intraosseous access is also sufficient at least initially. Burn wounds should be covered with clean dry dressings; saline/fluid-soaked dressings must be avoided to prevent hypothermia. Blankets and other warming devices should be used especially for patients evacuated by air.[10]

CARE AT ROLES II AND III

Initial stabilization and evaluation will take place at the Role II or III facility. The initial focus will be on injuries that are immediately life-threatening—those that involve airway, breathing, hemorrhage, trauma brain injury, and traumatic amputations—before considering the burn wound. Transfusion of needed blood products or whole blood should be considered.

Burn resuscitation can begin once other life-threatening injuries are addressed. The Joint Trauma System burn care clinical practice guidelines utilizes the "Rule of Tens" to guide burn resuscitation in adults.[11–14] Several casualties could potentially deplete the limited supply of crystalloids at a Role II facility, reinforcing the need to stabilize casualties and expeditiously transport them up the evacuation chain. For combat casualties, serial neurovascular examinations will be difficult to do with fidelity so it is prudent to perform escharotomies them before transfer.

There are many options for wound care for burn patients. One must consider that burn dressings that require daily or twice daily dressing changes are not practical in this environment. During the conflicts in Iraq and Afghanistan, silver-impregnated nylon dressings were used. The advantage of these and other silver dressings is that they can remain intact for several days and provide reasonable antimicrobial protection.[15]

AEROMEDICAL EVACUATION

Once US and coalition burn casualties are stabilized, preparation should be made for aeromedical evacuation. One major advance of recent conflicts was that patients could be evacuated from POI to the continental US in less than 96 hours. Appropriate level of care must be maintained throughout the evacuation process. Success hinges on good stabilization at Roles II and III before fixed-wing evacuation. All life-threatening traumatic injures must be addressed and at least stabilized. Most important is the respiratory assessment because patients may experience significant respiratory compromise at altitude. Severe inhalation injury may preclude safe aeromedical evacuation.[16] There may be a small window to evacuate these patients to Role IV where advanced modes of ventilation and extracorporeal life support (ECLS) are available.

During recent conflicts, critical-care teams were used to transport patients from the theaters of Iraq, Syria, and Afghanistan to the Role IV US hospital at Landstuhl,

Germany, and then from that hospital to the United States. Critical Care Air Transport team (CCATT), a US Air Force asset, was utilized for the transport of patients from the combat zone to the Role IV hospital, and for transcontinental transport of patients with intermediate-severity burns. The most critically ill burn patients—those with large total body surface area burns (usually >40%) and/or moderate-to-severe inhalation injury— were transported by the US Army Burn Flight Team (BFT). The latter has critical-care-trained providers, nurses, licensed vocational nurses, and respiratory therapists who work full time in the Army Burn Center. Elements of the CCATT and BFT are assembled for ECLS support missions to the theater of operations.[17]

CARE OF HOST NATIONALS

Military medical units must prepare to care for host nationals on the battlefield. In any conflict, injury to host national civilians and military personnel should be anticipated. The host national medical system will likely be disrupted, making military medical units the most capable hospitals in the theater of operations. Many civilian casualties will be evacuated to these units but, unlike US and coalition casualties, they may require more definitive treatment before discharge. The initial evaluation and stabilization of the host national burn casualty is nearly identical to their military counterparts. One major difference is that host nationals with large surface area burns (>50% in the recent conflicts) were placed in the expectant category. One reason is that there are limited or no options for temporary wound coverage (eg, cadaver allograft or porcine xenograft).[18] Another reason was the operational imperative to keep facility beds open for the treatment of anticipated combat casualties, whereas burn care is labor-intensive, resource-intensive, and time-intensive. However, deployed US burn surgeons demonstrated their ability to provide definitive care to injured host national burn patients. Our approach was to keep the hospital leadership aware of the progress of the burn patient and the value of maximizing treatment outcomes.

Military medical units in the theater of operations must also be prepared to care for pediatric burn casualties. Children will present with injuries sustained from combat operations, and with nonbattle injuries such as cooking accidents, heating accidents, and so forth. Military medical units should have pediatric medical equipment available and providers and nurses with experience in pediatrics should be assigned to the unit. During war in Iraq, a program involving the Role III hospital in Baghdad and the Shriners Hospitals in the United States processed pediatric patients with large and/ or complex burn wounds for transfer to United States for medical care. The patients returned to Iraq once their treatments were completed.[19]

BURN DISASTERS

A burn mass-casualty disaster is an event in which a health-care system is overwhelmed by an influx of burn injuries, which exceeds capacity and thus engenders morbidity and mortality above usual expected outcomes.[20] Goals for planning and policy are fundamentally simple: set in place the health-care response to a surge in burn injuries such that the most lives can be saved when demand outstrips finite resources, by "degrading gracefully."[21,22]

Economic constraints. A simplistic question might be to ask "why don't we just increase baseline burn-care capacity?" Burn care and its component infrastructure and resource utilization are expensive—arguably one of the more expensive casualty diagnoses.[23] Any given polity has a finite fraction of total budget that can be spent on health care, and therefore, no realistic pathway exists to limitlessly expand burn-care resources in anticipation of a disaster.

Nonscalability. Under a mass-casualty event, material, knowledge, procedures, and manpower are not linear with respect to the care burden. Many of these aspects will experience geometric increase in needs, whereas others will be a "hard fail" when the system is stressed suddenly. Such nonscalable, nonlinear dynamics make civilian defense planning more difficult and underscore the pressing responsibility to plan sensibly.[24]

Knowledge deficit. Severely compounding mass-burn-casualty preparations is the lack of widespread knowledge of burn care. Huge strides in outcomes have been made during the past 60 years but at the expense of hyperspecialization by a tiny fraction of health-care professionals. In the United States, burn training has been removed from the syllabus for general surgeons, and plastic surgical training requirements have been minimized.[25]

The ABA Austere Guidelines for Burn Care, along with more recent guidelines from the International Society for Burn Injuries and the Technical Working Group of the World Health Organization, were written to help address this fundamental burn-care knowledge deficit. They do not take the place of hands-on specialty training but are a critical link to better outcomes in times of disasters.[26] Another accommodation to address the knowledge deficit has been the preparation of just-in-time education—in response to the Russian invasion, in 2022, the American Burn Association and the Regional Disaster Health Response System Region 1 (New England) provided a syllabus of 13 burn-care videos for war surgeons in Ukraine.[26]

Three separate problems. In the United States, we have found it useful to separate potential future scenarios into 3 distinct categories (200, 2000, and 20,000 burn patients) because a cogent response to each magnitude of calamity takes on very different implications. There are roughly 2000 burn beds in the United States, with a typical occupancy rate of roughly 80%. In an event with 200 simultaneous burn casualties, the entire capacity of any one region would be consumed. A 2000-casualty event would require a whole-of-nation effort. Modeling of a nuclear device strike on a population center informs planners of an epicenter of complete obliteration, surrounded by a ring of perhaps 20,000 living individuals suffering from flash burns. This last scenario invokes drastic crisis standards of care and totally upends expectations on what can and cannot be done in the aftermath for burn victims.[27]

Crisis standards of care are a well-established concept in disaster medicine. There is an ethical imperative to optimize the most good for the most people in a resource-constrained scenario.[20] All polities must acknowledge and embrace this concept as sensible planning for mass-casualty disasters; deliberate premeditated rationing of care is infinitely preferable to no overarching strategy once in the midst of an actual response.

A sensible preparation for response to mass-burn casualties is arguably one of the most difficult problems facing stakeholders. A winning approach will only be achieved by harnessing a whole-of-society approach. Therefore, cogent plans and policies must be an airtight collaboration between the health-care system and the government.[28]

CONCEPT OF OPERATIONS

All disasters are local. The unfolding of a burn mass-casualty disaster and the most sensible set of responses has infinite permutations, all directly influenced by the uniqueness of each municipality, each geography, each polity's strengths and weaknesses, and so forth. Therefore, all scholarly work on disaster medicine (and burns in particular) must speak in wider principles so as to maintain relevance.[29,30]

Self-sufficiency. Every jurisdiction in the aftermath of a disaster becomes, for some time, an island. Typically, best practice (in well-resourced countries) assumes that there are at least 72 to 96 hours of isolation before any sort of outside help arrives. Each locality should contemplate how supplies can be shared, patients load-balanced, and practices modified to prevent a hard failure during this window of isolation.[31,32]

Situational awareness. Any cogent burn mass-casualty plan must incorporate reiterative assessment of situational awareness—how many casualties, their distribution, what is the loss of infrastructure and care capacity, what is the surge capacity of unoccupied burn-care assets. Things change—get better or worse—and therefore repeat assessments are critical.[33]

Secondary triage. Burn care is extreme specialty care, and initial triage during the confusion of a mass-casualty response will be inaccurate. This generates a requirement for secondary triage to match individual and population needs to ever-changing resources. This reallocation exercise must be built into response plans.[33]

Interface with other providers. In the United States, there are perhaps only 300 burn surgeons nationwide. Following a burn disaster, the only recourse is to enlist closely allied health-care professionals to fill the gap, armed with just-in-time education on burn-care fundamentals. These personnel include emergency medical system (EMS), emergency medicine teams, and trauma surgeons.[34]

Moving patients versus moving teams. One unanswered fundamental question in disaster medicine is the relative wisdom of bringing in specialty-care teams into the epicenter of a disaster versus transporting patients out of the epicenter. During the 9-11 attacks in New York and Washington DC, providers were brought into the epicenter with gallant intent but (in hindsight) uncertain impact. This question has still to be answered definitively, and currently both approaches are part of the fabric of preparations in the United States.[35]

MEDICAL MANAGEMENT

Life-saving interventions. In the first 6 hours postburn, proximal threats to life and limb are airway loss and (in a minority of patients) circumferential third-degree burns compromising limb perfusion or respirations. All other threats fall under the rubric of concomitant trauma.[36]

Burn shock becomes a proximal cause of death in later hours with burn sizes roughly greater than 20% to 30% total body surface area, colored by significant past medical history, presence of smoke inhalation, and/or frailty at the extremes of age. Intravenous fluid management of burn shock will likely be unavailable in large burn disasters, and oral fluid resuscitation plays a central role under these circumstances.[36]

Combined injuries. Any calamitous event that would engender burn injuries measured in the hundreds or greater is likely to be extremely violent, meaning that burns will be found paired with severe traumatic injuries. Sensible planning will include multidisciplinary care teams, with all the trauma subspecialties included.[37]

Time smearing. If there is one bedrock conceptual facet of medical management in burn disasters, it is to "time smear" the must-do tasks in the care of each patient who is one of many who need finite resources. The strategy is to do the minimum required to keep large numbers of burn victims from losing life or limb until (1) redistribution, (2) ramp-up of supplies and capacity, and (3) high fidelity situational awareness can be achieved. What is typically done for a burn patient in the first week during normal times might have to be degraded, metered out, and modified to span a time-smeared 3-week response window.[27]

Degrading gracefully. As described above, the response to a burn disaster must execute a time-smearing strategy to save as many lives as possible with the finite resources on hand. The next step is to invoke premeditated rationing of resources, and changes to the injury severity that falls under expectant/comfort care only. The ABA v.3 Actionable Triage Tables present a family of tables, each tailored to the previously mentioned broad categories of North American burn mass-casualty contingency planning, namely 200, 2000, or 20,000 concurrent burn casualties.[38]

Medico-legal and ethical considerations. The ethical implications of triage and rationing have been considered in a scholarly fashion during the past decade.[21] The intersection of medico-legal thought and crisis standards of care is an active topic at the National Academy of Sciences, with legal scholars deeply embedded in the discussions. The nascent US approach to "degrading gracefully" is informed by the latest discussions in this authoritative body.[39]

TRANSNATIONAL CONSIDERATIONS

The role of nongovernmental organizations. A recent publication aimed to catalog nongovernmental organizations (NGOs) working in the burn-care space.[40] This study was a response to the chaotic international response to the Haiti Earthquake in 2010. The response to the Sierra Leone burn disaster in November 2021 seems to have gone much more smoothly.

Cross-border decompression. The Russian invasion of Ukraine resulted in the displacement of large civilian populations, many of whom were grievously injured. There is evidence of decompression of casualties to neighboring Poland for medical assistance.[41]

Of all segments in burn care, pediatric care is arguably the most highly specialized and concentrated into the smallest group of experts. The Shriners Hospitals have been in the van for decades providing care for pediatric burn victims from around the globe, often in the aftermath of small mass-burn-casualty events. The US Army Institute of Surgical Research (Army Burn Center) also has a long history of globe-spanning humanitarian burn care, with both adult and pediatric patients. Thus, there is a strong, multidecade precedent of deeply resourced programs to offer global transport of burn victims that eclipse local resources. It remains to be seen whether we will be graced with a progressive enlargement of such laudable efforts and organizations from around the globe.[42]

SUMMARY

In summary, the modern battlefield is a dynamic environment. Roles II and III personnel should be trained in the care of burn patients to include pediatric burn patients, which they should anticipate encountering. Long-range aeromedical evacuation of combat casualties has greatly evolved during recent conflicts; much experience has been gained from the intercontinental transport of burned combat casualties.

Similarly dynamic is the planning for and response to burn disasters, with a clear emphasis on the former. Sensible planning as outlined will allow a polity's healthcare system to "degrade gracefully" in the face of overwhelming concurrent burn casualties.

DECLARATION OF INTERESTS

The authors have nothing to disclose. The opinions or assertions contained herein are the private views of the authors and are not to be construed as official or as reflecting the views of the Department of the Army or the Department of Defense.

REFERENCES

1. Cancio LC, Horvath EE, Barillo DJ, et al. Burn support for Operation Iraqi Freedom and related operations, 2003 to 2004. J Burn Care Rehabil 2005; 26(2):151–61.
2. Ramasamy A, Hill A, Clasper J. Improvised Explosive Devices. Pathophysiology, Injury Profiles and Current Medical Management. BMJ Military Health 2009;155: 265–72.
3. Koutras A, Syllaios A, Tsilikis I, et al. Dealing with burn patients in war zones. Disaster Med Public Health Prep 2021;15(1):15–9.
4. Belmont PJ Jr, McCriskin BJ, Sieg RN, et al. Combat wounds in Iraq and Afghanistan from 2005 to 2009. J Trauma Acute Care Surg 2012;73(1):3–12.
5. Rankin IA, Webster CE, Gibb I, et al. Pelvic injury patterns in blast: Morbidity and mortality. J Trauma Acute Care Surg 2020;88(6):832–8.
6. Marshall TJ Jr. Combat casualty care: the Alpha Surgical Company experience during Operation Iraqi Freedom. Mil Med 2005;170(6):469–72.
7. Mozingo DW, Smith AA, McManus WF, et al. Chemical burns. J Trauma 1988; 28(5):642–7.
8. Mozingo DW, Smith AA, McManus WF, et al. Chemical burns. J Trauma 1988; 28(5):642–7.
9. Lairet KF, Lairet JR, King BT, et al. Prehospital burn management in a combat zone. Prehosp Emerg Care 2012;16(2):273–6.
10. Mabry RL, Apodaca A, Penrod J, et al. Impact of critical care-trained flight paramedics on casualty survival during helicopter evacuation in the current war in Afghanistan. J Trauma Acute Care Surg 2012;73(2 Suppl 1):S32–7.
11. Chung KK, Salinas J, Renz EM, et al. Simple derivation of the initial fluid rate for the resuscitation of severely burned adult combat casualties: in silico validation of the rule of 10. J Trauma 2010;69(Suppl 1):S49–54.
12. Ennis JL, Chung KK, Renz EM, et al. Joint Theater Trauma System implementation of burn resuscitation guidelines improves outcomes in severely burned military casualties. J Trauma 2008 Feb;64(2 Suppl):S146–51 [discussion: S151-2].
13. Salinas J, Drew G, Gallagher J, et al. Closed-loop and decision-assist resuscitation of burn patients. J Trauma 2008;64(4 Suppl):S321–32.
14. Cartotto R, Greenhalgh DG, Cancio C. Burn State of the Science: Fluid Resuscitation. J Burn Care Res 2017;38(3):e596–604.
15. Driscoll IR, Mann-Salinas EA, Boyer NL, et al. Burn Casualty Care in the Deployed Setting. Mil Med 2018;183(suppl_2):161–7.
16. Beninati W, Meyer MT, Carter TE. The critical care air transport program. Crit Care Med 2008;36(7 Suppl):S370–6.
17. Renz EM, Cancio LC, Barillo DJ, et al. Long range transport of war-related burn casualties. J Trauma 2008;64(2 Suppl):S136–44.
18. Jeevaratnam JA, Pandya AN. One year of burns at a role 3 Medical Treatment Facility in Afghanistan. J R Army Med Corps 2014;160(1):22–6.
19. Schmidt PM, Sheridan RL, Moore CL, et al. From Baghdad to Boston: international transfer of burned children in time of war. J Burn Care Res 2014;35(5): 369–73.
20. Sheridan RL, Friedstat J, Votta K. Lessons Learned from Burn Disasters in the Post-9/11 Era. Clin Plast Surg 2017;44(3):435–40.
21. Hanfling D, Hick JL, Stroud C, eds. Crisis standards of care: a Toolkit for Indicators and Triggers. Washington, DC: National Academies Press (US), 27.

22. Dai A, Carrougher GJ, Mandell SP, et al. Review of Recent Large-Scale Burn Disasters Worldwide in Comparison to Preparedness Guidelines. J Burn Care Res 2017;38(1):36–44.

23. Mathews AL, Cheng MH, Muller JM, et al. Cost Analysis of 48 Burn Patients in a Mass Casualty Explosion Treated at Chang Gung Memorial Hospital. Injury 2017 Jan;48(1):80–6.

24. Kao HK, Loh CYY, Kou HW, et al. Optimizing mass casualty burns intensive care organization and treatment using evidence-based outcome predictors. Burns 2018;44(5):1077–82.

25. Gamelli RL. Who will follow? J Burn Care Res 2006;27(1):1–7.

26. Jeng JC. A Quartet of American Burn Association Clinical Guidelines for Austere Condition Burn Care: Gestation, Collaboration, Future Impact, and Post Humus Dedication. J Burn Care Res 2017 Sep/Oct;38(5):e883.

27. Barrera-Oro J. BARDA Thermal Burn Medical Countermeasures Program. Washington, DC: US Department of Health and Human Services 2018. Available at: https://www.medicalcountermeasures.gov/BARDA/Documents/BID2018_Presentations/BarreraOro_BID18_ThermalBurns.pdf. Accessed December 23, 2022.

28. Jeng JC. North American Burn Care Community + Ukraine War Surgeons Just-in-Time Education Burn Grand Rounds Lecture Series. Presented the International Society for Burn Injuries 21st Congress, August 28-September 1 2022, Guadalajara, Mexico.

29. Binkley JM, Kemp KM. Mobilization of Resources and Emergency Response on the National Scale. Surg Clin North Am 2022;102(1):169–80.

30. Thomasian NM, Madad S, Hick JL, et al. Hospital Surge Preparedness and Response Index. Disaster Med Public Health Prep 2021;15(3):398–401.

31. Ray J. Federal declaration of a Public Health Emergency. Biosecur Bioterror 2009;7(3):251–8.

32. Adams RM, Karlin B, Eisenman DP, et al. Who Participates in the Great ShakeOut? Why Audience Segmentation Is the Future of Disaster Preparedness Campaigns. Environ Res Public Health 2017;14(11):1407.

33. Chuang S, Woods DD, Ting HW, et al. Coping With a Mass Casualty: Insights into a Hospital's Emergency Response and Adaptations After the Formosa Fun Coast Dust Explosion. Disaster Med Public Health Prep 2020;14(4):467–76.

34. American Burn Association. Disaster Response. Available at. https://ameriburn.org/quality-care/disaster-response/. Accessed December 23, 2022.

35. Jordan MH, Hollowed KA, Turner DG, et al. The Pentagon attack of September 11, 2001: a burn center's experience. J Burn Care Rehabil 2005;26(2):109–16.

36. Kearns RD, Conlon KM, Matherly AF, et al. Guidelines for Burn Care Under Austere Conditions: Introduction to Burn Disaster, Airway and Ventilator Management, and Fluid Resuscitation. J Burn Care Res 2016 Sep-Oct;37(5):e427–39.

37. Cancio LC, Sheridan RL, Dent R, et al. Guidelines for Burn Care Under Austere Conditions: Special Etiologies: Blast, Radiation, and Chemical Injuries. J Burn Care Res 2017;38(1):e482–96.

38. Kearns RD, Bettencourt AP, Hickerson WL, et al. Actionable, Revised (v.3), and Amplified American Burn Association Triage Tables for Mass Casualties: A Civilian Defense Guideline. J Burn Care Res 2020;41(4):770–9.

39. Hodge JG Jr. Revisiting Legal Foundations of Crisis Standards of Care. J Law Med Ethics 2020 Mar;48(1):221–4.

40. Fabia R, Gallagher J, Wheeler KK, et al. Efforts to catalogue non-governmental organizations with a role in global burn relief. Burns 2020;46(4):804–16.

41. Anonymous. "The war changed everything": Surgeons Share Lessons Learned from Ukraine. Chicago: American College of Surgeons; 2022. Available at. https://www.facs.org/for-medical-professionals/news-publications/news-and-articles/press-releases/2022/the-war-changed-everything-surgeons-share-lessons-learned-from-ukraine/. Accessed December 23, 2022.
42. Fuzaylov G, Anderson R, Knittel J, et al. Global health: burn outreach program. J Burn Care Res 2015;36(2):306–9.

Radiation Injuries

Randy D. Kearns, DHA, MSA, FRSPH[a],*, William L. Hickerson, MD[b],
Jeffery E. Carter, MD[c]

KEYWORDS

- Radiation injuries • Acute radiation syndrome • Localized radiation injury
- Cutaneous radiation syndrome • Burns • Disaster planning • Surge Capacity

KEY POINTS

- Contamination occurs when radioactive material is present in or on a person. Exposure (irradiation) occurs whenever an individual has been in the presence of radioactive materials.
- Although ionizing radiation is more dangerous, there are risks associated with both ionizing and nonionizing radiation.
- Life-, limb-, and vision-saving care is the priority and should not be delayed for the decontamination of radioactive materials. The order of decontamination should be (1) wounds, (2) facial orifices (to include eyes), and (3) intact skin.
- Any patient with a radiation source exposure should be evaluated for acute radiation syndrome and for a localized radiation injury, also known as cutaneous radiation syndrome.

INTRODUCTION

Injuries involving radiation are rare but can be catastrophic for the patient while also exposing clinicians to significant risk.[1] This article focuses on radiation-related injuries and on thermal burns produced by a nuclear reaction. This work also addresses radiation injuries that may or may not have burn characteristics.[2]

Radioactive forms of elements are called *radionuclides*. There are more than 60 radionuclides found naturally in the environment, and others are manmade.[3] Although the smaller category, manmade sources play a significant role in causing radiation-associated injury. Inherently unstable atomic structures are termed *radioactive* due to their natural tendency to release excess energy or mass to attain states of greater stability. These emissions are called *radiation*.

[a] University of New Orleans, College of Business Administration, 347 Kirschman Hall, 2000 Lakefront Drive, New Orleans, LA 70148, USA; [b] University of Tennessee Health Science Center (Retired), G30 Jesse Turner Burn Center, 890 Madison Avenue, Memphis, TN 38103, USA; [c] Louisiana State University Health Sciences Center New Orleans, UMC Burn Center, University Medical Center New Orleans, 2000 Canal Street, New Orleans, LA 70112, USA
* Corresponding author.
E-mail address: rkearns@uno.edu

Surg Clin N Am 103 (2023) 539–550
https://doi.org/10.1016/j.suc.2023.01.011
0039-6109/23/© 2023 Elsevier Inc. All rights reserved.

surgical.theclinics.com

Radiation is a general term that simply refers to the emission of energy in the form of waves or particles. Radiation can be classified into 2 types: nonionizing and ionizing. Radio, microwave, and ultraviolet radiation are called *nonionizing radiation* because they lack the energy necessary to remove an electron from a target atom. On the other hand, *ionizing radiation* has enough energy to strip an orbiting electron from an atom. The remaining atom becomes positively charged. As a result, ionizing radiation poses a significant biologic threat (**Fig. 1**).[4]

IRRADIATION VERSUS CONTAMINATION

The term *irradiation* describes exposure of the human body to penetrating radiation emitted from radioactive materials or a radiation-generating device.[5] *External contamination* occurs when radioactive materials are deposited on the body surfaces, such as the skin. *Internal contamination* occurs when radioactive materials enter the body (eg, through inhalation, ingestion, absorption, or via wounds). Exposure to radioactive materials (irradiation) is not an absolute indication that an individual was also contaminated. This is an essential point, because the risk of contamination determines the need for personal protective equipment (PPE). The presence of contamination and the identity of the contaminating radionuclide should be determined as soon as possible, preferably before transport. However, lifesaving medical care should not be delayed based solely on contamination concerns.

During prehospital and emergency care, it is essential to differentiate between contamination and irradiation. An irradiated but uncontaminated patient poses no direct threat to the clinician, the transport vehicle, or the receiving facility.[6] By contrast, a contaminated patient takes radioactive material with them, so care must be taken to minimize contaminant spread during treatment or transport; this can include clothing removal or simply covering the patient with a sheet during transport. Even if the patient is not decontaminated at the scene, removal and bagging of the patient's clothing is reasonable so long as it does not affect patient care. Turnout gear, surgical clothing, and even paper coveralls may be adequate PPE for contamination events.

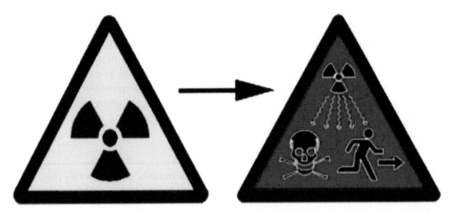

Fig. 1. In February of 2007, the United Nations introduced a supplemental symbol to augment the yellow background symbol. The new symbol (red background) was created to help reduce accidental exposure to large radioactive sources. The new icon is aimed at improving awareness regarding the potential dangers of being close to a large source of ionizing radiation. The new symbol will not be visible under normal use, but only if someone attempts to disassemble a device that is a source of dangerous radiation. It will not be located on building access doors, transportation packages, or containers.

TYPES OF IONIZING RADIATION

Both alpha and beta radiation are particulate in nature, whereas X rays and gamma radiation are electromagnetic. Gamma rays and X rays behave identically, so they will be considered together. Neutrons are emitted from a few radionuclides when there is a criticality or a nuclear detonation.

Alpha particles contain 2 protons, 2 neutrons, and a 2+ charge. They have minimal penetration capability, can be shielded by a piece of paper, and thus, as a rule, do not penetrate the stratum corneum. Although alpha particles do not pose a significant external threat to humans, alpha emitters can be hazardous if taken internally, such as through wound contamination, inhalation, or ingestion.

Beta particles are moderately penetrating (can penetrate human skin to the innermost layer of the epidermis, where new keratinocytes are produced) and can typically be shielded by materials such as aluminum foil or several sheets of paper. The term is used for high-energy electrons emitted from a nucleus. Beta particles are usually not a problem if they do not stay in contact with the skin for long periods. Depth of penetration is a function of their energy measured in mega-electron volts (Mev). As an example, a 0.1 Mev particle will penetrate 0.15 cm into tissue and a 5.0 Mev particle will penetrate 5.0 cm into tissue. Thus, beta particles can be an external hazard to the skin and lens of the eye. The radiation dose to the target organ must also be considered if internalized.

Gamma rays and *X rays* are highly energetic and penetrating and thus require dense materials, such as lead, to shield them. Although gamma rays and X rays differ in origin, they pose the same hazards via external irradiation.

Neutron radiation is rarely encountered; this is the only type of radiation that can make something else radioactive, a process referred to as neutron activation.

QUANTIFYING RADIATION EXPOSURE AND EFFECTS

The amount of radiation delivered to the body and the biological effects of that dose on the body are 2 different but related concepts and are measured differently. The gray (Gy) is an SI unit for the amount of energy absorbed by tissue. 1.0 Gy is equal to an absorbed dose of 1 J/kg. An absorbed dose of 0.01 Gy means that 1 g of tissue absorbed 100 ergs of energy (a small but measurable amount) because of exposure to radiation. 1.0 Gy = 100 rad; rad is a historical US unit.[6]

Grays and rads measure energy absorption but do not measure biological effects. A common way to quantify biological radiation damage and to estimate a resulting risk profile is an SI unit, the Sievert (SV), or a US unit, the Roentgen Equivalent Man (rem). These units of measurement are referred to as *dose equivalents*. These units are equal to the delivered radiation dose (rad or Gy), multiplied by a dimensionless weighting factor that benchmarks resultant biological damage to a hypothetical exposure from a common radiation source (usually gamma or X rays). In other words, the rem is defined as the dosage of a particular radiation type (measured in rad) that will cause the same degree of biological injury as 1 rad of either gamma or X rays.[6]

RISK ASSESSMENT

Radiation sources can be commonly found in many hospital and industrial settings. Industrial uses of radiation can range from instrumentation required to measure the density of soil being compacted during road construction to radioactive sources used for the nondestructive analytical testing of materials.

Two significant events involving nuclear power plants have occurred over the last 35 years, including substantial uncontrolled radiological releases at Fukushima in

2011[7–9] and at the Chernobyl Nuclear Power Plant in 1986.[8,10,11] Both events resulted in major uncontrolled releases of radiation and had a significant long-term impact on the environment in the immediate area of the plants.

According to a report published in 2004 by the US Federal Emergency Management Agency,[12,13] the most significant foreseeable risks of a mass-casualty event associated with radiation center on terrorism and military action. Scenarios outlined in that text include radiological dispersal devices, radiological exposure devices, and military-grade nuclear weapons:[14–31]

- *Radiological dispersal device or "dirty bomb"* includes anything that disperses radioactive material through detonation of conventional explosives or other (nonnuclear) means. Examples include a crop-dusting airplane, a building's ventilation system, or wrapping radioactive material around a common explosive device (such as dynamite).
- *Radiation exposure device* relies on placing radioactive material in a location to expose a person or persons without their knowledge. For example, sources commonly used in industry, such as a soil density probe or a cancer brachytherapy source, could be placed under a seat on a bus or subway.
- *Nuclear weapons* range from small to enormous weapons.[14,15] The 1945 detonations generated not only widespread radiation fallout but also tens of thousands of survivors with thermal injury.[16] Modern nuclear-weapon technology uses highly enriched materials. Comparatively compact weapons can be built to provide a wide range of explosive capabilities.

PATHOPHYSIOLOGY: LOCAL RADIATION INJURY

Exposure to high-intensity ionizing radiation can cause a burn injury. The literature describes this type of burn injury as *local radiation injury* (LRI) or *cutaneous radiation syndrome* (CRS).[6,17,18] The term "radiation burns" has also been used. LRI describes the pathological syndrome that results from acute radiation exposure to the skin. Nevertheless, visible burns produced by ionizing radiation should also prompt an assessment for acute radiation syndrome (see later discussion).

Cutaneous exposure doses greater than or equal to 3.0 Gy may result in skin changes, although their development may be delayed up to 2 weeks following an event. Generally, thermal burns may be distinguished from LRI because thermal burns often can be visually identified immediately. Sequential images of an LRI that were obtained as the injury developed over time are presented in **Fig. 2**.[19]

LRI occurs when the basal cell layer of the skin is damaged by radiation; inflammation, erythema, and dry or moist desquamation may occur. Furthermore, hair follicles may be damaged, causing epilation. Within a few hours after irradiation, a transient and inconsistent erythema (associated with itching) may occur. Depending on the site, condition of the skin (preexposure), and the dose of exposure, a latent phase may occur and last from a few days up to several weeks; this is visibly characterized by intense reddening, blistering, and ulceration of the irradiated site. In most cases, healing occurs by regenerative means; however, very large skin doses can cause permanent hair loss, damaged sebaceous and sweat glands, atrophy, fibrosis, decreased or increased skin pigmentation, and ulceration or necrosis of the exposed tissue.[20]

PATHOPHYSIOLOGY: ACUTE RADIATION SYNDROME

Acute radiation syndrome (ARS), previously known as "radiation sickness," is an acute illness caused by irradiation of most (or the entire) body by a high dose of penetrating

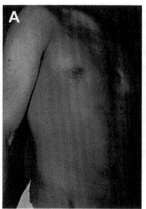
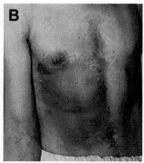
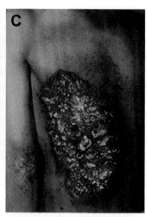

Fig. 2. (*A–C*) Localized radiation injury (LRI) caused by exposure to ionizing radiation. This patient found an unshielded 185 GBq Ir-192 source used for industrial radiography and placed it in his shirt pocket. (*A*) Day 6 after injury; (*B*) day 12; (*C*) day 15. He also showed early signs of ARS. The patient survived the injury. (INTERNATIONAL ATOMIC ENERGY AGENCY, The Radiological Accident in Gilan, IAEA, Vienna (2002).)

radiation; this typically is only a brief exposure (minutes), but the results can be devastating. The major mechanism of ARS is depletion of immature parenchymal stem cells in specific tissues. Any patient presenting with LRI or who suffers known exposure to a significant radiation source should be evaluated for the development of ARS. The organ systems that are most affected by ARS include those with either the highest rates of cellular turnover (eg, gastrointestinal, hematopoietic) or the least resilience to injury (eg, neurovascular). ARS is most likely associated with a large radiation dose (>0.7 Gy). The dose is typically external; the radiation must be penetrating (X rays, gamma rays, or neutrons); the entire body (or almost all the entire body) must have received the dose, and the dose must have been delivered in a short time.[20] There are 3 major ARS syndromes.

- *Hematopoietic or bone-marrow syndrome*: this syndrome presents with mild symptoms for doses as low as 0.3 Gy, and with more acute symptoms for a dose greater than 0.7 Gy. The greater the dose, the greater the destruction of bone marrow, resulting in infection and hemorrhage.[20]
- *Gastrointestinal syndrome*: this syndrome presents with mild symptoms for doses as low as 6.0 Gy, and with more acute symptoms for a dose greater than 10.0 Gy. Mortality is quite high for patients with acute symptoms (indicating exposure > 10.0 Gy), leading to dehydration and electrolyte imbalance.[20]
- *Cardiovascular/central nervous system (CNS) syndrome*: if doses are greater than or equal to 20.0 Gy, some cardiovascular or CNS symptoms may occur. Rapid onset of acute symptoms will occur if the dose is greater than or equal to 50.0 Gy. With either mild or acute symptoms, death is likely within 72 hours of exposure due to collapse of the circulatory system and increasing intracranial pressure.[20]

ACTIONS AT THE SCENE

Standard PPE does not protect the wearer from exposure to penetrating radiation; PPE only mitigates contamination. Potential contamination threats can be managed with many of the same principles commonly employed for more common hazardous materials. Effective methods of limiting radiation exposure include limiting time spent in the area of the radiation source, identifying the source location and maintaining a safe distance from it, and creating effective shielding of the source. Another management principle includes what is referred to as ALARA (As Low as Reasonably Achievable). The principles of ALARA are as follows: limit the time spent in the presence of radioactive materials, maximize the distance from radioactive materials, and maximize shielding from radioactive materials.[21]

DECONTAMINATION

Patients with known or suspected radioactive exposure should be decontaminated, with particular attention to skin injuries and open wounds. Lifesaving medical or surgical treatment of a casualty should not be delayed pending decontamination.[21] Care should be taken to minimize contaminants in ambulances and health care facilities. Interventions indicated by primary assessment findings should not be delayed for extensive decontamination efforts. Decontamination should include the following:

- Removal of clothing (bag and label with personal identification). When possible, this should be delivered with the patient to the hospital and can be quite valuable in determining the source of the radiation.
- Discarded dressings, bandages, cleaning materials, and clothes should be bagged and labeled.
- Whenever possible, take the steps necessary to minimize contaminants in transport vehicles and receive health care facilities.

The Armed Forces Radiobiology Research Institute states that radiological decontamination is very similar to chemical decontamination.[17] The key differences include the following. Chemical decontamination is an emergency, whereas radiological decontamination is not. Furthermore, for certain chemicals, the aim is chemical neutralization, whereas with radiological decontamination, the aim is the physical removal of the contaminants. Because this is not an emergency, containment is a reasonable strategy until the patient can be appropriately decontaminated. Wet decontamination (showering) may spread contamination and worsen the situation. Nevertheless, if there are multiple contaminants present (in addition to a radiation source), local procedures and best care practices may dictate the need for wet decontamination as well.

If wet decontamination is indicated, great care should be taken not to abrade or otherwise breach intact skin.[6] A conventional process for wet decontamination uses the method of rinsing affected patients with copious amounts of warm or cool water (not cold or hot). This process may include using a commercial decontamination shower, fire department booster hose, hand line (minimal pressure), or other realistic and safe means to facilitate access to copious amounts of water for thorough decontamination.

The order of decontamination should be (1) wounds, (2) facial orifices (to include eye irrigation), and (3) intact skin.[6]

INITIAL ASSESSMENT

Initial assessment and management of radiation-injured patients should address the following 4 issues.

- *ABCs and collateral injury:* initial assessment must include a primary survey (the ABCs). Injuries that are immediately apparent will be the result of collateral injuries, such as thermal injuries[22] or traumatic brain injury from blunt-force trauma. Treat these collateral injuries as indicated.

- *Qualify the exposure:* determine the exposure type—irradiation, external contamination, or internal contamination.
- *Quantify the dose:* determine the exposure dose, generally measured in grays (Gy). Data may be available from those on-site who have appropriate monitoring equipment. The presence of radiation is determined by a radiation meter, such as a Geiger-Mueller meter with a pancake probe. Readings of greater than 2 times background in counts per minute (cpm) are considered positive for contamination.[21] Do not delay transport to acquire this information.
- *Quantify the biological effect:* determine the interval between exposure and time-to-emesis (TE) (**Fig. 3**).[17,21] Delayed onset or absence of nausea and vomiting (emesis) is associated with a greater likelihood of survival. TE is a good indicator but not the sole determinant of prognosis.[17] In addition to TE, other early signs/symptoms of acute radiation syndrome include the onset and intensity of headache, core temperature (hyperthermia/hypothermia), diarrhea, neurological/cognitive deficits, and hypotension.[23]

DIAGNOSIS OF LOCALIZED RADIATION INJURY/ACUTE RADIATION SYNDROME

Assessment of the skin should start with determining the involvement of a radiation source, a thermal source, or both. If it is determined that a patient has been exposed to a radiation source, assessment should include the nature of the source as well as an estimation of the absorbed dose. Depending on the dose received, LRI can be manifested by epilation (hair loss), erythema, desquamation, ulceration, or even frank necrosis.[6,17,18]

For LRI, time-to-onset is an important dose-dependent phenomenon and can help estimate exposure magnitude. Sometimes, a radiation injury may take weeks or even months to become manifest. If a burn injury is readily visible in the immediate aftermath of a radiation exposure, the burn injury was probably produced by a heat rather than by irradiation. (For details regarding the estimation of early internal and external dose magnitude, see **Fig. 4**).[24]

Without knowledge of the exposure or of the radioactive source, the diagnosis of ARS can be difficult. Furthermore, depending on the dose, the prodromal stage

Physical injury without irradiation	Expected changes in triage categories after whole-body irradiation		
	<2 Gy Vomit >4 h	2–6 Gy Vomit 1–4 h	>6 Gy Vomit <1 h early erythema
Uninjured	Ambulatory monitoring	Ambulatory monitoring, Administer cytokines and delay hospitalization	
Minimal	Minimal	Delayed	
Delayed	Delayed		
Immediate	Immediate	Variable	
Expectant			Expectant

Fig. 3. Triage categories, taking into account the physical injury with exposure to radiation. (*From* Goans RE. Medical Management of Radiological Casualties, Fourth Edition. Armed Forces Radiobiology Research Institute (AFFRI). July 2013. *Available at* http://operationalmedicine.org/TextbookFiles/4edmmrchandbook.pdf; with permission.)

Skin Injury Thresholds vs. Acute Doses

Dose	Effect	Timing[a] (time post exposure)
3 Gy/300 rads	Epilation	14–21 d
6 Gy/600 rads	Erythema	Early, then 14–21 days later
10–15 Gy 1000–1500 rads	Dry Desquamation	2-3 Wk
15–25 Gy 1500–2500 rads	Wet Desquamation	2-3 Wk
>25 Gy >2500 rads	Deep Ulceration/Necrosis	Dependent upon dose

Fig. 4. Relationship between dose and effect for localized radiation injury (LRI). [a]At higher doses the time to onset of signs/symptoms may be compressed. (*From* Sugarman SLS. Early Internal and External Dose Magnitude Estimation. Dose Estimation Resources. Oak Ridge Institute for Science and Education (ORISE). July 2017. Available at https://orise.orau.gov/resources/reacts/dose-estimation-resources.html; with permission.)

may not emerge for hours or days following the exposure. Alternatively, the patient may already be in the latent stage by the time of initial assessment. At that point, the patient may seem otherwise well and report no significant symptoms. If a patient received more than 0.05 Gy and 3 to 4 complete blood counts (CBCs) are taken within 8 to 12 hours of the exposure, a dose estimate can be made relying on the Andrews Lymphocyte Nomogram (**Fig. 5**).[20,25] If initial CBCs were not taken, the dose can still be estimated by using CBC results over the first few days.[20]

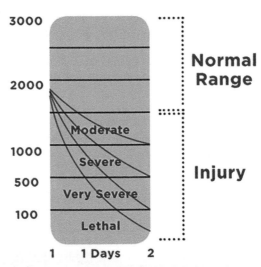

Fig. 5. Andrews lymphocyte nomogram. This graph correlates changes in the lymphocyte count with mortality risk during different time intervals following exposure to a radiation source. (INTERNATIONAL ATOMIC ENERGY AGENCY, ANDREWS, G.A., AUXIER, J.A., LUSHBAUGH, C.C., "The importance of dosimetry to the medical management of persons accidentally exposed to high levels of radiation", Personnel Dosimetry for Radiation Accidents, Proceedings of a Symposium Held in Vienna, Austria, 8-12 March 1965, IAEA, Vienna (1965) 3–16.)

If radiation exposure is not initially suspected, but an unexplained history exists of nausea and vomiting, ARS should be considered. Other indications of ARS are bleeding, epilation, or decreased white blood count and platelet counts several days or weeks following a bout of unexplained nausea and vomiting. Again, consider CBC and chromosome analysis and consultation with radiation experts to confirm diagnosis.[20]

On the other hand, if radiation exposure is initially suspected, a CBC (with particular attention to the lymphocyte count) should be performed every 2 to 3 hours for the first 8 hours after exposure and every 4 to 6 hours for the next two days.[20]

TREATMENT OF LOCALIZED RADIATION INJURY/ACUTE RADIATION SYNDROME

The underlying principle in the treatment of isolated LRI/ARS remains supportive care; this may include treatment of nausea and vomiting, intravenous fluids (lactated Ringer solution), and airway/breathing management.[26,27] Injuries of the skin are initially treated with clean dry dressings. A preferred hospital destination is one that routinely manages patients with cancer (ie, has experience with radiation therapy) or, when available, a treatment facility in the Radiation Injury Treatment Network (RITN).[18,28] Patients with burn injuries should be triaged to a burn center if possible or to a trauma center if a burn center is not readily available. With LRI/ARS, a health physicist should be involved as soon as possible to begin dose assessment and to help inform medical management.

Specific to the radiation injury, blood samples should be obtained for a CBC. The CBC should be repeated every 2 to 3 hours for the first 8 to 12 hours after exposure and every 4 to 6 hours for the following three days, to assess for lymphocyte depletion. Treat contamination as needed. Sequential changes in absolute lymphocyte counts over time are essential in understanding the lethality of the doses[25] (see **Fig. 4**).

With appropriate care, the LD_{50} is approximately 4.0 Gy to 6.0 Gy; without medical care, the LD_{50} is 3.5 to 4.0 Gy. A nonsurvivable whole-body dose is generally considered greater than 10 Gy. In severe cases, optimal care for ARS may include stem-cell transplant.[18,29,30]

A triage table (see **Fig. 2**) has been included to reflect combined burn, trauma, and radiation injury when the number of patients exceeds local resources.[31]

IODINE AND POTASSIUM IODINE

Increased risk of tactical-nuclear strikes or nuclear-power-plant attacks raises the concern of nuclear fallout and the risks of radioactive iodine. Nuclear or radiological events could release radioactive iodine into the air, which could contaminate local food and water supplies. To reduce the risks of radioactive iodine absorption by the thyroid, potassium iodide supplementation has been recommended.[32] Supplementation does not block ingestion or contamination or reverse the adverse effects of previously absorbed radioactive iodine. KI is available in most countries where nuclear power is a source of energy. In the United States, the Food and Drug Administration has approved 2 forms for oral supplementation. Allergy to iodine or certain skin or kidney disorders may preclude use.

SUMMARY

A rational approach to radiation events must facilitate the safe and comprehensive identification of potential radiation sources, the rapid determination of patient exposures, and the efficient and effective management of resources. This process includes sound triage principles while continuously maintaining the critical steps necessary to mitigate ongoing or evolving risks relevant to patients and clinicians.

CLINICS CARE POINTS

- Any patient with radiation-source exposure should be evaluated for ARS and LRI, also known as a CRS.
- The onset of signs and symptoms of radiation exposure may be delayed by hours, days, or up to 2 weeks.
- If a patient seems to have a burn almost immediately after an exposure, the injury is more likely to be a thermal burn, but the patient should still be evaluated for ARS and LRI.
- Patients with vomiting 1 to 4 hours following a potential radiation exposure should be evaluated for ARS. Patients with vomiting and/or diarrhea less than 1 hour after a known exposure typically have poor outcomes.
- Perform repeated CBC monitoring for suspected patients with ARS, looking for a decline in lymphocytes. Compare data with the Andrews Lymphocyte Nomogram.
- Key resources include the hospital health/medical physicist and local, state, and federal radiation experts such as the Radiation Emergency Assistance Center/Training Center (REAC/TS) and the RITN.

DISCLOSURE

R.D. Kearns and W.L. Hickerson have nothing to disclose that is relevant to this content. J.E. Carter: Consultant, Avita Medical Ltd, PolyNovo Ltd, and Spectral MD; Stockholder, Spectral MD.

REFERENCES

1. Christensen DM, Jenkins MS, Sugarman SL, et al. Management of ionizing radiation injuries and illnesses, part 1: physics, radiation protection, and radiation instrumentation. J Am Osteopath Assoc 2014;114(3):189–99.
2. Christensen DM, Iddins CJ, Sugarman SL. Ionizing radiation injuries and illnesses. Emerg Med Clin North Am 2014;32(1):245–65.
3. Eisenbud M, Gesell T. Natural Radioactivity. In: Eisenbud M, Gesell T, editors. *Environmental Radioactivity.* Academic Press; 1997. p. 134–200.
4. International Atomic Energy Agency. Drop It and Run. IAEA. Available at: https://www.iaea.org/sites/default/files/publications/magazines/bulletin/bull48-2/48202087072.pdf. Accessed Oct 10, 2022.
5. Radiation Emergency Assistance Center/Training Site. Basics of Radiation. 2022. Available at: https://orise.orau.gov/resources/reacts/guide/basics-of-radiation.html. Accessed Oct 9, 2022.
6. Radiation Emergency Assistance Center/Training Site. The Medical Aspects of Radiation Incidents (4th ed.). Oak Ridge, TN: REAC/TS. 2017. Available at. https://orise.orau.gov/resources/reacts/documents/medical-aspects-of-radiation-incidents.pdf. Accessed 14 Dec 2022.
7. Becker SM. Learning from the 2011 Great East Japan Disaster: insights from a special radiological emergency assistance mission. Biosecur Bioterror 2011;9(4):394–404.

8. Stalpers LJ, van Dullemen S, Franken NA. [Medical and biological consequences of nuclear disasters]. Ned Tijdschr Geneeskd 2012;156(20):A4394.

9. Sugimoto A, Krull S, Nomura S, et al. The voice of the most vulnerable: lessons from the nuclear crisis in Fukushima, Japan. Bull World Health Organ 2012; 90(8):629–30.

10. Dallas CE. Medical lessons learned from Chernobyl relative to nuclear detonations and failed nuclear reactors. Disaster Med Public Health Prep 2012;6(4): 330–4.

11. Takamura N, Yamashita S. Lessons from chernobyl. Fukushima J Med Sci 2011; 57(2):81–5.

12. FEMA. National Planning Scenarios. 2013. 2018. Available at: http://www.hsdl. org/?view&did=683091. Accessed Oct 10, 2022.

13. Howe D. Planning scenarios: executive summaries: created for use in national, federal, state, and local homeland security preparedness activities. Washington, DC: Homeland Security Council; 2004.

14. Centers for Disease Control and Prevention. More information on types of radiation emergencies. 2018. Available at: http://emergency.cdc.gov/radiation/ moretypes.asp. Accessed Oct 10, 2022.

15. Takada J. [Chernobyl nuclear power plant accident and Tokaimura criticality accident]. Nihon Rinsho 2012;70(3):405–9.

16. Zirkle RA, Walsh TJ, Disraelly DS, et al. A new methodology for estimating nuclear casualties as a function of time. Health Phys 2011;101(3):286–98.

17. Armed Forces Radiobiology Research Institute. Medical Management of Radiological Casualties (4th ed.). Bethesda, MD: Armed Forces Radiobiology Research Institute. 2013. Available at: https://afrri.usuhs.edu/sites/default/files/ 2020-07/4edmmrchandbook.pdf. Accessed 14 Dec 2022.

18. Ross JR, Case C, Confer D, et al. Radiation injury treatment network (RITN): healthcare professionals preparing for a mass casualty radiological or nuclear incident. Int J Radiat Biol. Aug 2011;87(8):748–53.

19. International Atomic Energy Agency. The radiological accident in gilan. Vienna: Non-serial Publications, IAEA; 2002. Available at: https://www.iaea.org/ publications/6284/the-radiological-accident-in-gilan. Accessed 14 Dec 2022.

20. Centers for Disease Control. A brochure for physicians: acute radiation syndrome. Atlanta, GA: CDC; 2017. Available at: https://www.cdc.gov/nceh/ radiation/emergencies/pdf/ars.pdf. Accessed 14 Dec 2022.

21. Cancio LC, Sheridan RL, Dent R, et al. Guidelines for burn care under austere conditions: special etiologies: blast, radiation, and chemical injuries. J Burn Care Res 2017;38(1):e482–96.

22. Kearns RD, Cairns CB, Holmes JH, et al. Blast injuries & burn care. EMS world 2013;42(5):34–40.

23. Thim T, Krarup NH, Grove EL, et al. Initial assessment and treatment with the airway, breathing, circulation, disability, exposure (ABCDE) approach. Int J Gen Med 2012;5:117–21.

24. The Radiation Emergency Assistance Center/Training Site. Early internal and external dose magnitude estimation. Oak Ridge, TN: REAC/TS; 2017. Available at. https://orise.orau.gov/resources/reacts/documents/rapid-internal-external-dose-magnitude-estimation.pdf. Accessed 14 Dec 2022.

25. Andrews GA, Lushbaugh CC, Auxier JA. The importance of dosimetry to the medical management of persons accidently exposed to high levels of radiation. Oak Ridge, TN: Oak Ridge National Laboratory; 1965.

26. Kearns RD, Cairns CB, Holmes JHT, et al. Thermal burn care: a review of best practices. What should prehospital providers do for these patients? EMS World 2013;42(1):43–51.

27. American Burn Association. Advanced burn Life support course provider manual. 2018 update. Chicago, IL: American Burn Association; 2018. Available at: https://ameriburn.org/wp-content/uploads/2019/08/2018-abls-providermanual.pdf. Accessed 14 Dec 2022.

28. Case C Jr. 10 years of preparedness by the radiation injury treatment network. Curr Hematol Malig Rep 2017;12(1):39–43.

29. DiCarlo AL, Horta ZP, Aldrich JT, et al. Use of growth factors and other cytokines for treatment of injuries during a radiation public health emergency. Radiat Res 2019;192(1):99–120.

30. Veenema TG, Moran TP, Kazzi Z, et al. Radiation injury treatment network medical and nursing workforce radiation: knowledge and attitude assessment. Disaster Med Public Health Prep 2022;16(1):170–6.

31. Hick JL, Barbera JA, Kelen GD. Refining surge capacity: conventional, contingency, and crisis capacity. Disaster Med Public Health Prep 2009;3(2 Suppl): S59–67.

32. Ilias I, Rizzo M, Meristoudis G. Potassium Iodide in nuclear accidents: give it timely, swiftly and judiciously. Endocr Metab Immune Disord Drug Targets; 2022.

Burn Care in Low-Resource and Austere Settings

Barclay T. Stewart, MD, PhD[a],*, Kwesi Nsaful, MBChB, FWAS[b],
Nikki Allorto, MBChB, MMed, FCS(SA)[c], Shankar Man Rai, MD[d]

KEYWORDS

- Low- and middle-income countries • Triage • Resuscitation • Austere • Burn

KEY POINTS

- The vast majority (more than 95%) of burn injuries and fatalities happen in low-resource and austere settings. Seventy percent of these are children.
- Relative austerity also exists in high-income countries during a disaster.
- Focusing on low-cost, core functions of multidisciplinary care (triage, resuscitation, wound care, surgery, anesthesia, nutrition, therapy) can improve outcomes.
- Many innovations developed in low- and middle-income countries out of necessity (eg, enteral resuscitation, leverage of lay personnel for care) can be adapted to higher resource settings, particularly in a mass-casualty incident.

INTRODUCTION

More than 95% of the 11 million burns that occur annually happen in low-resource settings, and 70% of those occur among children (**Fig. 1**).[1] Although some low- and middle-income countries (LMICs) have well-organized emergency care systems, many have not prioritized care for the injured and experience unsatisfactory outcomes postburn despite exhausting efforts by individual clinicians.[2]

Patients in low-resource settings are commonly treated by nonspecialist providers, outside of burn centers. Care is often delayed, inappropriate, and insufficient. Further, early rehabilitation is extremely limited, and follow-up is difficult. Burn patients may be discharged without completion of treatment due to the lack of services or inability to pay for basic supplies. However, there are simple and cost-effective actions we can take to improve burn care globally (**Table 1**). Much of burn care is the same regardless of

Funded by: DOD, Grant number(s): W81XWH-21-1-0364.
a University of Washington, UW Medicine Regional Burn Center, Harborview Medical Center, Seattle, WA, USA; b Department of Plastic, Reconstructive Surgery and Burns Unit, Ghana Navy, 37 Military Hospital, Accra, Ghana; c Head Pietermaritzburg Metropolitan Burn Service, Pietermaritzburg, KwaZulu Natal, South Africa; d National Academy of Medical Sciences, Nepal Cleft and Burn Center at Kirtipur Hospital, Kathmandu, Nepal
* Corresponding author. Harborview Medical Center, 325 9th Avenue, Seattle, WA 98104.
E-mail address: barclays@uw.edu

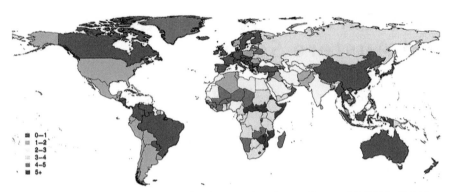

Fig. 1. Map of estimated age-standardized burn-related mortality per 100,000 in 2017 from the Institute of Health Metrics and Evaluation, University of Washington.

resources—triage, resuscitation, wound management, infection control, rehabilitation and reconstruction, and community reintegration. However, the ways in which these services are delivered do change with the availability of resources. The World Health Organization (WHO), American Burn Association, International Society for Burn Injuries, and Interburns have produced complementary documents that outline the necessary infrastructure and processes required to build emergency systems, perform essential burn care, and maintain quality improvement programs regardless of resources.[3–8]

EMERGENCY CARE AND RESUSCITATION

The LA_{50}—the total body surface area (TBSA) burned that results in a 50% mortality rate—for burn-injured young adults is 55% to 75% TBSA in high-income settings versus 20% to 45% TBSA in Africa and South Asia.[9] Less than 5% of patients with burn injuries larger than 40% TBSA survive in many low-income countries, even with access to essential services.[10] Effective triage requires local understanding of burn care capabilities and cultural nuances about specific care strategies (eg, palliative care) and death. All triage decisions are local, but key principles should be applied.

Triage and primary/secondary surveys should focus on (1) detection of life-threatening injuries and (2) general estimation of burn severity (ie, TBSA and inhalation injury). Usual primary and secondary surveys for injured patients as detailed by Advanced Trauma Life Support, Primary Trauma Care, or WHO Basic Emergency Care are performed. Burn-specific evaluation, such as outlined in Advanced Burn Life Support or Essential Burn Care, should occur concurrently.

Airway and Breathing

Most burns are small and not associated with airway injury or smoke inhalation. However, burns that occur during conflict, disaster, mass casualty incident (MCI), and in LMICs are more likely to be larger, caused by flames and/or extreme heat, and co-occur with smoke inhalation.[11] In patients who survive the initial injury, airway loss is the earliest cause of death. Initially, position the patient to optimize their airway. Sit the patient upright if there are no concerns for other injuries and provide oxygen. In austere settings where multiple providers are not available to assist with airway management (eg, during long transport with only one driver), it may be necessary to forego inline cervical stabilization and use of a rigid cervical collar.[12,13] If the risk of airway loss is most concerning and there are not resources to comanage these risks, position

Table 1
Issues in burn prevention and care derived from the Interburns Consensus Meeting on operational standards for burn care in low-resource settings

Issues	Opportunities
Lack of primary prevention activities	Implement awareness and advocacy campaigns; facilitate legislative efforts; ensure enforcement of evidence-based interventions (eg, building codes)
Very high incidence of burn injuries and burn-related disabilities	Reduce burn injuries through prevention initiatives; strengthen burn care capacity across the health care system
Limited knowledge of first aid	Increase awareness of both prevention and first aid at the community level; leverage respected community members
Limited burn care capabilities outside of major cities	Strengthen burn care capacity in first-level hospitals; develop referral criteria specific to the health care system
Late presentation of patients for acute and rehabilitative care	Improve awareness of the importance of early care seeking; reduce barriers to care
Poor communication and interhospital transportation infrastructure	Create and track effects of interhospital transfer policies
Insufficient burn care education and training	Promulgate courses like Essential Burn Care
Shortage of human resources, particularly in government hospitals	Educate diverse cadres on burn care
Poor uptake of guidelines for burn care	Incentivize high-quality care in accordance with evidence-based practices
Negative attitudes toward burn-injured patients and providers	Create a positive culture and community around burn care
Challenges of working with poor, undereducated patients	Ensure training in trauma-informed care; advocate for social services and philanthropic support
Corruption and political interference in health system	Leverage crises and key figures to advance messaging
Lack of coordination between different levels of health care facilities	Facilitate a regional quality improvement process
Lack of effective patient follow-up	Leverage tele-health, mobile devices, and local first-level hospital providers
Too many visitors	Limit visitors and train them in helping with basic care (eg, mobility, feeding, cleaning, hygiene)
Little or no systematic data collection or quality improvement initiatives	Use registries to inform resource needs, quality measures, antibiogram, and so forth
Lack of relevant research	Participate in professional societies, research courses, and partnerships to improve evidence-based burn care

children in sniffing position (ie, neck flexion with upper cervical extension and a roll under the shoulders and neck) and use chin-lift or jaw-thrust for adults with or without basic airway adjuncts (eg, Guedel or nasal airway). In addition, it may be necessary to place patients in recovery position (ie, semi-prone) to maximize airway patency when advanced airway maneuvers are either unavailable or inappropriate given broader resource availability. The use of nebulized epinephrine (5 mg per dose) can reduce airway swelling without causing significant side effects. Conversely, steroids are not helpful in reducing swelling from inhalation injury, particularly in the acute setting.[14]

Patients with deep head and neck burns, prolonged exposure to hot or superheated gases, significant inhalation injury, concomitant burn injury and other trauma, and/or large injuries (eg, ≥30%–50% TBSA) are likely to require a definitive airway. The appropriateness of advanced airway maneuvers should be considered before placing a definitive airway. Consideration should include survivability of the patient and availability of mechanical ventilation. Anticipating the duration of need for a definitive airway is useful given that short courses of mechanical ventilation (eg, <72 hours) can be lifesaving in some patients (eg, small burn size with upper airway injury). Dissociating the need for a protected airway with the need for mechanical ventilation may be necessary.[15] For example, a simple t-piece device delivering blow-by oxygen attached to the endotracheal tube may be sufficient for a short time for some patients. When ventilators are not available, lay persons (eg, nonclinical staff, family) can be rapidly trained in bag-mask ventilation.[16] Last, the conversion of endotracheal intubation to tracheostomy for those who require persistent use of a definitive airway and/or frequent reintubation/procedural sedation (eg, multiple returns to the operating theater) can lessen the demands on resources.

Resuscitation for Burn Shock

Timely resuscitation to treat shock after large (eg, ≥10% TBSA in children, 15%–20% TBSA in adults) is vital. Particularly in settings without availability of frequent or accurate laboratory testing or renal replacement therapy, the risk of death from progressive shock and acute kidney injury is high. In addition, careful resuscitation may prevent the progression of burn depth and forestall the need for excision and grafting.[3,17–19]

For patients with less than 10% to 20% TBSA injuries, drinking ad libitum is usually sufficient resuscitation. The administration of oral fluids to those with injuries ≥10% to 20% TBSA can be easily initiated until circumstances and resources allow for more formal resuscitation, beginning with accurate estimation of TBSA injured. The estimation of TBSA by inexperienced providers is surprisingly difficult and notoriously inaccurate. As a result, burn care organizations have advocated for the use of initial starting fluid rates after recognizing that a patient has a "major burn injury" (ie, ≥10%–20% TBSA). As example, adults can begin resuscitation at 500 mL/h, larger children 6 to 13 years at 250 mL/h, and smaller children less than 5 years at 125 mL/h.

An intravenous cannula should be placed peripherally as soon as possible. However, this is often challenging.[20] In cases where intravenous cannulation is not readily achievable, intraosseous access can facilitate timely resuscitation. Some providers recommend venous cutdown (eg, saphenous vein cutdown and direct catheterization). However, the relative complexity of this procedure combined with need for sterile technique, challenging operational environments, variable areas of burned skin, and frequent dislodgment make venous cutdown a procedure of limited benefit. Central venous cannulation is ideal in people with major burn injuries as it allows durable and multiport access for resuscitation and other medications. However, the supplies and expertise for safe central venous cannulation may not be available in low-resource settings.

Enteral Resuscitation

Given the challenges of securing intravenous access in austere settings, enteral resuscitation can be lifesaving.[3,21,22] It involves fluid administration through drinking or a nasogastric tube.[23] For other hypovolemic conditions (eg, acute watery diarrhea), enteral resuscitation has proven to be highly effective.[24] The small intestine can absorb 9 L/d normally and up to 20 L/d when needed; the large intestine can absorb 2 L/d normally and 9 L/d when needed—totaling 29 L/d or 1200 mL/h.

Enteral resuscitation is operationally superior to intravenous resuscitation for several reasons. WHO oral rehydration salts/solution (ORS) is supplied in small sachets of glucose and electrolytes (eg, sodium, potassium, chloride) in a specific ratio that, after reconstitution with clean water, maximizes the rate of intestinal fluid absorption. Through glucose-stimulated sodium absorption, WHO ORS is able to restore blood volume more efficiently than water or saline solution alone.[25] WHO ORS sachets are ubiquitously available, low in weight/cube, and can be kept for long periods of time. Supply chain and logistics needs to ensure timely availability of many bags of sterile crystalloid solution are not required. When ORS sachets are not available, ORS can be made locally with 1 L of clean water (eg, boil filtered water and let it cool), 0.5 to 1 teaspoon of table salt (3 g), and 6 teaspoons of sugar (18 g or 9 sugar cubes) (**Fig. 2**). Other solutions have been used for burn resuscitation based on local resources and familiarity (eg, rice water with salt, broths, gruel, rehydration drinks, coconut water, and tea).[26,27] However, all of these solutions have significant limitations and risks, mostly related to their relative sugar and electrolyte compositions. Another technique for resuscitation is proctoclysis (rectal infusion).[27] Proctoclysis is challenging to manage in any setting.

There is growing evidence that enteral resuscitation promotes gut blood flow and may mitigate several negative pathophysiological changes to the gut during burn shock, including shifts in the microbiome, loss of mucosal barrier integrity, and bacterial translocation.[23,28–34] Although there is limited guidance on how enteral resuscitation should be performed or operationalized, our experience provides some key considerations (**Box 1**).[29,35,36]

Resuscitation Monitoring and Endpoints

The enduring endpoint of goal-directed resuscitation for burn shock is urine output (0.5 mL/h or 30–50 mL/h in adults; 0.5–1.0 mL/h in children). When no urinary catheters

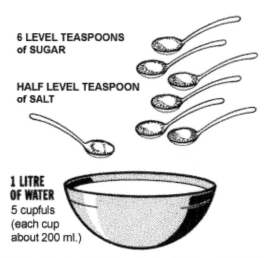

6 LEVEL TEASPOONS of SUGAR

HALF LEVEL TEASPOON of SALT

1 LITRE OF WATER
5 cupfuls (each cup about 200 ml.)

Fig. 2. World Health Organization (WHO) oral rehydration salts/solution can be used for enteral resuscitation or homemade solution can be used. (*From* The Mother and Child Health and Education Trust. Homemade Oral Rehydration Solution Recipe. Rehydration Project. Available at http://rehydrate.org/solutions/homemade.htm; with permission.)

Box 1
Operationalizing enteral resuscitation

1. Start with ORS at a rate identical to the recommended intravenous fluid resuscitation rate

2. ORS is generally more palatable with citrus flavor and at room temperature to slightly cooler than room temperature

3. Leverage the patient, family/friends, or other lay providers to mix and administer ORS by drinking or nasogastric instillation via gavage or a gravity bag

4. Use a nasogastric tube when the patient is very young or very old, has hand injuries, and/or during the night when resting

5. Continue to let the patient eat and drink as they would like and ensure early and consistent feeding when able

6. Use intravenous or intraosseous access to augment the resuscitation when resuscitation goals are not met (eg, low urine output; increasing heart rate; decreasing blood pressure; worsening laboratory markers consistent with hemoconcentration, hypovolemia, and/or acute kidney injury) or when patient experiences gastrointestinal intolerance (eg, refractory nausea, vomiting, diarrhea)

7. Maintain head of bed ≥30° to mitigate the risk of aspiration

8. Attempt to restart feeding and enteral resuscitation at half or full rates once gastrointestinal intolerance has subsided (usually 1–2 h).

Abbreviation: ORS, oral rehydration salts/solution.

---

are available, the use of physical examination (eg, changes in capillary refill, heart rate, blood pressure, pulse pressure) and laboratory data trends (eg, hemoconcentration, lactic acidosis) are used as endpoints. For example, monitoring of hemoconcentration with serial finger-stick blood samples spun in capillary tubes can be used.[27]

HOLISTIC BURN CARE
Infection Prevention and Control

Infections are the leading cause of death among patients who survive burn shock. Most facilities in LMICs were not designed with infection control in mind. Environmental exposure (eg, open windows, lack of weather stripping), use of organic surfaces (eg, wood benches, cloth dividers), unfiltered water supply, and layouts that promote contamination are common. In addition, widespread use of antibiotics for livestock, ease of availability at local shops, limited adherence to best practices (eg, antibiotic prescriptions for nonbacterial infections, not narrowing antibiotics when appropriate), and poor quality antibiotics have led to extensive antibiotic resistance in LMICs.[37] Raising awareness, refurbishing units to minimize environmental and other exposures (eg, closed windows and air filtration, water filtration, changes to human traffic flow, adding donning and doffing areas), and other practical strategies like those proposed in **Box 2** can reduce colonization and infections with drug-resistant pathogens.[38,39]

Burn Wound Management

Great creativity and improvisation are required to optimally care for burn wounds given available materials/products, personnel, and surgical and anesthesia capabilities. Dressing changes should be done where they are safe (eg, warm, clean, sufficient equipment; supplies; and space for airway management during procedural sedation),

---

Box 2
Example strategies to prevent infections and control the spread of drug-resistant bacteria

Example Strategies

Promote importance of hand hygiene and provide hand hygiene stations (eg, sanitizer dispensers, soap and water with paper towels or cloths that are not used from one wash to the next).

Use reverse isolation practices for high-risk patients.

Create and enforce protocols for surface cleaning, particularly in wound care areas.

Cover wooden benches and other organic surfaces with an impervious liner than can be cleaned and exchange cloth dividers for plastic or rubber ones.

Clean wounds with gloves, gowns, and soap and water; manage contaminated areas last; reduce time with open wounds.

Avoid overcrowding in dressing areas.

Additional filtration of taps in the burn unit and scrub sinks/tanks, and maintenance of drainpipes and pans.

Create rounding protocols that promote careful use and narrowing of antibiotics.

Collect local data on antibiotic sensitivity to inform appropriate empirical antibiotic therapy.

Disinfect patient beds while they are elsewhere (eg, tank for wound care, operating theater, walking, in a chair).

Promote enteral nutrition and the use of pre- and probiotics to avoid pathologic changes in the gut and wound microbiomes and endogenous bacterial spread.

---

convenient (eg, minimize patient transport times), and private when able. A process for daily wound examination by experienced providers should be established to make wound care and surgical plans and identify infection early. Performing dressing changes with sterile technique is usually not required, but teams should do all possible to perform wound care in clean environments and with antiseptic technique (eg, clean from cleanest areas to least clean areas, change gloves and supplies once soiled, avoid patient–patient transmission by practicing reverse isolation). Antibiotics should only be administered if there is suspected or confirmed burn wound infection, open fractures, delayed presentation greater than 6 hours for people with blast injury wounds, or inability to surgically debride a grossly contaminated blast wound in a timely fashion due to operational constraints.[40]

Daily dressings for partial-thickness injuries include a layer of nonstick material (eg, plastic or cellulose mesh, fine-mesh gauze treated with petroleum jelly/mineral oil) and antibacterial ointment or silver sulfadiazine depending on the location of injury, risk of multidrug-resistant organisms, and wound depth. Other options include a layer of nonstick material with bulky dressings soaked in dilute sodium hypochlorite solution (ie, Dakin's solution—0.5% bleach buffered with 4% boric acid), hypochlorous acid, acetic acid (ie, dilute white vinegar), 0.5% silver nitrate, or mafenide acetate. Dakin's solution is inexpensive, easily prepared, and has broad antimicrobial activity.[41–43] It is short-acting once exposed to oxygen and requires soaking through the dressings multiple times per day to be effective. Powdered mafenide acetate has a long shelf life and can be reconstituted in a 2.5% to 10% aqueous solution. Mafenide acetate has excellent efficacy against Gram-negative organisms, penetrates full-thickness eschar and other poorly vascularized wounds, and has been successfully used in the treatment of combat wounds for decades. Alternating topical antimicrobials (silver sulfadiazine and mafenide acetate) are highly effective at preventing burn wound infection but come at the cost of more complex and frequent dressing changes that might not be feasible. For first aid only, another option is polyethylene wrap (eg, cling wrap). Honey has been used since ancient times as a topical antimicrobial. Other home-made dressing materials have been described (eg, banana leaves, mashed papaya) but are not effective antimicrobials.

Multiday silver-impregnated dressings are particularly useful for the care of clean and partial-thickness wounds. However, there is a tendency for providers to place too much trust in these dressings and for unrecognized wound colonization to ensue. Bacterial resistance to silver occurs with increased exposure. In addition, silver-impregnated dressings are rather expensive. Their utility must be examined in light of their cost.

In settings where early excision and grafting is not possible, dressings that create a dry, leathery eschar for full-thickness injuries are often used. This may be achieved with silver nitrate, cerium nitrate, or iodinated tinctures. Wet eschar, particularly at areas of autolysis, is cut away each day and meticulously cleaned and treated with a desiccant solution. Some groups augment this technique with fans, hair dryers, or warm air guns to ensure desiccation. As the eschar separates and lifts, a granulating wound base is left that can be autografted. It should be noted that invasive wound infections are common with this approach and extraordinary vigilance with daily wound management and "pruning" of the lifting eschar is required for this technique to be successful.

Surgical Burn Care

Surgical Prerequisites

Extensive excision and grafting procedures are major operations that cause considerable physiologic stress, blood loss, and risk to patients when not well planned and executed. System requirements include excellent anesthesia and perioperative care, transfusion capabilities, wound coverage options (eg, xenograft, allograft, and autograft), critical care capacity, and nutritional supplementation. In many locations, these capabilities exist only in part, and surgeons must consider the strengths and weakness of their system in relation to specific patient needs.

Minimizing Intraoperative Blood Loss

Blood loss during tangential excision of burn wounds can be significant and result in the need for massive transfusion, which may not be possible in austere settings. Techniques to avoid major blood loss include the use of early excision when able, staged procedures, epinephrine tumescence/clysis, forced limb exsanguination and tourniquets, systemic and/or topical tranexamic acid, epinephrine-soaked gauze, and quick hemostasis with sutures and/or electrocautery if available. Whole blood or blood products are necessary for large excisions. In austere settings, the lack of blood product availability is often a limiting factor in ability to perform large excisions.

Temporary Wound Coverage

One of the major gaps in burn care in austere settings is the lack of affordable and effective temporary wound coverage. Xenografts from porcine or fish skin are cost prohibitive in much of the world.[44] Skin allograft banks have been developed in low-resource settings, but remain limited due to high costs, cultural challenges to donation, and logistical hurdles.[45] Although typically discouraged given donor morbidity, allografts can be lifesaving for temporary coverage in small children (eg, 10%–40% TBSA). When applied to a healthy wound bed and maintained with good wound care and nutrition, they can temporize excised wounds, whereas the child undergoes serial excisions and autografting to limit the overall metabolic insults. Human amnion has also been used with moderate success and is available globally. Some burn centers in LMICs have developed birthing centers to facilitate timely availability of sufficient and affordable amnion.[46]

Delayed Excision

In settings where large early excision and reconstruction is not safe, or transport to a burn center is not possible, priorities focus on supporting healing of partial-thickness injuries and actively managing the eschar of full-thickness wounds as described above. Wound contracture can be managed by keeping patients either involved in active or passive stretching or splinted and positioned in positions of extension (eg, shoulders, hips, elbows, knees, neck) or function (eg, wrists, ankles, fingers). Similarly, eyelids, lips, mouth, and genitals should be included in stretching routines. Limbs that are nonviable or nonfunctional should be amputated. After 2 to 3 weeks, partial-thickness injuries will have healed, and full-thickness injuries will have started to granulate. The granulating wounds can be tangentially excised to reduce biofilm and grafted in stages to avoid major physiologic insults and blood loss.

Reconstruction

Given that deep partial-thickness injuries and grafted wounds experience scar contracture, surgeons should be familiar with contracture release and reconstruction techniques. These procedures should occur with patients engaged in a therapy/exercise program and be complementary to stretching, splinting, positioning, and compression efforts; surgery does not negate the importance or necessity of these therapies. Severe contractures are seen more commonly in settings with lower quality acute burn care. Scar releases and reconstructions alongside splinting, positioning, and functional activity training should be done by providers comfortable in these procedures and with established follow-up systems whenever possible.

Nutrition

Malnutrition and weight loss can be mitigated through the frequent provision of high-calorie and protein-rich foods that are locally available, palatable, and culturally acceptable (**Table 2**). Of note, the comparatively small glycogen stores and high metabolic rates of burn-injured children place them at very high risk of hypoglycemia and starvation ketosis. Therefore, children less than 30 kg should always have a sugar

| Table 2 | |
| Nutritional strategies for people with burn injuries in low-resource settings | |
Burn Size	**Nutritional Strategy**
<10%–20% TBSA without significant inhalation injury	Increased oral intake of regular foods and high-calorie, high-protein drinks (eg, porridge, kefir, whey, milk, nuts)
≥10%–20% TBSA, significant inhalation injury, large donor sites, and/or malnourished on admission	Increased oral intake and supplementation with enteral feedings via a nasogastric tube with commercially prepared formulations or blenderized staple foods (eg, lentils, cereals, eggs, milk) with the addition of oils, dairy, soy, and/or sugars. The latter should be prepared under clean (not necessarily sterile) conditions but not stored for prolonged periods of time to avoid infectious enteritis.

Abbreviation: TBSA, total body surface area.

Box 3
General acute rehabilitation considerations to mitigate postburn injury contractures

Elevate limbs to prevent edema.

Position shoulders away from body (abduction) and elbows straight (extension).

Position hands with objects that prevent fisting (resting hand).

Position legs away from body (hip abduction) with hips flat (extension) and knees straight (extension).

Position ankles at right angles (dorsiflexion).

Stretch affected joints, wound, skin and grafts at least twice daily (patients and families should be encouraged to do so hourly while awake).

Sit out of bed and walk as soon as possible.

---

source administered (eg, dextrose maintenance fluids during resuscitation, enteral feedings). The use of mid-upper arm circumference can be helpful in assessing children for malnutrition and can be followed to assess effectiveness of nutritional supplementation even in children with burn injuries.[47] Weights should be measured and tracked weekly to monitor progress and prompt intervention if weight begins to near 90% of their admission weight.

In many austere settings, patients often arise with pre-injury anemia, helminth infections, protein–calorie malnutrition, and/or micronutrient deficiencies. Work-up, and/or empirical treatment if capacity for work-up is not available, should be started as soon as possible. Additional efforts to conserve blood should be used when patients are anemic on presentation (eg, optimize red blood cell mass, minimize blood loss, manage anemia). Children and young women are at particular risk of malnutrition and anemia in many settings.

Rehabilitation

Supporting rehabilitation activities is the responsibility of each member of the care team in concert with the patient and their family (**Box 3**). Low-cost and readily available equipment and supplies can be used to create splints (eg, plaster, polyvinylchloride pipes, thermoplastic) and positioning aids (eg, pillows, foam). Safe range of motion exercises and mobility can be supported by lay providers and family with minimal education. When appropriate, engaging patients in measured and self-directed stretching, range of motion, and ambulation regimens can mitigate wound, scar and graft contractures, particularly when patients are managed without early excision and reconstruction. Strength and coordination exercises and functional retraining often require more skilled therapy and should be prioritized when resources allow. Compression therapy can be performed regardless of resource availability (eg, custom or noncustom compression garments or wraps that aim to achieve a pressure of 25 mm Hg) and should be used early to prevent edema and discomfort and maximize mobility.

Community health workers, local care providers, and disability organizations should be aware of the manifestations of burn injury, scar complications, people living with burn injury in their catchments, and how to reengage health care services when required.

SUMMARY

In low-resource settings, all team members are responsible for the multiple dimensions of burn care, identifying opportunities to deliver services more efficiently and caring for one another in stressful times. With planning and organization, patients can achieve satisfactory outcomes.

CLINICS CARE POINTS

- Airway management should be aligned with patient need, clinical capabilities, and situational capacity

- Resuscitation can be simplified using validated strategies and/or be enterally based when resources are limited

- Tenets of safe surgery and multidisciplinary burn care can be adhered to regardless of resources with planning and organization

---

REFERENCES

1. James SL, Lucchesi LR, Bisignano C, et al. Epidemiology of injuries from fire, heat and hot substances: global, regional and national morbidity and mortality estimates from the Global Burden of Disease 2017 study. Inj Prev 2020; 26(Supp 1). i36-i45.
2. Gupta S, Wong E, Mahmood U, et al. Burn management capacity in low and middle-income countries: A systematic review of 458 hospitals across 14 countries. Int J Surg 2014;12(10). 1070-3.
3. Hughes A, Almeland SK, Leclerc T, et al. Recommendations for burns care in mass casualty incidents: WHO Emergency Medical Teams Technical Working Group on Burns (WHO TWGB) 2017-2020. Burns 2021;47(2):349-70.
4. Young AW, Graves C, Kowalske KJ, et al. Guideline for Burn Care Under Austere Conditions: Special Care Topics. J Burn Care Res 2017;38(2):e497-509.
5. Cancio LC, Barillo DJ, Kearns RD, et al. Guidelines for Burn Care Under Austere Conditions: Surgical and Nonsurgical Wound Management. J Burn Care Res 2017;38(4):203-14.
6. Cancio LC, Sheridan RL, Dent R, et al. Guidelines for Burn Care Under Austere Conditions: Special Etiologies: Blast, Radiation, and Chemical Injuries. J Burn Care Res 2017;38(1):e482-96.
7. Potokar T, Bendell R, Chamania S, et al. A comprehensive, integrated approach to quality improvement and capacity building in burn care and prevention in low and middle-income countries: An overview. Burns 2020;46(8):1756-67.
8. Falder S, Potokar T, Bendell R. Essential burn care. Swansea, UK: Interburns; 2016.
9. Seyed-Forootan K, Karimi H, Motevalian SA, et al. LA50 in burn injuries. Annals of burns and fire disasters 2016;29(1):14-7.
10. Karki B, Rai SM, Nakarmi KK, et al. Clinical Epidemiology of Acute Burn Injuries at Nepal Cleft and Burn Centre, Kathmandu, Nepal. Ann Plast Surg 2018;80(3 Suppl 2):S95-7.
11. Atiyeh BS, Gunn SW, Hayek SN. Military and civilian burn injuries during armed conflicts. Annals of burns and fire disasters 2007;20(4):203-15.
12. Maschmann C, Jeppesen E, Rubin MA, et al. New clinical guidelines on the spinal stabilisation of adult trauma patients - consensus and evidence based. Scand J Trauma Resuscitation Emerg Med 2019;27(1):77.
13. Sundstrom T, Asbjornsen H, Habiba S, et al. Prehospital use of cervical collars in trauma patients: a critical review. J Neurotrauma 2014;31(6):531-40.

14. Greenhalgh DG. Steroids in the treatment of smoke inhalation injury. J Burn Care Res 2009;30(1):165–9.

15. Kearns RD, Conlon KM, Matherly AF, et al. Guidelines for Burn Care Under Austere Conditions: Introduction to Burn Disaster, Airway and Ventilator Management, and Fluid Resuscitation. J Burn Care Res 2016;37(5):e427–39.

16. Halpern P, Dang T, Epstein Y, et al. Six Hours of Manual Ventilation With a Bag-Valve-Mask Device Is Feasible and Clinically Consistent. Crit Care Med 2019; 47(3):e222–6.

17. Driscoll IR, Mann-Salinas EA, Boyer NL, et al. Burn Casualty Care in the Deployed Setting. Mil Med 2018;183(suppl_2):161–7.

18. Butler FK Jr. Fluid Resuscitation in Tactical Combat Casualty Care: Yesterday and Today. Wilderness Environ Med 2017;28(2S):S74–81.

19. Chang R, Eastridge BJ, Holcomb JB. Remote Damage Control Resuscitation in Austere Environments. Wilderness Environ Med 2017;28(2S):S124–34.

20. Lairet JR, Bebarta VS, Burns CJ, et al. Prehospital interventions performed in a combat zone: a prospective multicenter study of 1,003 combat wounded. J Trauma Acute Care Sur 2012;73(2 Suppl 1):S38–42.

21. Leclerc T, Potokar T, Hughes A, et al. A simplified fluid resuscitation formula for burns in mass casualty scenarios: Analysis of the consensus recommendation from the WHO Emergency Medical Teams Technical Working Group on Burns. Burns : journal of the International Society for Burn Injuries 2021;47(8):1730–8.

22. Committee IPG, Steering S, Advisory S. ISBI Practice Guidelines for Burn Care. Burns 2016;42(5):953–1021.

23. Kramer GC, Michell MW, Oliveira H, et al. Oral and enteral resuscitation of burn shock the historical record and implications for mass casualty care. Eplasty 2010;10.

24. Milner SM, Greenough WB 3rd, Asuku ME, et al. From cholera to burns: a role for oral rehydration therapy. J Health Popul Nutr 2011;29(6):648–51.

25. Binder HJ, Brown I, Ramakrishna BS, et al. Oral rehydration therapy in the second decade of the twenty-first century. Curr Gastroenterol Rep 2014;16(3):376.

26. Peck M, Jeng J, Moghazy A. Burn Resuscitation in the Austere Environment. Crit Care Clin 2016;32(4):561–5.

27. Jeng J, Gibran N, Peck M. Burn care in disaster and other austere settings. Surg Clin North Am 2014;94(4):893–907.

28. Gomez BI, Harrington BK, Chao T, et al. Impact of oral resuscitation on circulating and splenic leukocytes after burns. Burns : journal of the International Society for Burn Injuries 2019;46(3):567–78.

29. Burmeister DM, Little JS, Gomez BI, et al. Operational Advantages of Enteral Resuscitation Following Burn Injury in Resource-Poor Environments: Palatability of Commercially Available Solutions. J Spec Oper Med 2019;19(3):76–81.

30. Gomez BI, McIntyre MK, Gurney JM, et al. Enteral resuscitation with oral rehydration solution to reduce acute kidney injury in burn victims: Evidence from a porcine model. PLoS One 2018;13(5):e0195615.

31. Hu S, Lin ZL, Zhao ZK, et al. Pyruvate Is Superior to Citrate in Oral Rehydration Solution in the Protection of Intestine via Hypoxia-Inducible Factor-1 Activation in Rats With Burn Injury. JPEN J Parenter Enteral Nutr 2016;40(7):924–33.

32. Hu S, Liu WW, Zhao Y, et al. Pyruvate-enriched oral rehydration solution improved intestinal absorption of water and sodium during enteral resuscitation in burns. Burns : journal of the International Society for Burn Injuries 2014;40(4):693–701.

33. Bao C, Hu S, Zhou G, et al. Effect of carbachol on intestinal mucosal blood flow, activity of Na+-K+-ATPase, expression of aquaporin-1, and intestinal absorption

rate during enteral resuscitation of burn shock in rats. J Burn Care Res 2010; 31(1):200–6.

34. Hu S, Che JW, Du Y, et al. Effect of carbachol on intestinal mucosa blood flow and absorption rate of glucose-electrolyte solution during enteral resuscitation. Zhongguo wei zhong bing ji jiu yi xue = Chinese critical care medicine = Zhongguo weizhongbing jijiuyixue. 2008;20(3):167–71.

35. Mehta K, Nakarmi K. A single-center effectiveness-implementation randomized trial of enterally based versus intravenous resuscitation for major burn injuries in Nepal In:2022.

36. Gyedu A, Mehta K, Baidoo H, et al. Preferences for oral rehydration drinks among healthy individuals in Ghana: A single-blind, cross-sectional survey to inform implementation of an enterally based resuscitation protocol for burn injury. Burns 2022.

37. Chokshi A, Sifri Z, Cennimo D, et al. Global Contributors to Antibiotic Resistance. J Glob Infect Dis 2019;11(1):36–42.

38. Aguilera-Saez J, Andreu-Sola V, Larrosa Escartin N, et al. Extensively drug-resistant Pseudomonas Aeruginosa outbreak in a burn unit: management and solutions. Annals of burns and fire disasters 2019;32(1):47–55.

39. Bowen-Jones JR, Coovadia YM, Bowen-Jones EJ. Infection control in a Third World burn facility. Burns : journal of the International Society for Burn Injuries 1990;16(6). 445-448.

40. Stewart B, Gyedu A, Agbenorku P, et al. Routine systemic antibiotic prophylaxis for burn injuries in developing countries: A best evidence topic (BET). Submitted to International Journal of Surgery 2015. 168-72.

41. Ottesen TD, Qudsi RA, Kahanu AK, et al. The Continued Utility and Viability of Dakin's Solution in Both High- and Low-resource Settings. Arch Bone Jt Surg 2020; 8(2):198–203.

42. Hirche C, Kreken Almeland S, Dheansa B, et al. Eschar removal by bromelain based enzymatic debridement (Nexobrid(R)) in burns: European consensus guidelines update. Burns 2020;46(4):782–96.

43. Boiangiu AM, Marinescu SA, Giuglea C, Mihai RI, Shoham Y. The use of NexoBrid in larger burns (over 15%) within or outside the label. Paper presented at: European Burns Association Congress2017.

44. Yamamoto T, Iwase H, King TW, et al. Skin xenotransplantation: Historical review and clinical potential. Burns 2018;44(7):1738–49.

45. Roberson JL, Pham J, Shen J, et al. Lessons Learned from Implementation and Management of Skin Allograft Banking Programs in Low- and Middle-Income Countries: A Systematic Review. J Burn Care Res 2020;41(6):1271–8.

46. Kesting MR, Wolff KD, Hohlweg-Majert B, et al. The role of allogenic amniotic membrane in burn treatment. J Burn Care Res 2008;29(6):907–16.

47. Grudziak J, Snock C, Zalinga T, et al. Pre-burn malnutrition increases operative mortality in burn patients who undergo early excision and grafting in a sub-Saharan African burn unit. Burns 2018;44(3):692–9.

Moving?

Make sure your subscription moves with you!

To notify us of your new address, find your **Clinics Account Number** (located on your mailing label above your name), and contact customer service at:

Email: journalscustomerservice-usa@elsevier.com

800-654-2452 (subscribers in the U.S. & Canada)
314-447-8871 (subscribers outside of the U.S. & Canada)

Fax number: 314-447-8029

Elsevier Health Sciences Division
Subscription Customer Service
3251 Riverport Lane
Maryland Heights, MO 63043

*To ensure uninterrupted delivery of your subscription, please notify us at least 4 weeks in advance of move.

Printed and bound by CPI Group (UK) Ltd, Croydon, CR0 4YY

03/10/2024

01040474-0002